A SPECIAL HELL

Institutional Life in Alberta's Eugenic Years

Using rare interviews with former inmates and workers, institutional documentation, and governmental archives, Claudia Malacrida illuminates the dark history of the treatment of "mentally defective" children and adults in twentieth-century Alberta. Focusing on the Michener Centre in Red Deer, one of the last such facilities operating in Canada, *A Special Hell* is a sobering account of the connection between institutionalization and eugenics.

Malacrida explains how isolating the Michener Centre's residents from their communities served as a form of passive eugenics that complemented the active eugenics program of the Alberta Eugenics Board. Instead of receiving an education, inmates worked for little or no pay – sometimes in homes and businesses in Red Deer – under the guise of vocational rehabilitation. The success of this model resulted in huge institutional growth, chronic crowding, and terrible living conditions that included both routine and extraordinary abuse.

Combining the powerful testimony of survivors with a detailed analysis of the institutional impulses at work at the Michener Centre, *A Special Hell* is essential reading for those interested in the disturbing past and troubling future of the institutional treatment of people with disabilities.

CLAUDIA MALACRIDA is a professor in the Department of Sociology at the University of Lethbridge.

T0314181

CLAUDIA MALACRIDA

A Special Hell

Institutional Life in Alberta's Eugenic Years

UNIVERSITY OF TORONTO PRESS
Toronto Buffalo London

© University of Toronto Press 2015
Toronto Buffalo London
www.utppublishing.com
Printed in the U.S.A.

ISBN 978-1-4426-4953-8 (cloth)
ISBN 978-1-4426-2689-8 (paper)

Library and Archives Canada Cataloguing in Publication

Malacrida, Claudia, 1953–, author
A special hell : institutional life in Alberta's eugenic years / Claudia Malacrida.

Includes bibliographical references and index.
ISBN 978-1-4426-4953-8 (bound).   ISBN 978-1-4426-2689-8 (pbk.)

1. Michener Centre – History.   2. People with mental disabilities – Institutional
care – Alberta – Red Deer – History – 20th century.   3. People with mental
disabilities – Education – Alberta – Red Deer – History – 20th century.   4. People with
mental disabilities – Abuse of – Alberta – Red Deer – History – 20th century.
5. Sterilization (Birth control) – Alberta – Red Deer – History – 20th century.
6. Alberta – Social policy.   I. Title.

HV3008.C32R43 2014   362.3'850971233   C2014-905898-5

This book has been published with the help of a grant from the Federation for the Humanities
and Social Sciences, through the Awards to Scholarly Publications Program, using funds
provided by the Social Sciences and Humanities Research Council of Canada.

University of Toronto Press acknowledges the financial assistance to its publishing program
of the Canada Council for the Arts and the Ontario Arts Council, an agency
of the Government of Ontario.

Canada Council   Conseil des Arts
for the Arts   du Canada

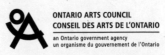

ONTARIO ARTS COUNCIL
CONSEIL DES ARTS DE L'ONTARIO
an Ontario government agency
un organisme du gouvernement de l'Ontario

University of Toronto Press acknowledges the financial support of the Government
of Canada through the Canada Book Fund for its publishing activities.

For those who lived it.

Contents

Figures and Tables

Figures

Tables

Acknowledgments

This book has been a long time in the making, and it has also been at many points a collaborative venture. My particular thanks go to Anne Hughson and Bruce Uditsky for bringing me on board over a decade ago to participate in a book project through Alberta Association for Community Living that involved oral histories with survivors, *Hear My Voice*. Their work has been an inspiration to me, and they have changed the lives of many community members for the better. For the funding on that leg of project, my gratitude goes to the Alberta Historical Resources Foundation.

I also thank the many undergraduate and graduate student assistants who have worked on this project over the years providing transcription, data coding, and document and archival searches, and who have read successive drafts of the manuscript. These students include Lynette Schick, Michelle Volkart, Tamara Larter, Gillian Ayers, Brad Robertson, and Tiffany Boulton; without their assistance I doubt I would have managed to get this book written. Ian MacLachlin of the Faculty of Geography at the University of Lethbridge graciously pitched in to provide population data, and sociologist Kimberly Mair gave a critical and informed eye to the final draft of the manuscript. My husband and partner, Carey Malacrida, has, as always, tolerated my withdrawal into the land of writing with grace and kindness; he too has read drafts and contributed through many discussions to the final product. Finally, partial funding of the project has come through a University of Lethbridge Research Fund grant.

I have been critical in this book of the policies that constrain archival research. However, the archivists at the Red Deer archives and at the provincial archives have been more than helpful. In particular, I want to acknowledge provincial archivist Anna Gibson, who clearly understood the project both historically and morally, and whose work made a strong contribution to the final product. I also recognize and appreciate the new leadership at Michener Centre and particularly Wayne Morrow, who facilitated my visit to the campus with good humour and generosity.

I also am particularly grateful to the three anonymous reviewers who provided their commentary to previous drafts of the manuscript. Their careful and extremely informed reading of the text enriched and strengthened the final version. Doug Hildebrand at the University of Toronto Press was an invaluable ally as the publication process unfolded. I would also like to acknowledge the generosity of Harold Hopp who provided permission for the use of his father, Bert Hopp's, aerial photograph of Red Deer.

This book would be nothing without the courage, patience, and spirit of those who survived institutional life. It is a shame that these people cannot be named for ethical reasons, as their accomplishments in surviving and thriving are truly deserving of public recognition. These are people who lived through much, yet in the interviews they were quick to forgive and slow to blame. I remain humbled by their stories and by their strength and generosity of spirit. Likewise, those ex-workers and the one mother who shared their stories are to be praised; it is quite courageous to speak about these historical practices, and the willingness of these folks to provide a candid description of the institution and their roles is laudable. Finally, any errors or omissions in the following remain entirely my own.

A Note on Language

In this book, when dealing with historical data, I use historical terminology that includes, but is not limited to, terms such as *mental defective, feeble-minded, idiot, moral taint,* and *moron*. While I eschew the use of quotation marks or italics, for the most part, when using this language, I want to be clear that my use of the terminology does not indicate my acceptance or endorsement of it. Rather, I use this terminology so as not to whitewash the violence embedded in much of the historical language.

On a related note, while the advocacy movements of the 1990s, particularly in Canada, adopted a people-first language relating to disability, current academic and advocacy literature is moving away from language that describes people as living with disabilities. The arguments against people-first language include that it is perceived as grammatically awkward and that it makes disability seem to be a natural part of the individual. In this literature, describing people as *disabled people* should be considered as a political statement that conveys that disability is not an embodied or a natural phenomenon but is instead primarily a set of social practices that marginalize and stigmatize people (Barnes, 2003; Thomas, 2007). In this book, I take the position that the debate on this issue is ongoing, and so I use both people-with-disabilities and disabled-people terminology.

A SPECIAL HELL

Institutional Life in Alberta's Eugenic Years

Chapter One

Introducing the Michener Centre

In the early twentieth century in Alberta, children deemed to be intellectually disabled were left at home without services, interned alongside people labelled as insane, or sent to a specialized institute for children in Brandon, Manitoba, almost a thousand kilometres from the Alberta border (Alberta Social Services and Community Health, 1985). By 1923, the Alberta Government had built an institution to house those it called mental defectives at Oliver, just north of Edmonton. However, at the last moment, the government decided instead to place those labelled as insane in the new Oliver facility and to move the children it deemed to be mental defectives into an empty facility on the outskirts of the small town of Red Deer, Alberta. The impressive three-storey brick building that was to become the Provincial Training School (PTS)[1] for mental defectives[2] had originally been built as a short-lived private girls' school and was then purchased by the government to accommodate shell-shocked soldiers returning from World War I. By 1923, this function was no longer necessary, and in October, PTS began operations as an institution for the residential care and training of mentally defective Albertans.

When it opened, PTS housed 108 residents and consisted of a single building. By 1970, the complex comprised 66 buildings on approximately 130 hectares of land, with a resident population that exceeded 2300 individuals (Alberta Social Services and Community Health, 1985). The phenomenal growth of the institution does not reflect general population growth in Alberta but is instead tied to the increasing normalization of segregating individuals with intellectual disabilities[3] in the West during the early twentieth century (Kevles, 1995; McLaren, 1990; Rafter, 1997). It should also be noted that although the institution's initial designation as a training school implied that education, training, and a return to community living were central institutional goals, as will be made clear from survivors' stories, the institution operated less as a school than as a life sentence. In reality, individuals who were interned there as children were typically not released when they became adults or their schooling ended. Indeed, in an official history produced in 1985, the government itself noted that although the mandate of the institution was ostensibly for the training and reintegration of children, less than 20% of all children admitted were provided with any formal education, let alone provided training that would permit them to reintegrate into the community (Alberta Social Services and Community Health, 1985). Instead, residents were typically provided with short-term or part-time schooling and transferred at 18 years of age from the school side of the campus to Deerhome, a long-term-care facility for adults. In practice, many individuals lived in the institution virtually their entire lives, from childhood to adolescence, through adulthood to death; those who have participated in this study eventually left the institution because of a wave of public and professional distaste over the excesses of institutionalization that culminated in the 1970s deinstitutionalization movement.

Although training and education were the given reasons for the existence of PTS (renamed the Michener Centre in 1977), in fact, eugenic concerns played a central role in establishing and sustaining the institution. During the first half of the twentieth century, a belief that "feeble-mindedness" could be attributed to genetic inheritance prevailed in the minds of social reformers, government officials, and medical and scientific practitioners throughout the Western world (McLaren, 1986, 1990; Smith, 1985). At PTS/Michener Centre, institutionalization, segregation, and eugenics were intimately linked. The lifelong internment of "mental defectives" in a virtual fortress set at distance from a small rural town, and the reportedly almost obsessive sex segregation within the institution, functioned as a passive form of eugenics; defective individuals segregated in these ways posed little risk of polluting the social body with their presumed genetic taint.

More overt eugenics programs also operated within the institution. In 1928, just five years after the opening of the Provincial Training School, the Province of Alberta implemented the Sexual Sterilization Act and established the Alberta Eugenics Board. The Board regularly met at PTS, and although things started slowly with only 16 sterilizations performed in 1930, by the time the Board disbanded, it was approving between 30 and 40 involuntary sterilizations per year, most of them on PTS/Michener residents (Alberta Social Services and Community Health 1985; Park & Radford 1998). Although the eugenics doctrine swept the Western world during the first half of the twentieth century, Alberta's (and the Michener Centre's) eugenics program was unique, operating openly and longer than many others, only ceasing with the repeal of the Sexual Sterilization Act in 1972 (Grekul, 2002; Grekul, Krahn, & Odynak, 2004;

McLaren, 1986, 1990; Smith, 1985). The individuals whose stories are told in the following pages were, for the most part, survivors of both institutionalization and eugenic sterilization.

Institutionalization and Eugenics in Context

According to the institution's own historiographer, when it opened, PTS was seen as very progressive because it segregated the "mentally retarded from the mentally ill," moved children closer to their families, and purportedly shifted the focus from psychiatric treatment to education and from incarceration to re-entry into community life (Alberta Social Services and Community Health, 1985, p. 2). In this chapter I examine the international, national, and local forces that, by the early twentieth century, made institutionalization and, ultimately, eugenic sterilization seem to be a natural and proper response to children labelled mentally deficient. In so doing, I want to make it clear that the benign motives described in the institution's history were firmly embedded within broader and more draconian discourses concerning the segregation, devaluation, and eugenicization of people who were deemed to be deficient. In this chapter I also begin to examine the actual practices at PTS/Michener Centre concerning admission and retention, concluding that while education and rehabilitation may have been the founding principles of the institution, in practice, people who entered the institution were rarely provided these services.

Economics, Productivity, and Exploitation

It has been difficult for historians to construct a balanced history of the treatment of individuals with mental differences; such individuals are typically either erased from the record, or their stories are told through the voices of helpers, authorities, professionals, and those who saw them more as categories than as people of value or interest in their own rights (Digby, 1996; Hubert, 2000). That being said, historians have created a body of work outlining how, in the past century and a half, individuals who have been characterized as being less than mentally competent have often seen their fortunes change in concert with broader social and economic shifts. During industrialization, with its attendant need for an increasingly productive and skilled workforce, children who were deemed intellectually different were not consistently excluded from normative notions of the productive citizen. Rather, in ways that echo the inclusion of women in the paid labour force, these children's treatment varied according to economic exigencies. Thus, in the prosperous mid-nineteenth century in America, a small network of asylums for voluntary patients was established, where individuals who were then referred to as educable idiots could learn productive life skills in an atmosphere of kindness and community, reflecting optimism concerning both the robust economy and the ability of all members of society to contribute to it, and mirroring a general optimism stemming from the great humanist and progressivist narratives of the early modern period (Bailey, 1997; Trent, 1995). These asylums were based on a home or cottage model and had a focus on education and reintegration into society; their programs, drawing on methods from the humanitarian French reformers Pinel and Seguin, were founded on a belief that mental defectives could, with gentle patience, be cured and be made into productive citizens (Jordan, 1993; Rafter, 1997; Trent, 1994). In contrast, the American Civil War brought with it tremendous social upheaval, mass destitution, and significant fears about race and impurity; the social reformers of the mid-nineteenth century responded by shifting their focus from rehabilitation and a strong belief in the ability of kindness to develop human potential to either releasing all their charges because of financial restraint or keeping their inmates inside the institutions to protect them from the chaos of the outside world. Either way, the relatively benign and hopeful period of small, home-based, educational facilities gave way to larger, long-term institutions (Trent, 1995). Across North America during the late nineteenth and early twentieth centuries, the cautious optimism of the followers of Pinel and Seguin was replaced by pessimism about the curability of idiots and an increasing belief that few institutional inmates would ever be fit to return to their communities. Calls for segregation and long-term institutionalization of the feeble-minded became the norm (Osgood, 2001; Rafter, 1997; Trent, 1994).

Further fluctuations in the fortunes of individuals with mental defects occurred in Europe in the early to mid-twentieth century, again reflecting both social and economic shifts. In Germany, during the deprivations of World War I, supporting people in institutions came to be seen as a luxury; it is estimated that approximately 30% of the pre-war asylum population, which included individuals labelled as mentally ill and those labelled as mentally deficient or incurable idiots, died from starvation either in the institutions themselves or in the outside world, having been summarily expelled from the institutions into the chaos of a war-torn and impoverished country (Burleigh, 1994, 1997). The profound economic depression of Germany after World War I did not improve matters for vulnerable people, and "long before the National Socialist government appeared on the scene, some psychiatrists advocated or countenanced, killing this permanent reminder of the limits of their own therapeutic capacities and permanent burden upon the nation's scant resources" (Burleigh, 1997, pp. 116–17).

Thus, individuals who failed to live up to the rehabilitative ambitions of the helping professionals became particularly vulnerable, and their fate was closely tied to their productivity and the costs attached to their care. Long before any discussions of solutions to what the National Socialists called the Jewish Question, Aktion T4[4] called for the elimination of burdens on the state based on a chilling economic analysis that weighed the costs of disinfection (or mass death) against the costs of maintaining mental patients, cripples, and long-term asylum residents (Burleigh, 1994; Proctor, 1995). Indeed, the killing machine that terminated the lives of some 70,000 (by the Nazis' count) to 275,000 (by more recent historians' counts) German citizens deemed to be mentally defective or incurably insane operated as a test case for later genocide in the Nazi regime (Burleigh, 1994, 1997; Kuhl, 1994; Weikart, 2004).

Throughout the history of institutionalization, economic concerns operated in multiple ways. Individuals were institutionalized often precisely because of fears that they would not be able to take care of themselves or contribute economically, and the rationale for the institutions themselves rested on the promise that such institutions could train people to become productive. When these training efforts failed to produce economic independence, budgets within institutional walls tended to be mercilessly reduced (Trent, 1994). Thus, once these institutions were established, institutional goals and policies tended to shift from educational investments to ensuring that the institutions were economically viable in themselves, placing no burden on society at large (Jordan, 1993; Rafter, 1997; Scheerenberger, 1983; Trent, 1994). The shifting treatment of individuals with disabilities can be understood as a side effect of the development of modern capitalist nation states, through the lens of what Andrew Scull (1984) has termed *social junk*. Scull uses this term to refer to individuals who refuse or are unable to participate fully in the demands of the capitalist system. Thus, old people, poor people, and particularly people with mental illnesses or disabilities become disposable in a system that does not benefit from their exploited labour. These people pose no particular threat to the social order, so they can be regulated and contained rather than punished or rehabilitated; in other words, they can be forgotten. Such people become commodified under a system that only values productivity (Scull, 1984). They are used either to work on their own behalf or as the objects of production for workers who gain wages and employment in servicing them. In this model people with intellectual disabilities are both a burden and a resource, a topic that I explore further in Chapter Seven, on work and training in the institution.

In light of this historical trajectory, PTS's stated philosophy at its establishment in the 1920s was something of an anomaly; the institution opened with a population of only 108 children, and its mandate of education and rehabilitation echoed the philosophy of an earlier, gentler time in the history of treating mental defectives. When other North American institutions were giving up on rehabilitation and building increasingly large empires within a network of similar institutions (Trent, 1994), PTS seemed to be espousing principles that harkened to earlier philosophies of educating children who were different for eventual reintegration into productive community life. Nevertheless, despite its ambitions to be a training and rehabilitation facility, concerns about the productivity of the institution and its inmates were central to the goals of the Michener Centre from its very beginning. For example, in its 1923 inaugural annual report, the institution's medical superintendent, Dr William McAlister, took considerable pains to describe the ways that maintenance costs had been obtained for inmates of the facility. On the positive side of the ledger, he listed payments from private family members, transfer funds from the residents' home municipalities, proceeds from the sale of inmates' clothing, and the contributions of inmates to both the renovation of the facilities and the generation of produce from the facility farm. In addition, he expressed concern about those unfortunates whose home municipalities either refused to pay or were incapable of paying for the inmates' sustenance (McAlister, 1924, p. 2), worrying that since these people were lacking support, they may not receive the same level of care as inmates from wealthier municipalities. Two years later, economic concerns were highlighted again when McAlister noted that the wait lists for admission were filled with people whose families had been unable to secure municipal funding, and he fretted that this might place too heavy a burden on the ability of the institution to support itself and its inmates (McAlister, 1926, p. 11). In both of these comments, McAlister makes it clear that care for inmates was tied to their ability to cover its costs; we might speculate that even at this early stage, those who did not have the means to pay their own way received less than optimal treatment.

The government to whom the superintendent reported also seems to have placed a high value on inmates' productivity, almost to the extent of economic exploitation. In a question and answer period just before the opening of PTS, when Member of the Legislative Assembly Louise McKinney asked if service was required of patients in asylums in the province, the response was that occupation was considered an important and necessary part of treatment, and, in some cases, this treatment permitted payments that were "made for the same on cost of maintenance" (McAlister, 1924, p. 2). Thus, inmates were expected to work for their keep, and, in some unspecified cases, the benefits the state accrued from their labour would be used to mitigate the debt owed by the institutionalized workers for their own care.

Residents were expected to pay their way not only through transfer funds from their municipalities or through their labour within the institution but also through their families or their estates. Records filed annually by the Public Guardian indicate that, at least until 1940, properties belonging to inmates were held in trust, leased out, and actively farmed, with the resulting income used to offset institutional costs (Low, 1939; Wilson, 1940). Government documents dating as late as 1958 show that this practice persisted: an individual who had a disability and was resident in an "institution for the care of incurables ... may be paid the [state disability] allowance if he is paying or there is being paid on his behalf by a member or members of his family ... [funds to cover] the whole or the greater part of his accommodation" (Manning, 1958, p. 288). In other words, an annual pension for disability would be paid to those in the institution only if their institutional upkeep was being covered through other means; otherwise, these funds would be transferred directly to the institution.[5] Note that these financial arrangements stood outside the everyday exploitation of inmates through their unpaid or occasionally underpaid labour while in the institution, as I will discuss more fully later. Thus, although concerns about inmates' lack of preparedness for a productive life may have brought them into the institution, once they were institutionalized, residents were expected to be productive and to pay their way, whether through interests and rents on estates, monies derived from their home municipalities or their family members, or their labour inside the institution and in its surrounding community.

As I discuss throughout this book, survivors' interviews indicate that economic considerations played a role in their institutionalization in three ways. First, helping professionals' and public officials' anxieties about the failure of disabled children and young people to contribute to society, either through attending school or through productive employment, were among the core concerns that led officials to institutionalize many of the children and young people at PTS. Second, within the institution, inmates' work performance and evidence of industry on rare occasion provided them with in-house rewards and on even rarer occasions enabled inmates to prove themselves capable enough to be released from the institution. Finally, rhetoric about training and education was used to justify the economic exploitation of residents. The languages of occupational therapy and vocational rehabilitation were used to rationalize practices in which inmates provided unpaid or very poorly paid labour under the guise of training and education both inside the Michener Centre and in the farms, businesses, and homes in the Red Deer community.

Compulsory Schooling and Social Exclusion

While the institutionalization of individuals identified as mentally deficient was tied to economic trends and attitudes about the necessity for productivity among such people, economics were not the sole factor in the development of institutionalization. As we read earlier, the optimism of very early educational reformers about the capacity of intensive education to overcome developmental disabilities led to an early establishment of small, cottage-based training facilities. When these failed to produce the desired results, institutions ceased to be seen as short-term interventions and began to take on more long-term and less enlightened practices, shifting their primary purpose from educating individuals to warehousing them. In addition to the failure of the early special educational programs, the advent of compulsory education in general may have had a stronger effect on the growth of institutions. This is because public schooling brought children with intellectual differences to the attention of authorities in ways that were previously hidden when children were tutored at home or schooled through private means.

In Canada, universal education arose from the humanitarian and compassionate efforts of the primarily female social reformers who had witnessed the hardships endured by children during the industrialization and urbanization of eastern Canada during the nineteenth century. These women sought to reduce child labour and increase health and literacy through establishing publicly funded universal education (Rooke, 1983; Sutherland, 1976; Vallance, 1983). Other, less compassionate grounds also provided the impetus for educational reform. In the first instance, the needs of business and government meant that Canada required an increasingly literate and technologically savvy workforce to help with nation building (Rooke, 1983; Sutherland, 1976; Vallance, 1983). In addition, the displacement and disruption of families coming to urban centres seeking work resulted in a broad range of social problems, such as unruly and underemployed youth, troubled families, addictions, and illness and disability relating to poverty, and these concerns gave rise to moral panics about a new dangerous underclass (Rooke, 1983). These displacements and social problems were both exaggerated and protracted in the Canadian west. They were exaggerated because in the west, migrations of settlement originated not only from outside the country but also from within Canada as people hoped to make their fortunes in the western frontier. The social problems were protracted because these waves of migration continued well into the mid-twentieth century, causing social disruption much later than in other, more developed parts of the country. Further, the standardized scientific charity child welfare systems that developed in the eastern Canadian provinces in the first decades of the twentieth century were adopted in Alberta only in the mid-1940s. Following a number of exposés in the popular press, the Imperial Order Daughters of the Empire (IODE), a Canadian women's charitable organization whose mission focuses on improving the quality of life for children and youth, commissioned a survey of child welfare conditions across the province. They found that services were both arcane and haphazard, and pushed for the centralization, routinization, standardization, and professionalization of child welfare services in Alberta (Rooke, 1983).

As with child welfare services, the implementation of compulsory schooling occurred in Alberta somewhat later than in much of Canada. In Canada, the combination of social ills arising from urbanization, industrialization, and displacement, coupled with an increasing demand for literate workers, ultimately led to the establishment of compulsory education in the late nineteenth century. In 1873, Canada amended the Public School Act to state that children who were no younger than 7 and no older than 14 were required to attend school (Government of Canada, 1872). By way of comparison, in 1901, Alberta only required children between the ages 7 and 12 to attend school, and then for a maximum of 16 weeks, 8 of which were to be consecutive (Government of Northwest Territories, 1901). Alberta joined the Dominion of Canada in 1905 and in theory came under Canada's compulsory education laws at that time. However, the Alberta Truancy and Compulsory School Attendance Act was enacted only in 1910, and it was some years later that regulation and enforcement of compulsory education came to be uniformly applied across the province (Oreopoulos, 2005). Nonetheless, by the mid-1930s, compulsory education and the policing of truancy were well established in Alberta (Oreopoulos, 2005).

The rise of universal education in Western societies has had particularly profound effects on individuals deemed to be outside the bounds of "normal," resulting in systemic exclusion of individuals with intellectual differences (Porter, 1997). Angus McLaren, in his survey of western Canadian eugenics, notes that the feeble-minded were created and consolidated as a category when education became free and compulsory. This labelling occurred not only because compulsory education meant that children's bodies were congregated and scrutinized but also because education became increasingly medicalized through the establishment of school health nurse visits and the implementation of in-school screening programs (McLaren, 1990). Compulsory education raised the profile of children deemed to be feeble-minded in three important ways. First, before compulsory education, children with intellectual differences were likely to remain in their homes and their communities without coming to the attention of public authorities; after the advent of compulsory schooling, children were subject to truancy laws and were readily identified as delinquent or as having behavioural problems simply through their non-attendance in the classroom. Second, children's intellectual differences were highlighted once all children were brought into public educational systems. Children were increasingly scrutinized in their collective classrooms through standardized tests, universal curricula, and regularized classroom expectations (Porter, 1997; Trent, 1994, 1995). Finally, children's health was closely examined through medical inspections, public health programs, and standardized psychological testing, all funnelled through public education systems (McLaren, 1990; Porter, 1997; Vallance, 1983). In short, public schooling became a vehicle for observing huge numbers of children, provided the means for comparing them against one another, and acted as a sorting house for children deemed to be unfit for the classroom.

Although the Alberta Government's own history of the Michener Centre (Alberta Social Services and Community Health, 1985) claims that the opening of PTS was an enlightened, progressive, and welcome development in services for children who were intellectually different, social historians offer more complex insight into these kinds of events, arguing that the establishment of special institutions did not arise from an urge to rescue children from social isolation, inadequate education, or incarceration in inappropriate mental health facilities, but instead was an unintended consequence of the legislation and professionalization of education (McLaren, 1990; Rafter, 1997; Trent, 1994). In this analysis, the sorting process that occurred in compulsory classrooms provided policymakers, helping professionals, and politicians for the first time with information about the extent of intellectual difference. These data, in turn, added fuel to ongoing moral panics about race suicide, moral degeneration, and the dangerous classes, topics I will turn to later. The data also contributed to a public perception that hordes of children were unable to meet the new and arbitrary norms of educational achievement, feeding into fears of a growing class of mental defectives who would not only fail to become productive and educated citizens but would also pose dangers on the streets because they did not fit in the classroom. Taken together, the increasing use of tests and sorting instruments, followed by moral panics about degeneration and challenges to education and training, helped to solidify the intellectual terrains of educational psychology and educators in general as arbiters of public intellectual capital (McLaren, 1990; Trent, 1994). And, of course, the fears raised by these professional judgments ultimately justified the establishment of segregated institutions for mental defectives (McLaren, 1990; Rafter, 1997; Trent, 1994).

It is clear from the institution's early annual reports that compulsory education provided at least some of the impetus for Michener's growth. While governmental operations, such as the welfare system and the juvenile court system, provided routes of entry for some inmates to the Michener Centre, teachers and public health nurses working through the schools were the main identifiers of mental defectives who were sent to live at the institution in its early years (McAlister, 1924). Further, it is clear that the institution's promise of training and education for the feeble-minded provided the justification to government and to the general public both for the opening of the Michener Centre and for its continued expansion. In its annual reports to the government for almost all years between 1924 and 1968 (after which, perhaps in response to considerable public and official criticism of the institution, the format of annual reporting was streamlined into simple one- or two-page tallies of admissions, paroles, sterilizations, and finances), considerable time is spent describing educational programs, outlining plans for training facilities, and pushing for additional staff and buildings to accommodate the needs of trainees. Nevertheless, these demands for additional staff to work with trainees and for additional trainee and staff housing, despite being couched in the language of education, are somewhat misleading. In fact, all residents of the institution were referred to as trainees, whether they were attending Low Grade training programs, such as "Sense Training";[6] High Grade options, such as vocational training; the limited academic schooling available to an extremely small minority of the residents; or even when – as was most often the case – they received no training or educational services at all. The insistence on calling patients or residents trainees, and of calling the institution "Provincial Training School" and at one point "Alberta School Hospital," reflects the centrality that education had in legitimating the institution's existence. The vocabulary also reflects a certain amount of window dressing; as we will hear from former inmates, education represented a very small portion of daily life for most children and virtually all adults in the institution. Even by the government's own account, less than 20% of Michener residents ever received any form of education (Alberta Social Services and Community Health, 1985).

I will discuss educational experiences within the institution more fully later, but for now it is sufficient to note that sense training was rarely a springboard to occupational therapy or a higher level of vocational training for inmates, and traditional literacy and numeracy education was a rare privilege afforded to only a few inmates. In addition, calling inmates *trainees* obfuscated the reality that little training occurred within the institutional walls; rather, much of what was counted as education – as I will examine more fully in the chapter on work and exploitation in the institution – was little more than repetitive, unpaid labour carried out under the rubric of vocational training. Vocational training, the most common of the advanced educational opportunities available to inmates, bore little relation to formal education and instead operated more as a workfare program. In its own history, the Michener Centre notes that vocational training provided students with skills that kept "permanent trainees constructively employed for part of each day" and gave trainees competencies in such activities as shoemaking and repairs, which were used for "the good of all trainees" since these skills were used to keep the institution running (Alberta Social Services and Community Health, 1985, p. 10). In addition, inmates were taught skills and given workfare opportunities in the community and in sheltered workshops, performing menial and undervalued work that had little effect in making them marketable as workers outside of these arrangements. In other words, the educational opportunity available to most inmates appears to have been geared toward educating workers for the local community labour under-market and to teaching inmates skills that would help to keep institutional costs down. Conversely, literacy and numeracy skills that might have fostered independence and preparedness for community living were typically not offered at the institution.

In later chapters, I discuss the role of education in the lives of the Michener survivors both before entering the institution and during their tenure as inmates, but for now it is enough to note that before admission and once inside Michener, education and training did not deliver on its promise of inclusion and improvement for these individuals. Instead, the survivors' experiences of marginalization and exclusion in their community schools often actively contributed to their institutionalization, and once inside the institution, the promise of educational opportunities led only to disappointment. Thus, even though the promise of more appropriate educational and vocational opportunities than those available in the public system acted as the central rationale for institutionalization, once inside Michener, most inmates' educational experiences were inadequate at best and exploitive at worst.

Normalization and the Growth of the Professions

The sorting of fit and unfit students within compulsory public schools was not only accomplished through standard curriculum and examinations but also facilitated by what Michel Foucault has termed the *normalizing judgment* (Foucault, 1995). Foucault describes the nineteenth-century prison, orphanage, clinic, and army as arenas in which new categories of normal and abnormal were constructed through the use of surveillance (sometimes called *the gaze*), through the implementation of disciplines of the body (which he terms *bio-power*), and through the application of judgments that created categorizations or typologies of people, all of which only became possible as a result of the congregation of large numbers of bodies in public, disciplinary spaces (Foucault, 1994, 1995). In these public spaces, bodies were measured, capabilities recorded, activities relentlessly routinized, and the data that resulted from these aggregated observations were collected and registered in central knowledge bases in ways that were made possible through the development of new disciplines, such as statistics, psychology, and demography. These new disciplines gave rise to professionals who analysed the data collected and then created categories that in turn were used to reinforce judgments on individual people and their varying abilities to measure up to the newly created norms (Foucault, 1977, 1995; Smart, 1985). Further, the management and interpretation of these new bodies of information demanded new kinds of knowledgeable actors; knowledge workers in medicine, the social sciences, and the helping professions both contributed to and shored up their own professional legitimacy by collecting, interpreting, and applying data collected from large populations. Hence, the births of the clinic, the prison, the school, and the asylum were accompanied by the growth of medicine, criminology, social work, education, psychiatry, and psychology (Armstrong, 1983; Foucault, 1994, 1995; Smart, 1985). Indeed, the growth of institutions for mental defectives, such as Michener, gave rise to a broad range of new professionals, including institutional superintendents, who formed an international professional association, established professional journals, and developed standards of practice and educational programs that operated to legitimate their status as educated knowledge brokers. These were also among the fiercest proponents of the larger, more centralized institutions (Trent, 1994). In addition to superintendents, specially trained nurses and caregivers developed professional status parallel to the development of institutions; for example, PTS offered its own two-year in-house postsecondary training to confer graduates with the designation of *mental deficiency nurse* (MDN). The growth of professional bodies, such as those for institutional superintendents and MDNs, relied on the institutions' capacities to categorize people as morons, imbeciles, and mental defectives, in turn producing an increasing demand for specialized, professional services.

The twinned developments of a system of normalizing knowledge, in which the categories of what was normal and what was not normal were to become increasingly detailed and routinized, and of a wide array of professional bodies authorized to administer the normalizing judgment had profound implications for children with intellectual differences. As we have already seen, the development of compulsory and universal systems of public education provided the arena in which children's characteristics were, for the first time, observable to the professional. David Armstrong (1983), using a Foucauldian framework to guide his analysis, notes that schools provided opportunities for surveillance and judgment not only to teachers but also to medical personnel. He notes that medicine and psychiatry in particular were closely involved in constructing normalcy in school systems; doctors and nurses visited schools on a regular basis, teachers reported their concerns to community health clinics, and children who might have otherwise escaped the monitoring of public health officials were no longer invisible (Armstrong, 1983). Thus, the daily scrutiny of children through compulsory schooling, the development of an increasing arsenal of assessment tools, and the interprofessional collaborations of education, medicine, and psychiatry all converged in the construction of typologies of pathology for an increasingly broad range of abnormal behaviours. Conversely, these practices, tools, and technologies not only added to professional knowledge but also legitimated the professions of education, medicine, and social work as appropriate to the intervention and management of abnormalcy.

The interprofessional collaboration and knowledge that constructed some children and their families as normal or abnormal, healthy or defective, was key to the establishment and expansion of the Michener Centre. From its inception, the Michener Centre was positioned under the umbrella of the Department of Public Health through the Division of Mental Health. This arrangement brought the institution and its professionals into contact with other mental health services, including the provincial mental hospitals in the small cities of Raymond and Claresholm, the provincial mental institute in Ponoka, the Mental Hygiene Clinics across the province, and the Alberta Eugenics Board that operated administratively out of the capital city of Edmonton (Alberta Department of Public Health, Mental Health Division, 1940). This interprofessional contact also increased the level of surveillance and facilitated knowledge production relating to mental difference across the province. It is apparent from reading the annual reports of the member institutions of the Mental Health Division, and from the stories told by the surviving inmates, that considerable exchange among these institutions occurred. Children who experienced mental health crises while in Michener were sent to Ponoka Mental Hospital, mental health patients from Ponoka were transferred to Michener as their situations stabilized, and the Eugenics Board held rotating meetings at Ponoka, Claresholm, Raymond, and, most often, at the Michener Centre in Red Deer. In addition, the Mental Hygiene Clinics that were established in major centres in the province, and that conducted travelling visits on a regular basis to outlying districts across the province, drew on referrals from schools, social workers, and local physicians and funnelled admissions to all the residential facilities serving children with mental health concerns or intellectual disabilities. Finally, the Eugenics Board occasionally conducted inspections of the various mental health facilities in the province and held its meetings regularly at the institutions, and the superintendents of the various institutions (particularly of Michener, whose superintendent was an unofficial standing member of the Eugenics Board) had significant influence on the proceedings of the Eugenics Board (Alberta Department of Public Health, Mental Health Division, 1940; Grekul, 2002; Grekul et al., 2004; Oreopoulos, 2005; Park & Radford, 1998).

The Mental Hygiene Clinics (later renamed as Guidance Clinics) in particular contributed to the surveillance, codification, and treatment of children deemed deficient. These clinics, which were established after the Provincial

Training School and continued to operate well into the 1960s, were maintained in the major centres and also provided visiting services to smaller towns and villages throughout the province. Their mandate of examining patients referred by physicians, social workers, and educators was a means of identifying mental health problems among Alberta citizens. Each year, between 90 and 100 such clinics were held, in areas both rural and urban, including isolated communities in the northern reaches of the province (Alberta Department of Public Health, Mental Health Division, 1938, 1940, 1961–1962). The medical practitioners involved in the clinics not only identified individuals who might be suited for admission to the institutions of the Mental Health Division but also conducted follow-up investigations of patients who had been released from the various institutions and made recommendations for actions, including directly putting cases from the community forward to the Eugenics Board. Thus, through the normalizing gaze of the Mental Hygiene/Guidance Clinics and the interprofessional exchange of knowledge produced by the various institutions in the province, the Mental Health Division became an entrenched and efficient bureaucracy for the relentless detection, classification, and treatment (including institutionalization and eugenic sterilization) of those who the clinics considered to be Alberta's mental defectives.

An instructive example of the sorting machine operating within Alberta's school-clinic-institutional-professional nexus can be understood in survivor Sam Edwards's story. In the late fall of 1969, 11-year-old Sam was generating numerous complaints by his teachers and was referred for an assessment with the staff of the visiting Guidance Clinic, who then recommended that Sam be placed in a residential program for children with behavioural problems operating at Linden House on the Michener campus. Sam's mother, Dorothy, left a cache of Michener-related documents to Sam on her death, including the following letter, written as part of a formal complaint filed with the provincial ombudsman, George McLellan, on 5 April 1970:

Dear Sir;
In the beginning my son Sam aged eleven years was misbehaving at school. Sam was never a problem at home and was never involved with the police. His behavior seemingly was not controllable by the teacher in charge. Consequently I was advised and pressured by the school counselors and by the Superintendent that the child be placed so that he would receive psychological attention. I was advised to place Sam at Linden House, a villa connected with the Alberta School Hospital[7] in Red Deer.
I inquired about the place by having an interview with the psychologist Mr. X. Mr. X assured me that the children were treated kindly. He told me that

everyone there was very fond of children and that every child had individual attention and the needs of each individual was attended to in a gentle manner. He told me that these children were never punished. He told me that the children were rewarded for good behavior. He assured me that there would be no sadism used in the form of sarcasm or any other derogatory action. He assured me that the children were never strapped.

I was quite impressed. I thought that if perhaps my son is emotionally disturbed they will surely find this out there, and that he would be treated with the utmost consideration. I placed him there on the second of January.

In this mother's letter, it is possible to see described not only the interchange between multiple government offices to identify, pathologize, and treat a specific child but also the way expert knowledge from multiple sources about the child's behaviour is used to trump the mother's own knowledge that her son was a good child without significant problems at home. This strategic and collaborative interprofessional use of expert knowledge seems to have been typical in pre-admission interactions with parents. Carl Semkow lived in Michener for 13 years. His mother, Mavis, who provided an interview for this project, described similar pressures from multiple state-employed professionals to institutionalize both her children (Carl's sister also lived in the institution for 13 years). This coercion occurred shortly after Mavis's husband abandoned the family, leaving her destitute and forcing her to seek the assistance of local family services, which then referred her to the local Guidance Clinic. Thus, it seems that contact with any helping professionals – teachers, social workers, welfare workers, psychologists, and physicians – could bring families into the net of the provincial institutional admissions machine.

While the Michener Centre was shaped through its interprofessional relations with other governmental bodies concerning the identification and treatment of mental defectives, the institution was not simply the passive recipient of patients funnelled through external knowledge brokers. Rather, the institution itself contributed to the legitimation of those processes through the development of its in-house specialist training program for MDNs. Michener also developed linkages to both universities in the province, which provided the institution with relatively cheap employees in the form of summer psychology interns to staff the institution as part of their field training. In turn, many of the graduates of both the in-house and the university programs moved into staff positions in community agencies and clinics that provided referrals to the Guidance Clinics.

In terms of credentialing, it seems the institution was as much a driver as a recipient of expert knowledge as a form of legitimation. In virtually all the annual reports filed for Michener, staffing concerns were mentioned as administrative challenges; however, as the institution itself grew and solidified, the tone of these comments also underwent significant shifts. In 1923, the director mentioned the difficulties in finding appropriate staff but seemed to place little value on credentials, noting instead "the need for an efficient, sympathetic type of an attendant – one who will place her own interests secondary to those of a defective, often repulsive, but a very helpless child" (McAlister, 1924, p. 16). By the mid-1930s, however, compassion and efficiency were no longer deemed sufficient, and by 1937 the Provincial Training School had instituted in-house training programs that included a three-year training certificate in mental deficiency nursing. Until the 1950s, employees were not required to obtain the MDN certificate, but by 1954, agreement to undertake certification became a condition of employment at Michener (Alberta Social Services and Community Health, 1985). Although the MDN program was dissolved in 1973, the training program not only raised the credentials and professional status of Michener employees but also elevated the institution from being merely an institution for mental defectives to being a postsecondary institution in its own right. In turn, this elevated status undoubtedly aided in legitimating the institution and provided evidence for outsiders that the staff at the Michener Centre were competent professionals, trained to judge, label, and treat abnormal individuals. It is worth noting that this trend toward certification did not necessarily translate into a truly highly trained or more compassionate professional workforce. In his provincially mandated review of mental health services Dr William Blair noted that 100 to 130 MDNs were being trained each year by one trainer who had no training beyond her or his own MDN certificate; the MDN program was discontinued as the review found it to be little more than an enhanced orientation program (Blair, 1969).

Psychology/Psychiatry and Normalization

Nikolas Rose (1990) explains normalization as the ways that the concept of the "normal" child has been constructed over the past two centuries through an increasingly detailed and expanding definition of what is abnormal. Rose notes that the advent of child welfare and child psychology arose not from a desire to protect children but from a perceived need to discipline, manage, and observe them. In particular, he traces the ways that IQ tests and similar psychological and educational assessment tools were able to expand the categorization of children as abnormal beyond those whose differences could be read easily on the body to include those whose differences were "located in the soul" (Rose, 1990, p. 137). Normalization, a core impetus in the growth of the medical and helping professions during the late nineteenth and early twentieth century, also contributed to the establishment and expansion of the institutionalization of mental defectives during that period. In particular, the development of Alfred Binet's IQ test in the early years of the twentieth century had profound implications for individuals with mental difference and the advancement of normalization.

In her book outlining the trajectory of the idea of the "born criminal" (more commonly described at the time as the "moral imbecile"), Nicole Hahn Rafter (1997) describes how the IQ test made the scientific construction of typologies of abnormal possible and how the use of IQ testing in turn legitimated psychology and "mental retardation" experts. Rafter notes that, early in the history of institutionalization, a core aim of the professionals working in the institutions for mental defectives was the search for a scientific measure to identify the feeble-minded. This search was motivated in the first instance by a desire to provide accurate assessments so as to separate the purportedly curable mentally ill from the presumably incurable mental defectives, but it was also tied up with the efforts of institutional superintendents to gain professional legitimacy. Until the turn of the twentieth century, medical practitioners had been ascendant in running the institutions; however, they had achieved little recognition or acceptance from the rest of the medical profession for their work (Rafter, 1997; Trent, 1994). Psychology, itself a new and ambitious discipline at the turn of the twentieth century, began producing professionals who found their skills well suited to institutional work, shifting the institutional superintendents' focus for professional alliances away from medicine and toward psychology. One such psychologist, Henry Herbert Goddard, established a research institution at the Vineland Training School for Feeble-Minded Boys and Girls in New Jersey, one of the largest and most prestigious institutions in North America. Goddard's research was driven by the perceived need to develop an assessment tool that could not only identify whether an individual was mentally deficient (as opposed to mentally ill) but also discern the level of such deficiency. On a research trip to Europe in 1908, Goddard learned of Binet's IQ test, and on his return, he presented his discovery at a professional meeting of the Association of Medical Officers of American Institutions for Idiotic and Feeble-Minded Persons (AMO) (Rafter, 1997). The AMO's members, in part motivated by a desire to move away from medical diagnostic tools, medical terminology, and medical control over their activities, were also impressed by the flexibility promised by Binet's IQ test.

Built on the repeated testing of large numbers of children ranging in age from very young to young adult, the test had been used to establish scales of "mental ages," producing easy (if inaccurate) standards by which to measure complex mental processes. As such, it permitted testing of younger children than medical diagnosis would permit, with a stronger ability to discern the level of defect (Rafter, 1997; Trent, 1994). Drawing on Binet's scales, Goddard developed his own instrument, which despite being criticized even then for being too inclusive, too easily administered, and too inaccurate, was used by the AMO in its member institutions and by eugenicists more broadly (Trent, 1994, p. 137). Goddard's instrument permitted a new set of categories based on Binet's mental age typology and a new level of statistical (if not conceptually sound) accuracy, and included the following labels and measures:

- *idiots:* individuals who tested at scores achieved by normal children who were less than one or two years of age
- *imbeciles:* individuals whose tests scores were within the range achieved by normal children between three to seven years of age
- *the feeble-minded:* those who tested at the normal 8- to 12-year-old level
- *morons:* those who somehow were able to pass for normal but who were degenerate, criminally inclined, sexually profligate, or otherwise arrested at the level of puberty

For Goddard and those who used his scale, this "upper-grade feeble-minded" or "moron" group was particularly dangerous because they were sneaky and difficult to detect through simple observation, and had adult capabilities, such as licentiousness, without possessing the morality to curb those propensities (Trent, 1994, p. 139).

The adoption of an easily administered psychological test that could scientifically and "accurately" detect both intellectual and moral defects was taken up enthusiastically, because it not only provided, as Nikolas Rose (1990) points out, a window onto the physical and medical character of the problem child or wayward adult but also widened the net by providing a diagnostic window onto the soul. Coincidentally, it also served to shore up the reputation of psychologists and institutional superintendents as rational, logical, and accurate practitioners in the burgeoning field of administering intellectual difference.

Since its introduction, the IQ test has been criticized as an arbitrary, culturally biased, and poorly conceptualized tool that not only is sloppy in its construction but also merely measures the ability to take tests rather than anything as complex and undefined as intelligence (Gould, 1981). Aside from the general inadequacy of the IQ tests, these concerns would have been particularly problematic for children who had never been included in educational settings and thus had not been given literacy skills, and the cultural biases embedded in the texts would have posed significant problems for children of immigrants, who, as we will see, were particularly overrepresented in the Michener population.

Despite a critique of IQ testing that began with Goddard's introduction of it to North America, at the Michener Centre, the use of the IQ test and its categories was enthusiastically taken up. In the centre's inaugural report to the minister of health, it was noted that of a population of 107, there were 43 idiots, 55 imbeciles, 7 morons, 1 constitutionally inferior individual, 1 psychopathic individual, and 1 mental defective psychopath (McAlister, 1924). By 1938, the categories had been collapsed from lowest to highest to include idiots, imbeciles, morons, and a final category of borderline individuals, whose characteristics would have positioned them in the difficult-to-assess category but whose IQ test scores nevertheless positioned them as defective. These categories continued to be used until 1968, the final complete[8] annual report available (LeVann, 1968a). The categorization of individuals at the Michener Centre and in the province more generally by their level of intelligence had profound ramifications; the largest group of Alberta citizens by far to be sterilized were people diagnosed as mental defectives, whose diagnosis was established by achieving an IQ score of 70 or lower (Grekul et al., 2004; Park & Radford, 1998). These numbers were undoubtedly aided by the 1938 amendment to the Sexual Sterilization Act, wherein consent by those people deemed to have an IQ below 70 was posited to be an oxymoron; such people, by dint of their IQ scores, were not believed to be capable of informed consent and hence did not have to provide it to be approved for eugenic sterilization.

At Michener, although the general diagnostic descriptor for all inmates was *mental deficiency*, in fact there were six possible classifications for admission to the institute: in addition to the grounds of being an idiot, an imbecile, or a moron, three other categories – psychopathic, mentally deficient, or constitutionally inferior – were used (Alberta Social Services and Community Health, 1985). Thus, not only intellectual capacities but also behavioural and psychological categories could be applied and used to sort the "fit" from the "fit to be removed" category, bringing a child to live at PTS/Michener Centre. The final category for admission – being deemed constitutionally inferior – draws directly on the eugenic notion that some people are not fit for full citizenship in their communities nor for a full sexual or reproductive life.

Eugenics, Race Suicide, and Gendered Panics

A final motivator in the push toward institutionalizing individuals with mental difference stemmed from the eugenics movements of the late nineteenth and early twentieth century. Worries prevailed concerning *degeneration*, the term used to described the widely believed phenomenon that while people of good stock (middle- and upper-class Anglo-Saxons) were committing *race suicide* because of their decreased fertility, those of tainted stock were flooding modernizing societies with their troubled offspring (Soloway, 1990). In most advanced and industrializing countries,[9] the social problems attached to urbanization and industrialization of the late nineteenth century gave rise to moral panics about dangerous classes who threatened the progress of these nations. Members of new immigrant groups, the poor, and single women were all disproportionately represented among those identified as socially or morally unfit (Brady, 2001; Dowbiggin, 1995; McLaren, 1986; Noll, 1998; Schoen, 2001). Women were particularly worrisome to eugenicists because it was widely assumed that being mentally deficient was tantamount to being morally deficient. The thinking was that not only would women who were intellectually unfit produce children who were likely to inherit their physical or mental conditions but because of their moral frailty, these women would be sexually profligate; in the eugenics discourse, the syphilitic, the alcoholic, the sexually precocious teenager, the mental defective, and the born criminal were commonly conflated (Brady, 2001; Noll, 1998; Schoen, 2001).

In North America particularly, general fears about the decline of good breeding stock were exacerbated by racial fears stemming from the immigration of non-British peoples. In particular, eastern European and southern Mediterranean citizens were viewed as a threat to the existing social order and a burden on developing countries that required strong, productive, and healthy citizens to establish themselves as nation states (Dowbiggin, 1995; McLaren, 1986, 1990; Reilly, 1991). Although not specifically mentioned in the eugenics rhetoric, colonial ambitions for race purity also extended to the treatment of First Nations peoples. Residential schools implemented programs of cultural erasure not only as a means of assimilating First Nations peoples to the dominant Anglo-Canadian world view of the Canadian national destiny, but also in an attempt to erase the presumed laziness, intransigence, and animal nature (which, in similar language to that concerning mental defectives, included the purported over-breeding in the form of sexual profligacy and promiscuity) among First Nations persons (Million, 2005).

These moral panics were both fuelled by and confirmed through the use of new social research tools, such as surveys, statistics, and censuses, and by knowledge constructed through the new disciplines of demography and psychology. Demographers and epidemiologists, armed with survey instruments and statistical tools and funded by governments wanting to quell the tide of social problems that came with modernization, were deployed to show that popular fears of an expanding mass of an unhealthy, antisocial, and unruly dangerous class could be scientifically proven (Rafter, 1997; Soloway, 1990). With these surveys and censuses came increasing moral panics about the poor physical and mental health of many citizens, fuelling eugenic fires (Hollander, 1989; MacNicol, 1992). The advent of psychology and the use of IQ testing also contributed to the increasing belief that degeneracy was rampant; the widespread IQ testing of army recruits in 1917 and 1918 caused a public uproar when it became known that a large number of recruits identified by IQ testing as defective had indeed been passing as normal (Gould, 1981; Trent, 1994). However, the new sciences of demography, psychology, and epidemiology did more than simply outline the breadth of social problems; instead, demographic findings were combined with other scientific developments in biology and genetics in ways that attributed the problems of poverty, ill health, and poor education to hereditary rather than social causes.

In the 1860s, Francis Galton, cousin to Charles Darwin, began to establish the discipline of genetics as a legitimate science. Galton noted that eminent men were often related to other eminent men, and he launched numerous studies using family histories to support his theory that this tendency was due to genetic rather than social causes. In a foundational study, he surveyed members of the Royal Society, Great Britain's most prestigious intellectual organization. Using questions devised by early sociologist Herbert Spenser, Galton found that the relatives of the 100 respondents to his study were disproportionately represented in elevated intellectual, commercial, and political circles. His findings led him to believe that humanity could improve its own species through a process he termed *eugenics* (literally meaning "wellborn") (Reilly, 1991). It is ironic that Spenser, considered by many to be one of the early proponents of sociology, should have argued a biodeterminist claim that people achieved excellence not as a result of privilege or social factors but as a result of their more advanced nature (Reilly, 1991). Nevertheless, he was a central contributor to the further development of eugenics through several books promulgating the idea of an evolutionary human society. For example, his *Social Statistics*, a book that received tremendous popular support and readership, expressed a survival of the fittest concept about human diversity, concluding that those who, by nature, were not "sufficiently complete" to thrive would – and indeed should – die out (Spenser as cited in Reilly, 1991, p. 4).

While early eugenic ideas were based on Francis Galton's idea that "like begets like" in terms of family inheritance of traits, they were later added to by renewed interest in the work of Gregor Mendel, whose agricultural studies provided evidence that not only does like beget like, but an individual with a recessive trait might also beget a defective child. With this understanding, it was no longer adequate to examine the individual herself or himself for potentially harmful defects; instead, eugenicists developed pedigree studies that purported to trace back the character traits of family lines so as to identify the hidden or recessive taint in seemingly normal people (Rafter, 1997; Reilly, 1991). Foundational among eugenicists promulgating the use of pedigree studies and eugenic sterilization was Henry Herbert Goddard, the American psychologist who, as mentioned earlier, imported Binet's IQ test, adapted it for use on mental defectives, and, through the use of such screening and a concomitant notion that such deficits were irremediable, contributed strongly to the growth of institutionalization in North America (Rafter, 1997).

In addition to being a booster of pedigree studies and the use of IQ testing, Henry Goddard made a major contribution to the field of eugenics by publishing several popular books on degeneracy and family pedigrees. In particular, Goddard's 1912 book outlining the pedigree study of one particular family, the Kallikaks, was both vastly popular and highly influential. Goddard's book built on the foundation laid in an earlier popular book written by Richard Dugdale, who was raised in England and the United States and educated in the arts and business rather than the sciences. Dugdale received a small inheritance, which "permitted him to pursue a zealous interest in social reform ... in New York City" (Reilly, 1991, p. 11), and he became a central figure in sociological societies and prison reform societies in New York. His work closely followed economist and demographer Thomas Malthus's concerns about overpopulation and criminologist and physician Cesare Lombroso's idea that criminality was related to heredity and could be detected by examining people's physical features. In the 1870s, under the umbrella of a New York Prison Association grant, Dugdale began a study seeking the causes of criminality through a survey of New York prisoners, during which he discovered six members of one family to be inmates of one prison. This finding prompted him to exhaustively study the family, seeking the roots of their "pauperism" and criminality. Members of this same family had previously been studied by Dr Elisha Harris, a physician and the registrar of New York's Board of Health, whose work had examined the plight of the Jukes, a large, impoverished, and deeply marginal family living in an isolated valley outside New York City (Carlson, 2001). Harris lent his authority to Dugdale's work by writing the foreword to Dugdale's 1877 book *The Jukes*, which became a bestseller, going through three printings in several months and contributing to the commonly held notion that pauperism and criminality were not only generational but inherited (Reilly, 1991, pp. 10–11). The book had both populist and academic appeal; indeed, Herbert Spenser and Francis Galton both referred to Dugdale's work, which served as a template for subsequent family degeneracy studies. Interestingly, Dugdale's view of evolution was not Mendelian but Lamarckian; he believed that inherited traits and genetic expression could be corrected over several generations if the environment were improved and permitted expression of and evolution toward more positive traits (Carlson, 2001).

Drawing on Dugdale's methodology and refining it by using his own pedigree study methods, Henry Goddard wrote his popular and populist book on the subject of blighted family trees. He focused on the family background of an inmate of the Vineland Training School whom he named Deborah Kallikak, a serene, attractive, and intelligent-looking young woman. This was a considered choice: through choosing such a normal-seeming subject, Goddard sought to show the hidden, seductive, and recessive qualities of feeble-mindedness (Rafter, 1997; Smith, 1985). In Goddard's highly successful book, he was able to "prove" the lines of heritability by going back to the patriarch of the family, one Martin Kallikak who, through a liaison with a feeble-minded barmaid had produced 480 illegitimate, alcoholic, epileptic, or criminal descendants, culminating in Deborah Kallikak, an institutionalized mental defective. Happily for Goddard, Martin Kallikak had later married a respectable woman whose line had produced 496 descendants, all of whom were "upstanding or even superior" (Rafter 1997, p. 143). By comparing these two lineages, Goddard was able to provide even more convincing proof of the heritability of "taint" than had previous studies. In the 1970s, critics of his work argued that the family histories were only based on hearsay and were not reliable, that Dugdale tampered with photographs of the Kallikak "bad" side of the family to exaggerate their degenerate look, and he questionably interpreted social problems of poverty and marginalization as biological issues rather than as the effects of social deprivation. However, because of a naivety in reading the new technology of photography that Goddard used to substantiate his claims and because of the eugenics-friendly climate in which Goddard's arguments were made, his work was enthusiastically accepted within the academy and by the general public (Gould, 1981; Smith, 1985). Perhaps some of his popularity came from the fact that Goddard's work followed the biologically determinist stream of Mendelian genetics, which argued that undesirable traits were the result of genetics expressions that were unaffected by environmental improvements. This kind of account provided simple explanations and opened the way for simpler responses to social problems; if these problems were indeed explained purely by genetics, then containing those genes was the obvious solution.

In developing nations, concerns over rampant immigration and immigrant hyperfertility were fuelled by worries over the race suicide or underbreeding of middle- and upper-class Anglo-Saxons. These, in turn, were coupled with worries over the rampant sexuality particularly of females of the lower classes, races, and nationalities, and circulating scientific and populist discourses about the heritability of degeneracy. Finally, the simplicity, certainty, and economic efficiency attached to Mendelian views on genetic inheritance were taken up enthusiastically by social reformers who sought simple answers to complex social problems. All these discourses combined to make the eugenic containment of problematic individuals seem an attractive and indeed necessary response. Finally, changes in the philosophical approach to the institutionalization of the feeble-minded from education to prevention, as outlined earlier, resulted in renewed interest in incarcerating mental defectives to keep them out of the breeding pool and ultimately resulted in support for the sterilization of institutional inmates.

Sterilization and the Institutions

Although eugenics discourse culminated in sterilization programs in Germany, Scandinavia, Japan, parts of Canada, and parts of the United States, the early arguments for eugenic containment were limited to passive eugenics through the segregation of those who were determined to be dangerous because of their tainted stock. In the United States, for example, the AMO pushed for increasingly large institutions, and increasingly longer institutional stays, so that institutional goals became custodial rather than rehabilitative (Rafter, 1997). In the United Kingdom, the 1913 Mental Deficiency Act was passed to allow the institutionalization of individuals deemed unfit for normal society, with the explicit aim of preventing the breeding of the feeble-minded (Walmsley, 2000). Although involuntary sterilization was never adopted legally in England, in the United States and Canada during the Progressive Era of the early twentieth century sterilization laws were passed in many states and provinces, often with the rationale that sterilization was more benign and more economical than the lifelong institutionalization of mental defectives (Leonard, 2003). James Trent (1993, 1994) notes that in addition to public concerns about institutional overcrowding and the economic advantages of sterilization over the enormous costs of long-term institutionalization, the institutions themselves supported sterilization. First, not all sterilizations were simple tubal ligations or vasectomies; sometimes orchidectomies (removal of the testes) and oophorectomies (removal of the ovaries) were recommended for particularly sexualized mental defectives. These more invasive operations were often recommended in the hopes of suppressing sexual activity, including masturbation, which seemed to be both an effect of the degrading conditions in the institution and an obsession of Victorian-era institutional superintendents and workers (Trent, 1993, 1994). Second, the unwanted effects of sexuality (pregnancy or sexually transmitted disease) were not unknown among inmates within the institutions; inmates were sexually active with one another and, as we will hear later from survivors, inmates were also vulnerable to sexual abuse by staff. Hence, from an institutional standpoint, sterilization in addition to segregation made sense.

In Alberta, as elsewhere, institutionalization also preceded sterilization, since the "success" of the institution ultimately made arguments for sterilization seem attractive. The higher rates of detection and admission made possible through interprofessional surveillance within the Mental Health Division, and the increasingly lengthy institutional stays that resulted from the ideology of segregation as an early form of eugenics, meant that the institution faced constant overcrowding. As in other jurisdictions, in Alberta it was argued that some inmates might be able to return to society without danger after being sterilized, and eugenic sterilization was sold as more benign than lifelong institutionalization (Park & Radford, 1998; Wahlsten, 1997). However, this was only a minor argument; the primary motivators for sterilization legislation rested in the intellectual and political climate in the broader society.

Angus McLaren (1990) has argued that the alacrity with which Alberta's elite were able to succeed in pushing for eugenic legislation was driven by very high rates of European immigration in the late nineteenth and early twentieth centuries, with newcomers arriving into a province of fewer than 200,000 Anglo-Saxon settlers; a survey of the province published in 1921 indicated that "social inefficiency and immorality" and mental deficiency were rampant and were expressed particularly among the Slavic subpopulation (McLaren, 1990, p. 99). In addition, the actions of a small but extremely powerful group of social reformers who were able to sway both public opinion and political will were remarkably effective. Emily Murphy and Nellie McClung, venerable figures in the Canadian suffragist and child-saving movements, along with members of the United Farmers of Alberta and particularly Margaret Gunn of the United Farm Women of Alberta, lobbied successfully both at the political and the grassroots levels through sensationalist publications and speeches on the issue (Grekul et al., 2004; McLaren, 1990). Drawing on the already-discredited theories of Henry Herbert Goddard concerning the heritability of feeble-mindedness, these social reformers argued that segregation was not adequate in containing the threat of degeneration and that sterilization offered a more effective and economically viable means of controlling the spread of mental deficiency (Park & Radford, 1998). Thus, in Alberta, the establishment of institutional segregation was closely tied to the later push for legalized eugenic sterilization.

Just five years after the opening of Michener, the Province of Alberta passed the Sexual Sterilization Act, and from that time forward, the relationship between the Eugenics Board and Michener was a strong one. As noted earlier, meetings of the Eugenics Board were held on-site in the institution, the Michener superintendent was a standing, if unofficial, member of the Eugenics Board, and the Eugenics Board assisted the Mental Health Division of the Department of Health by providing experts to inspect Michener operations at several points in its history (Grekul, 2002; Wahlsten, 1997). An example of the closeness of these two institutions and their influence on each other's practices is evidenced in Alberta's rather innovative use of IQ tests in eugenic sterilization procedures. In the early years of the Eugenics Board operations, a repeated concern was expressed over individuals who were put forward to the Board for sterilization but who could not be operated on because they or their guardians withheld consent for the operation; as the years progressed, so did the backlog (Grekul, 2002; Grekul et al., 2004). In 1937, however, a creative solution was found; after considerable lobbying on the part of the Eugenics Board and the Michener Centre superintendent, an amendment to the Sexual Sterilization Act was made by the then-ruling Social Credit Party so that once a patient was diagnosed as mentally defective, consent would no longer be necessary (Grekul, 2002, p. 118; Grekul et al., 2004). Thus, IQ testing on Michener inmates served two purposes; first, it sorted inmates by scientific categories of intellectual ability, and second, but more importantly, it made it possible for any inmate with an IQ score of 70 or less to undergo sterilization without consent. As a result, over its history, *mental deficiency* was the diagnosis for 55% of the cases sent before the Board and accounted for the vast majority of cases in which sterilization occurred without consent (Grekul, 2002).

Conclusion

In the preceding sections, I have outlined some of the philosophical, intellectual, and professional influences that contributed to the idea of "feeble-mindedness" as a biologically determined category and the acceptability of institutionalization and sterilization as meaningful social responses to the problem of mentally deficiency. Concerns about race purity, nationhood, and the social upheaval that accompanied settlement and industrialization were combined with the development of science, professional interests, and social improvement to create a climate of intolerance of difference, the entrenchment of surveillance and social control, and the naturalization of incarcerating and sterilizing people found to be deficient. In Alberta, these concerns were exaggerated and protracted because of immigration trends and efforts at nation building. As well, these concerns and practices were permitted to flourish because of the closed institutional circle of mental health services in the province. This tight circle of professionals and legislators was able to create draconian laws that permitted relatively easy incarceration of individuals in the Michener Centre and also permitted a system of performing eugenic sterilizations virtually without accountability or, often, even consent. In Chapter Two, I will outline briefly some of the qualities of the individual survivors whose narratives are included in this book, and I will connect those personal qualities to the broader themes of race, nationality, sex, social class, and educational experiences that were described here. As well, we will hear from survivors themselves about the circumstances that brought them into the institution and their early impressions of institutional life.

Chapter Two

Entering the Gulag, Leaving the World

In light of the close ties between the move to long-term institutionalization for mental defectives and the development of eugenics, it is reasonable to assume that certain race, class, gender, and ethnic categories were overrepresented in institutional populations, including those at the Michener Centre. Low IQ test scores or unsatisfactory educational performance were not the only traits that sent children into segregation and professional "care" for mental defectives. Rather, disproportionally large numbers of females and people who were impoverished, rural, or of First Nations, eastern European, or Mediterranean descent composed the institutional population (Grekul, 2002). This is the case for the survivors in this study as well – because people were not placed into the institution arbitrarily, this group of survivors' personal situations and characteristics reflect broader moral and social panics relating to race, sexuality, and eugenics. When asked why they thought they had been institutionalized, many survivors' responses revealed marginalization and lack of inclusion in their social worlds. Further, their family histories show countries of origin, family structures, and socio-economic issues that made them vulnerable in a routinized climate of segregationist and eugenic sensibilities.

In this chapter I examine the attention paid to eugenic concerns in the Michener Centre at an institutional level, moving then to consider how such eugenic ideas are reflected in the personal and demographic qualities of the Michener survivors who participated in the oral history part of this project. Finally, we begin to hear from the survivors about how it was for them to enter, and become adjusted to, life in the institution.

Eugenic Traits – The Institutional Record

In the early days of the Michener Centre, a central component of the institution's annual reporting included demographic information about inmates. The birthplaces of all inmates and their parents were noted; the salient categories included Canada, Alberta, British, and Foreign (in that order), with the majority of inmates falling into the last category. As well, the religions of inmates were listed and included Roman Catholic, Greek Catholic, Protestant, Hebrew, and Unknown (McAlister, 1924, 1926). The reporting of these categories can be read as a straightforward inventory; however, the categories also code race and ethnic status, and their inclusion references broader concerns about what kinds of individuals would be most likely to require internment and containment. The socio-economic status of parents, coded as Dependent, Marginal, Comfortable, or Unknown, was also included, mirroring circulating discourses about race degeneration and *pauperism*, which was the term then used to describe poverty, reflecting commonly held ideas that poverty was more a disease or a syndrome than a set of social circumstances and illuminating assumptions about the relationship of poverty to defectiveness. Finally, crude pedigree study data were presented in reports of the "Disease Incidence In Family History" of inmates; the reportable categories included Epilepsy, Insanity, Mental Defect, Neuroses, Alcoholism, Syphilis, and Tuberculosis (even then, a disease of poverty) (McAlister, 1924, 1926). Indeed, the rationale for including these categories was provided in clear eugenic terms in one report, where the description of the parental summary stated:

There is no question that in the large percentage of cases where feeble-mindedness is there will be found decadent stock, and where decadent stock is there the problems of dependency, pauperism, vice and crime are sure to be found presenting themselves as sources of worry and economic loss to the community and to the state. (McAlister, 1924, p. 6)

It is also clear that these ideas continued to be salient to the institutional philosophy; these kinds of sentiments were expressed even more clearly in official documents over the next few decades of operation. In the year before the outbreak of World War II, the annual reports still listed race, religion, and family history. Religions noted in the 1938 report included Roman Catholic and Greek Catholic, along with additional marginalized categories, such as Seventh Day Adventists and Mennonites (McCullough, 1938b). The reporting of the "Nativity" of admissions also persisted but with much more detail. Rather than simply "European," we see detailed listings of countries, ranked hierarchically, with England and Scotland at the top, Denmark and Belgium in the middle, and "Ukrania," "Galicia," and Russia at the bottom. The socio-economic status of families continued to be reported; however, the "Disease Incidence" of families had been abandoned, perhaps reflecting the more global discrediting of such pedigree studies. In its stead, a new category, the IQ test scores of both new and continuing inmates, was reported, signifying the incorporation of scientific normalization and standardization technologies, along with their eugenic implications, into the institutional routines.

It is perhaps not surprising that 1945, the final year of World War II, was the last year that the annual reports included full details about the Nativity, religion, and socio-economic status of inmates' parents. The discovery of the horrors practised under Germany's eugenic program in the camps of Europe did much to temper overt public acceptance of the eugenics movement (Kuhl, 1994; McLaren, 1990; Weikart, 2004) so that the usual zeal for tracing eugenic lineage in Michener's reports may have suddenly become unseemly. However, even after World War II undermined much of the intellectual, professional, and public acceptance of eugenics, the shadows of these early enthusiasms and the echoes of pedigree studies and notions of decadent stock initiated by the likes of Dugdale and Goddard decades earlier persisted at the Michener Centre and in the province of Alberta. This thinking was evidenced by the fact that Alberta's legal and publicly known involuntary sterilization program endured for almost three more decades, ending only in 1973 with the repeal of the Sexual Sterilization Act.

Most individuals who participated in this study entered the institution long after the purported debunking of eugenics discourse and practice in the Western world. However, in the Michener survivor group, latent eugenic assumptions about these individuals are evident, since many of their personal demographic qualities would undoubtedly have raised concerns in eugenically inclined officials about "race purity," immigration status, moral degeneracy, and tainted or degenerate stock. Although I am not arguing that these survivors are necessarily representative of the population at Michener or eugenic victims in Alberta, it is nevertheless clear that within this group are people with many characteristics that officials at the time would clearly have seen as polluting or degenerate. Further, significant evidence shows that the Alberta eugenics cases were predominately among people who came from single-parent families, families dealing with addiction or poverty, Catholics, new immigrants, and people of Aboriginal or Metis backgrounds (Christian & Barker, 1974; Grekul, Krahn, & Odynak, 2004). In the rest of this chapter, I explore issues of ethnicity, Nativity, family construction, and socio-economic status as they relate to the personal qualities of the Michener survivors and then-extant Alberta eugenic ideals.

Survivors' Eugenic Traits

The survivors who participated in this research were self-selected and, as I noted earlier, they are not necessarily representative of the general population within Michener. Nonetheless, it is clear that some characteristics of the survivors do relate to eugenic concerns about race purity and moral degeneracy and to the ethnic, racial, and social attributes that were then perceived as problematic. People with those attributes were overrepresented in the population involuntarily sterilized under the Act (Grekul, 2002). Of 22 survivors in this study, only 7 come from Anglo-Saxon backgrounds, while more than half of the survivors have central or eastern European backgrounds (Table 2.1). Further, 3 of the 22 survivors are Metis, having one First Nations parent and one (usually French) Caucasian parent. The Nativity of these survivors is reminiscent of the eugenic moral panics over the belief that eastern European immigrants and First Nations people were "overbreeding," posing a threat to Anglo-Saxon ascendancy in nascent North American societies (Dowbiggin, 1995; McLaren, 1990).

It is possible that eugenics concerns motivated the admissions of these survivors to the Michener Centre in other, more subtle ways than simply because of race or ethnicity. These individuals' stories indicate that they were often excluded from regular classrooms and were left to their own devices in communities that marginalized them; indeed, several survivors imputed their admission to the Michener Centre to professionals' worries about truancy and delinquency (Table 2.1). When we recall that early eugenic panics centred on the social fallout of urbanization and industrialization, where children who were neither in school nor at work were seen as a threat to the social order, we can speculate that similar concerns may have motivated the admissions of these survivors to Michener. Further, in the survivors' descriptions, we can see manifested the development of interprofessional collaboration in the normalization of people I outlined in the previous chapter. In these survivors' stories, a broad network of mental health professionals identified and coded these people as "fit to be removed" from mainstream society based on behavioural markers and educational or psychological assessments. The following examples illustrate the connections between public school exclusion and professional surveillance that often contributed to institutionalization.

Sean Hoskins had been removed from public school because of behavioural problems and was institutionalized when he was 12 years old, after an incident in which he "ripped up some clothes" at home, where he spent his days alone. He was first sent to reform school (a detention centre for juvenile delinquents) and from there to the Michener Centre. Michel Aubin came to Michener through a similar route, after being caught stealing some chickens when he was 15 years old; he spent two years in the reform school and was then transferred to Michener. Similarly, 12-year-old truant Jim Molochuk was picked up while bottle-picking during school hours in an alley near his home, and the resulting

Table 2.1 Eugenic Descriptors of Michener Survivors

Name/Pseudonym	Ethnicity[1]	Reason for Admission	Family Particulars[2]
Betty Dudnik	Ukrainian	Family could not cope	–
Beverly Buszko	Ukrainian	Polio, missed school, appropriate schooling	Alcoholic father, abusive parents
Bonnie Cowan[3]	–	Better care	
Carl Semkow[4]	Polish father	Mother could not cope, better care	Single mother, violent marriage; sibling in institution
Donald Graham	–	Not stated	–
Donna Bogdan	Ukrainian	Appropriate schooling	Orphaned by single mother, ward of the province
Gene Forzinsky	Ukrainian	Appropriate schooling	–
Gerta Muller	Polish German	Polio, missed school	–
Guy Tremblay	Metis	Hospitalized, missed school	Family poverty
Harvey Brown	–	Recommended by school, appropriate schooling	Single father, five children
Janice Holmes[3]	–	Better care	–
Jim Molochuk	Ukrainian	Truancy, seizure	–
Laura Smith	–	Father could not cope with disability	Single father, five children
Louise Roy	Metis	Appropriate schooling	Single, alcoholic mother
Mary Korshevski	Ukrainian	Polio, missed school, appropriate schooling	Single mother (widowed)
Michel Aubin	Metis	Truancy, delinquency	–
Paul Anjou	Metis	Delinquency, temper	Lived in separate province
Ray Petrenko	Ukrainian	Appropriate schooling	Sibling in institution
Sam Edwards[5]	–	Behaviour problems in classroom, appropriate schooling	Divorced mother
Sandra Karnak	Ukrainian	Appropriate schooling	Alcoholic, abusive mother

Table 2.1 Eugenic Descriptors of Michener Survivors (*cont.*)

Name/Pseudonym	Ethnicity[1]	Reason for Admission	Family Particulars[2]
Sean Hoskins	–	Truancy, delinquency	Divorced mother; sibling in institution
Tammy Burns[3]	–	Family could not cope	Family poverty

1. I note only ethnicities that would, in the cultural and historical context, have been associated with the "inferior classes."
2. I include only traits that have pertained to "troubled" or "dangerous classes," such as alcoholism, poverty, sexual profligacy as indicated by things like single parenthood, and the identification of another family member as "mentally defective." Where no information is provided, the family is described as headed by a heterosexual, married couple in unremarkable circumstances.
3. The person's history was written by a relative or friend (issues relating to poverty or family dysfunction may be underreported).
4. The oral history was provided in an interview with the mother of the institutional survivor. Carl was one of two of Mavis's children who were institutionalized.
5. Additional archival materials (letters, forms, institutional records saved by deceased mother of the survivor) were provided at the time of the interview.

concerns over his well-being led to his institutionalization. Paul Anjou described himself as a seven-year-old in trouble at school and in the community who was sent to multiple foster homes. He said he was a child with a "bad, bad temper, and the homes they sent me to couldn't handle me so they sent me away." In each of these stories, worries about keeping problem children off the streets and out of trouble may have led professionals to segregate these potentially difficult and vulnerable young people from the rest of the community. The narratives also intimate that the children's families were seen as doing an inadequate job in keeping their children from harm. In these survivors' stories, the reaction of multiple public officials, including school administrators, social welfare workers and health professionals, to the children's antisocial behaviour was to incarcerate these children, to hive them off from the rest of society, typically for their entire lives. This reaction is reminiscent of earlier moral panics about dangerous classes of moral degenerates (or *born criminals*) who professionals claimed needed to be segregated from society, not necessarily to protect the people themselves, but to protect society from them.

Often, these survivors, as children, became framed as dangerous or in danger as a direct result of the social or educational systems that failed them. In particular, lack of accommodation in schooling created situations that brought a number of these children to the attention of authorities. Several participants described schools that had failed them in a variety of ways. Jim Molochuk, who was put into juvenile detention for bottle-picking, described attending school only until the grade three, at which point he was sent home because "the teachers were saying that I was a slow, slow learner" who could no longer benefit from classroom attendance. Donald Graham, who entered Michener at nine years of age, also described the reasons in terms of a failure of the public school system to accommodate his needs, saying, "Teachers and doctors wanted to move me to Michener Centre. They said I was too blind and deaf, and I heard people call me crazy and stupid." Thus, school systems that failed to provide a place for these children operated to put them out of the classroom and onto the streets, where their presence was seen as dangerous to themselves and to the public. In an ironic twist, public school exclusion made the "protection" of these children through long-term institutionalization seem both natural and necessary.

Intellectual challenges or disabilities were not the only school-related issues that sent children into the institution. In addition, childhood illnesses and injuries that resulted in significant lost school time precipitated children's admission. Mary Korshevski, Beverly Buszko, and Gerta Muller all described attending regular schooling without much difficulty until each of them contracted polio and spent several years in hospital. For all three children, once hospitalization was no longer necessary, a return to the classroom became impossible, perhaps because, as all three women indicated, they had not received much schooling during their lengthy hospitalizations. For Mary and Beverly, admission to Michener was made directly from the hospital. In Beverly's case, this admission decision may have been precipitated by Social Services' concerns; Beverly described her father as a violent alcoholic and stated both parents were abusive to her. Gerta returned to her community after she recovered from polio, but she never pursued further schooling. This lack of education cost her; at age 25, uneducated and underemployed, Gerta was admitted for two years to the Michener Centre for vocational training during which time she was involuntarily sterilized. It is haunting to imagine what the lives of these three women would have been like had their illnesses been accommodated by the school system; it is also easy to understand that the presumed mental defectiveness that sent them into the institution was caused by their inadequate educations and troubled families rather than by any intellectual disabilities. I am, of course, not arguing that it was appropriate for any child to be incarcerated at the Michener Centre, but in the context of what might have counted at the time as a legitimate label for admission, these women were clearly not correctly categorized.

Indeed, the accuracy of the multiple and interlacing professional processes that led each of these survivors to be institutionalized was hardly accurate. In many of the interviews I held with survivors, it was clear to me that, despite many years of sensory and intellectual deprivation from life inside the institution, these were people whose "diagnoses" did not match their capabilities. For example, Sean Hoskins, Jim Molochuk, and Ray Petrenko learned to read and write as adults after leaving the institution, and several of the survivors lived independently, married, and had successful careers following their return to communities, intimating that their removal from society was not predicated on their inability to learn or on an intellectual "incapacity" to manage a full life in the community. As well, children like Sam Edwards, discussed briefly in the previous chapter, came to the Michener Centre for no reason except that they were perceived as children with behavioural or emotional problems whose needs were not being met adequately in their classrooms. Finally, Leilani Muir, who was admitted to Michener as a child who "seems intelligent – [so is thus] a moron" waited until four years after her admission to receive proper psychometric testing in 1957 (*Muir v. Alberta*, 1996, p. 9). The internally administered IQ test, conducted as part of the preparation for putting Ms. Muir's 1996 court case forward to the Alberta Eugenics Board, gave her a score of 64, which placed her in the mental defective category, deeming her as fit to be sterilized without her informed consent. In 1989, Ms. Muir was given an IQ test as a screening tool for participation in group therapy, and her score was 89, well within normal limits; not only was Ms. Muir not a "suitable" candidate for sterilization, but even by the standards of the time she also should not have been admitted to the Michener Centre in the first place (Wahlsten, 1997).

These examples indicate that the sorting machine that included Alberta's schools, Guidance Clinics, physicians' offices, psychologists, and social and child welfare workers seems to have been frequently inaccurate at best and obfuscatory at worst. Indeed, the system seems to have operated under American philosopher Abraham Kaplan's dictum: "Give a small boy a hammer, and he will find that everything he encounters needs pounding" (1964, p. 28). Children with behavioural problems, with learning difficulties, and, as we will see in the next section, with "problem" families were all treated in the same way (with admission to Michener) simply because that institution was such a commodious, multifaceted, and readily deployed hammer.

Survivors' Families' Eugenic Traits

When survivors explained their reasons for admission, in addition to classroom problems, truancy, and their own troublesome behaviour, they often cited family problems as contributory or even central motivators for their institutionalization. Harvey Brown was raised, along with four siblings, by his single father in extremely impoverished conditions. He said his father's decision to institutionalize him was necessary because his father "couldn't cope with the pressures of raising a large family" and supporting a disabled child on his own. Harvey says his family doctor convinced his dad that life inside Michener would be better for Harvey than it was at home and in his community, and he also argued that Harvey's institutionalization would help to provide respite for the rest of his family. Similar grounds for admission were reported by several other survivors and in the two records (one an interview and the other letters written to the institution in the mid-1970s) provided by mothers who decided to put their children into care; it is clear that families with limited resources were not provided with support to keep their children at home and were instead convinced by doctors, social workers, and educators that the institution would be best for the child and for the rest of the family. Thus, social problems, such as poverty or family stress, were not responded to with social assistance; instead, families were offered further family breakdown and shame in the option of institutionalizing a child.

In addition to these pathologizing responses to social problems, institutional admissions appear to have operated from a belief in a more biologically founded or eugenic focus relating to family "taint." Thus, three of the survivors in this study also had siblings who were placed in the institution, indicating that these families were perhaps seen to be inadequate to the task of providing care for their children or to having children at all. As well, surrendering families displayed moral or degenerate attributes that might have contributed to the likelihood of the children's admissions. As can be seen in Table 2.1, Harvey Brown was not the only child among the survivors who was raised by a single parent. Indeed, of 21 survivors interviewed, 8 came from families headed by lone parents. Although today this figure might not raise many eyebrows, in the 1950s to 1970s, when most of the survivors were admitted, divorce and single parenthood were highly stigmatized social attributes, and such families could readily be seen as immoral, incompetent, or inadequate. Such characterizations certainly would strengthen the argument that the institution could do a better job of raising these children than the families could. Drawing on the eugenics discourse, divorce or single parenthood also carried a significant moral load; such parents may have been seen as morally lacking and their children as problematic simply because of the family's presumed moral status. In Table 2.1, troubling family traits are almost as clearly linked to the children's admissions as are the more legitimate reasons, such as the purported availability of appropriate educational opportunities available at Michener Centre.

Many of the survivors' families were characterized by isolation, poverty, abuse, and addiction, qualities that then identified them as degenerate or as coming from tainted stock. Beverly Buszko's father was an abusive alcoholic. Bonnie Cowan's mother drank and was violent with the children. Donna Bogdan was born out of wedlock, lived in an orphanage until she was 16 years old, and was then transferred to Michener Centre once she was old enough to leave formal schooling, basically because there was no other solution for what to do with her during the daytime. In her interview, Carl Semkow's mother, Mavis, described her married years as chaotic; her husband was both a heavy drinker and physically abusive to her, and the family lived in extreme poverty as a result of his difficulties in maintaining a job. Mavis separated from Carl's father when Carl was only four years old, and Carl, his sister (who was also institutionalized but whose story is not included in this study), and his mother continued to live under destitute conditions. In each of the stories, we can understand how such children might come to the attention of authorities and why the intervention of physicians, social workers, and helping professionals might be necessary. If, however, we were to apply the lens of an earlier era to these stories, we might not see troubled families suffering from the social problems associated with poverty and being underprivileged; instead we might see families that authorities might characterize as "degenerate," whose offspring needed not protection but containment. Thus, by examining the moral qualities of the families of the survivors, we can see that deep-seated attitudes about what constituted the "wrong" kind of family and an unwavering belief in segregating people of problematic stock continued to play a role in the admissions of children to the Michener Centre well into the early 1970s.

Institutionalization, Education, and Eugenics

In the last chapter, I explained that institutions for mental defectives were originally and optimistically conceived of as places that would offer short-term stays and specialized learning opportunities for children and young people with intellectual disabilities. However, as institutionalization became increasingly normative for individuals with intellectual disabilities, so too did the idea of lifelong internment. Rather than offering short institutional stays with a focus on remedial education, the institutions of the twentieth century came to focus more on long-term segregation and eugenic containment, as evidenced by shifts in the organizational and physical operations on the campus.

Although PTS opened as a school for the training of primarily young children with a modest starting population of around 105 children, by the time the individuals involved in this study were interned at Michener, the facility had grown tremendously, and its operations had become increasingly geared toward segregation rather than short-term interventions. The population had grown steadily since the institution's opening, and with the 1949 appointment of an ambitious new medical superintendent, Dr Leonard Jan LeVann, the campus population exploded from 293 in 1950 to 1433 in 1959, and by the end of Dr LeVann's tenure in 1974, the population had risen to more than 2300 residents (Alberta Social Services and Community Health, 1985). This increase in the institutional population required the building of some new classrooms, a new ward for girls, three new children's "villas" (each of which was designed to house almost 250 residents on three floors), a power house, an infirmary, and a home for Superintendent LeVann (Alberta Social Services and Community Health, 1985, p. 11). The period also saw the separation of adult and children's services, with the implicit recognition that many of the institution's inmates were not going home once they were no longer of school age. Thus, in addition to construction projects on the children's side of the campus during LeVann's early tenure, between 1955 and 1957, another major building project, Deerhome, was undertaken on the north side of the campus. Deerhome began as a complex of three three-storey dormitories for residents who had reached the age of 18 (to which 335 residents were immediately admitted on opening), a separate utilities building, and a kitchen. Over the next decade, Deerhome itself expanded to included "eight residential/dormitory buildings, a recreational hall, two nurses' residences, and administration building and various structures housing support services" (Alberta Social Services and Community Health, 1985, p. 11). In short, what was originally a small, educationally focused single-building facility became, during the decades of LeVann's tenure, more like a small town with all the usual services to provide for a self-contained population.

The survivors interviewed for this study tell stories that realistically reflect an institutional philosophy of lifelong internment rather than one of short-term educational interventions. These survivors came into the PTS/Michener institution at the height of its legitimacy and in the heyday of the ambitious Dr LeVann's tenure as superintendent, and their stories provide evidence of the ideology of containment and segregation, despite the "educational opportunities" rationale given for their institutionalization. Almost half (9) of the 22 survivors explicitly stated that one of the primary motivators given for their internment was the belief, conveyed to parents and caregivers by educational, medical, or psychological professionals, that the Michener Centre would provide the children with an appropriate education, presumably because their local schools were unable or unwilling to accommodate their classroom "problems" (Table 2.1). However, those promised educational opportunities or short-term stays for schooling were not the norm among the individuals in the study. This discrepancy can be best understood by an examination of the ages and durations of stay of the survivors (Table 2.2).

Of the 22 individuals interviewed,[1] the average age at admission was 12, and all admissions except one were made during the children's school years. This young admission age supports the survivors' claims that the promise of a suitable education for children with learning disabilities or emotional and behavioural challenges was a component of their admission to the Michener Centre. Conversely, although almost all the survivors entered the institution during their school years, the survivors' average age at leaving was nearly 27 years, with a range between 18 and 39 years of age. Clearly, inmates who reached adulthood (18 years of age in Alberta) were no longer there to receive an education. Further, although a number of these survivors left the institution in their late teens and early twenties, it is possible that, because of the timing of their discharge, they left early as compared with previous generations. Most of these survivors left the institution during the 1970s and 1980s, a period of strong outside pressures on the Michener Centre to achieve deinstitutionalization.

In 1969, following significant media coverage of abuses and irregularities in the mental health system in Alberta, William Robert Nelson Blair, then president of the Alberta Psychological Association, published the massive government-commissioned Blair Report. This report provided a comprehensive review of mental health services in Alberta and offered the government guidelines for addressing the problems that plagued the mental health system. A central recommendation was the closure of long-term facilities for housing people with developmental disabilities; in short, Blair recommended the closure of the Michener Centre (Blair, 1969). Although almost 45 years later this recommendation has still not been fully achieved, the Blair Report and the significant media and popular outcry that accompanied its publication contributed to a deinstitutionalization and Community Living groundswell among family members, community members, and disability advocacy groups. In addition, 1974 was the last year of LeVann's tenure as superintendent, after 25 years at the helm; his leaving heralded the end of aggressive and ambitious expansion on the Michener campus.[2] This combination of public outcry, governmental enquiry, public activism, and change in internal leadership meant that even in the face of actions to keep the institution operating (for a fuller discussion, see Chapter Ten), during the 1970s and 1980s the Michener Centre saw significant numbers of inmates discharged.

As can be seen in Table 2.2, all survivors participating in this project left the Michener institution after the Blair Report and its fallout. We can presume that without this strong movement to deinstitutionalization, these individuals would have probably stayed even longer, perhaps even for their entire lives. As it is, the people in this study spent an average of almost 13 years in the institution, and one person interviewed spent more than 30 years inside. Further, most of the

Table 2.2 Institutional Stay, Sterilization Data on Survivors

Name/Pseudonym	Admitted	Departed	Ages	Duration	Sterilized
Sam Edwards[1]	1969	1970	11–12	6 months	No
Gerta Muller	1972	1972	25–27	2 years	Yes
Gene Forzinsky	1971	1975	15–19	4 years	Yes
Bonnie Cowan[2]	1971	1976	13–18	5 years	Not stated
Harvey Brown	1965	1971	13–19	6 years	Yes
Sandra Karnak	1968	1974	12–18	6 years	Yes
Sean Hoskins	1979	1986	12–19	7 years	Not stated
Beverly Buszko	1969	1977	10–18	8 years	Not stated
Betty Dudnik	Not stated	Not stated	7–18	11 years	Not stated
Louise Roy	Not stated	Not stated	12–23	11 years[3]	Not stated
Donna Bogdan	1969	1981	16–28	12 years	Yes
Carl Semkow[4]	1970	1983	8–21	13 years	No
Donald Graham	1966	1980	9–23	14 years	Not stated
Tammy Burns[2]	1971	1986	18–33	15 years	Not stated
Ray Petrenko	1959	1975	10–25	16 years[3]	Yes
Paul Anjou	1967	1985	7–25	18 years[3]	Not stated
Michel Aubin	1957	1976	13–32	19 years	Not stated
Laura Smith	1970	1990	9–29	20 years	Yes
Mary Korshevski	1955	1976	15–36	21 years	Yes
Jim Molochuk	1949	1974	12–37	25 years	Yes
Janice Holmes[2]	1960	1986	11–37	26 years	Yes
Guy Tremblay	1956	1986	9–39	30 years[3]	Yes

1. Additional archival materials (letters, forms, institutional records saved by deceased mother of the survivor) were provided at the time of the interview.
2. The person's history was written by a relative or friend (issues relating to poverty or family dysfunction may be underreported).
3. Some dates are approximate, as these survivors were very young upon admission and were not certain of the dates, particularly of their admissions. Approximations, where necessary, were based on the grade-levels at which children were taken out of regular schooling, their age at discharge, and their date of discharge.
4. The oral history was provided in an interview with the mother of the institutional survivor. Carl was one of two of Mavis's children who were institutionalized.

participants described living in wards on the South Campus/Alberta School Hospital (ASH) or the children's side of the Michener campus and then being moved across to the adult North campus/Deerhome side of the institution, once they were 18 years old. In the end, survivors' lengthy stays and multiple residences on both campuses in Michener do not support the institution's claims that children were committed for education and reintegration but instead reflect practices more akin to lifelong internment.

The long-term cordoning off of children and adults deemed to be mentally defective in institutions like Michener was an effective way to preclude their sexuality and procreation, and it worked as a covert or passive form of eugenics. There is a significant body of literature indicating that the fears of overbreeding that fuelled segregationist and eugenic efforts were unduly levelled at "wayward" girls and women. Immorality and lack of moral control were presumed to be associated with feeble-mindedness both because such young women were naturally hypersexual and, in classic blame-the-victim thinking, because of assumptions that they were more likely to be preyed on (Brady, 2001; Noll, 1998; Schoen, 2001; Walmsley, 2000). At the Michener Centre, the ratio of female to male patients did not consistently reflect this bias; indeed, for most of the institution's history, male inmates slightly outnumbered females (Alberta Social Services and Community Health, 1985; Grekul, 2002). A recent survey of epidemiological studies on intellectual disability concluded that across diagnoses, males are more common than females, and in cases of mild disabilities, "males have about a 1.5-fold greater prevalence" than females (Maulik & Harbour, 2013, Gender section, para. 1). Thus, the incarceration rates at Michener, rather than being truly reflective of prevalence rates more generally, saw females being overrepresented. Further, females were more likely to be presented to the eugenics board for sterilization, so that "58% of all the people sterilized under the direction of the Eugenics Board were women" (Grekul, 2002, p. 107).

Among the survivors in this study, the gender ratio is split between males (11) and females (11) so that females may be very slightly overrepresented in the survivor group as compared with the general institutional population and people generally who are identified as having an intellectual disability. Five of the women (45%) and four of men (36%) in this study stated that they had been involuntarily sterilized while residing in the Michener Centre. These numbers are, however, somewhat misleading. Five women and four men declined to answer this question, reflecting the sensitivity of the topic. These responses may indicate the survivors' shame and the residual trauma attached to the sterilization experience; although some of the survivors clearly were angry about this violation of their persons, others expressed some shame at what had happened to them, and these feelings may have kept some survivors from disclosing their sterilization status. In addition, all the individuals for whom life stories were written either by a family member or a worker declined to disclose sterilization status, which may say as much about the people who wrote the life stories as about the individuals' actual histories. It may be that these writers felt the topic to be taboo, or they felt some discomfort about their possible roles as guardians in placing their children in an institution where such abuses occurred. Only Mavis, a mother of a survivor who provided an interview on her son's behalf, unequivocally stated that her son had not been sterilized. Despite this assertion, it is not absolutely certain that the people in this study who believed that they had not been sterilized were necessarily correct, because of the protocols for consent attached to the Alberta eugenics program.

Given the way that sterilizations were handled in the institution, Mavis's consent would not necessarily have been sought for her son's sterilization, nor would she have been informed of the operation after the fact. Because of difficulties in obtaining consent for sterilizations from individuals that the Alberta Eugenics Board deemed "fit for sterilization," the Eugenics Board got off to a sluggish start, with a backlog of people approved for the operation but not having agreed to undergoing it. To increase its scope and to deal with the pesky problem of recalcitrant candidates, in 1938 the Board successfully petitioned the Alberta Government for an amendment to the Sterilization Act. Thus, after 1938, the Board was able to proceed with sterilizations without obtaining consent on people who were deemed to be mental defectives: those who obtained an IQ score lower than 70 (Grekul, 2002; Grekul et al., 2004). Speculatively, Mavis's son could have been sterilized without his or his mother's knowledge. This experience – of not knowing one's medical background – is not unusual among survivors of Michener Centre; in her landmark lawsuit against the provincial government for wrongful sterilization (discussed more fully in Chapter Nine), Leilani Muir only learned that she had been sterilized after she had left the institution, married, and experienced difficulties getting pregnant (*Muir v. Alberta*, 1996; Wahlsten, 1997). It is thus possible that information provided by the survivors about their sterilization histories may also be underreported, reflecting this secretive aspect of the Alberta Eugenics Board's practices.

Going to Live at Michener

The 22 people who told their stories entered the institution for diverse reasons, yet their stories also share remarkable similarities. They were sent because their communities and their schools could not or would not accommodate them. They went because their families were, or were perceived to be, unable to provide adequate care for them. They went because they had been sick, isolated, troubled, and under-served by a social safety net in their homes and communities. Often, they went because their homes were themselves troubled. However, one thing is common to all the stories these survivors tell about why they were sent to the institution: they went because they or their families were told that life inside the institution would be better for them than life outside. They went because they were promised that the institution would provide more to them than their families, their schools, and their communities could do. In short, they went because they and their loved ones believed that going to Michener was for the best.

What must it have been like for these children to arrive and enter the institution? How did these children experience admission? How did their families manage the transition? And what were the first few weeks like after the children were admitted? In this section of the book, we will hear much more from survivors themselves about their experiences inside the Michener Centre, beginning with their descriptions of entering the institution.

Recall that according to Michener's own historiographers, in 1923 in Alberta, the establishment of an institution specially built for the housing of mental defectives was seen as both progressive and beneficial because the institution segregated the "mentally retarded from the mentally ill" and, perhaps more importantly, because it moved children closer to their families than previous arrangements had permitted (Alberta Social Services and Community Health, 1985, p. 2). However, for all the survivors in this study, the institution was not close to their homes. Almost all the survivors' Michener stories begin with a long, cheerless drive through the expansive Alberta countryside. Among the 22 survivors, not one came from Red Deer and its surrounding area: instead, these children came from Alberta's two major cities, each 150 kilometres away, or from rural communities up to 500 kilometres from Red Deer. One survivor, Guy Tremblay, came from another province; his parents lived almost 1000 kilometres from the place that Guy would call home for 30 years.

As well, almost all the Michener stories begin with deceit; only one or two children recalled hearing anything about Michener before their arrival, but for most, this long, tense drive and their arrival at the imposing red brick administrative building on the Michener campus occurred without any real preparation and without any clear explanation. Mavis, the mother of two children placed in the Michener Centre, concentrated her narrative on the story of Carl, her eldest child. She provided insight into the ways that admission occurred in her description of the day she took her son to the institution:

I ended up getting a letter, and there was a date, something like that, that we had to have him up there. It took us almost four hours – it was a terrible winter. We took him up ourselves. I don't remember if I told him where he was going or not. They didn't give me a tour or anything. I even had to leave him in that big red brick building ... I didn't know where he was going to, which building he was going to be in. He just went with them. I don't think he – I don't know. He just went with them.

From Mavis's story, we can understand how little information was provided to her or, in turn, to her son before admission. Like others, Mavis described a silent drive, perhaps fraught with feelings of guilt or hope over relinquishing family members, and certainly laced with doubt and uncertainty for the children who were being committed. If any survivors did recall being told anything about their move to Michener, they remembered only a general comment promising that at Michener they would be getting some better schooling or better care than they could hope for in their homes. The lack of information and the surprise and sorrow that accompanied the pre-admission process were virtually universal; most survivors described knowing nothing or very little about the Michener Centre itself, nor did they remember being told how long they were to stay there.

Some, like Gerta Muller, described scenes that seem almost cinematic in their darkness. Gerta, having lost several years of school because she contracted polio, described languishing at home once she was released from hospital. One day, as she played outside, "a big black car" made the long, dusty drive up to her rural farmhouse. A man and a woman stepped out and spoke with Gerta's mother. Her mother went in the house, brought out a suitcase, and told Gerta that she would be going away "for a little while" to get some proper vocational training and that this new school was going to be a good opportunity for her. Gerta entered the car alone and left her family home for two years. Gerta's memory of the situation might be sharper than those of the other survivors since she was 25 when she entered the institution; for most of the other survivors, these admission scenarios played out much earlier, when they were still children. However, almost all the survivors had vivid childhood memories of the day they went to the Michener Centre.

On arrival at the institution, typically little was said or done to reassure the children. Mary Korshevski, who was 15 years old when admitted to Michener, provides a typical description of the survivors' first impressions of the institution that was to become their new home:

I really didn't know why I couldn't stay home, you know? I went to Michener Centre April 15, 1955, and when I got there all I could see was a big, great big, brick building. You know? And I kind of thought, "No. What is it? What is this? What is it going to be for me?" ... I sensed that I would not go back home with my family.

For Mary, like most of the survivors, the first glimpse of the imposing red brick clinical building of the Michener Centre remains a stark and sobering memory; that was when they first began to sense that something unimaginable and terrible was about to happen to them. In retrospect, the survivors described being unsure why they were going to the Michener Centre, what they could expect when they got there, when they would next see their families and friends, and when (or even whether) they would leave the institution to return home.

Parental Abandonment

On arrival at the clinical building, children were permitted little opportunity to speak about their concerns or even to say goodbye to their family members. Instead, parents were whisked into the main office to sign papers and complete formalities, while children were removed to separate waiting rooms to await their fate. As Louise Roy, who was 10 years old when she first went to Michener, explained:

> What happened was when I first went, there was my mom and a staff. I was told to sit down and wait in the hallway with a suitcase by my chair, and then the staff came and took my arm and my suitcase and put me in this bedroom by myself with the suitcase and shut the door. I didn't even get to say goodbye to my mom.

The lack of explanation or farewell and the sense of abandonment pervades the survivors' stories. The admission process seems to have been organized in a way that would, ostensibly, minimize parent–child interactions, reducing guilt and keeping emotions at bay. However, although this procedure might have been helpful to parents and staff, the survivors' recollections indicate that the partings were very traumatic for the children. As Ray, who was so young that he can no longer recall his exact age at the time of his admission, described, "The hardest thing for me was when I was first put in Red Deer, to see my family drive away and me being left behind. It was a scary experience." Undoubtedly, being left alone at the institution was terribly frightening, but it was more than that; with the exception of Donna Bogdan, who came to the institution from an orphanage, these experiences also mark the first, and for most of the survivors, the final break in the children's relationships with their parents. Separated from

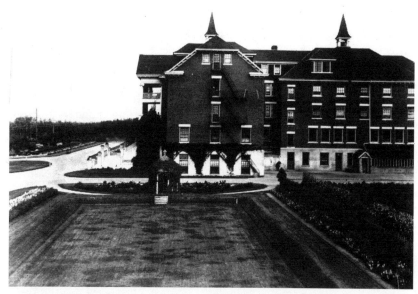

Figure 2.1 Main Michener administration building, circa 1955. Note the highly manicured grounds. Courtesy Red Deer and District Archives (N5412).

family, in a strange place, the children's reactions were predictable: they felt frightened, sometimes betrayed, always hurt. Louise Roy described how, after learning that her mother had gone without saying goodbye, she was left "wondering why she did that to me because I felt that she didn't want me anymore." For Louise, and for the other children who lived this experience, admission was overwhelmingly characterized by confusion, loss, and profound trauma.

It is not unreasonable to ask why parents would behave in such seemingly callous ways. Although we might presume that some of the parents were indeed relieved to have the long, tense drive and the wrenching decision-making process behind them, it is also fair to assume that many of the parents would have liked to have said goodbye and behaved in a more humane fashion during the admission process. It seems, both from the observations made by survivors and from the description provided by the one mother, that the institution itself encouraged this abrupt and harsh separation of children and parents, and also encouraged a distinct break between the children and their former lives. A number of the survivors indicate that they were not permitted to have visitors for the first year of their stay in Michener and that this was a part of the routine policy of the Michener Centre.

This policy was, in fact, enshrined in the admission process. Recall that Sam Edwards's mother had placed him at the Provincial Training School (PTS) because of behavioural problems in his classroom and that she left a cache of PTS/ Michener documents to him on her death. Among these was the pamphlet provided to parents on admitting children. In it are directives concerning visits. In addition to limiting visiting to "Wednesdays, Saturdays and Sundays, between 2 and 4 p.m." and excluding siblings under 16 years of age, who were not permitted to visit "on the Villas," the policy stated:

> We try to make it a general rule for children not to be visited for the first month or six weeks to accustom them to a new environment where they will be encouraged to make friends with other children and get to know their teachers, occupational and recreational therapists and the geography of the School generally.
>
> It may well be that a child who has made rapid adjustment, will not require this length of time to adjust to being away from home, in which case the parents are usually notified that they may visit sooner. (Government of Alberta, n.d., p. 3)

Thus, the policy limited the kinds of visitors, the times of visits, and the frequency of visits, and established an early intervention of separating children from their homes and families, all under the guise of permitting children to adjust to institutional routines. However, the brief adjustment time does not match the survivors' tales of only rarely being visited by parents and of having to wait up to a year to see their parents after being admitted.

Some insight as to why the visits were infrequent can be seen in the papers left behind by Sam Edwards's mother, Dorothy. In two letters written to his mother during the first few months of his time in Michener, Sam spoke longingly of coming home to visit. By February (three months after being admitted), he wrote, "I hope I can come home next week. So I'm going to be a good boy so I can. How are the pets? Are they o.k.?" In her letters to Superintendent LeVann, through whom all communications with children or staff members were to be directed (Government of Alberta, n.d.), Dorothy repeatedly asks when she can see Sam and when he will be coming home to visit. On 20 March 1970, more than four months after Sam's admission, LeVann replies that "Sam appears to be well and happy. He is doing fairly well but has not earned sufficient stars to enable him to go home for the week-end" (LeVann, 1970a). Although the manifest reason given for Sam's isolation was initially adjustment and then disciplinary control, it also seems that Dorothy felt herself to be disciplined by these procedures. Once she removed Sam from the institution, she began a formal complaint with the provincial ombudsman, to whom she wrote the following:

> To help Sam overcome his first break away from home I wrote twice a month. This was frowned upon for some reason unknown to me and I was asked not to write so often. All my letters to Sam were censored and all Sam's letters to me were censored. In fact, I never received many of the letters that Sam wrote. Is this necessary? (Edwards, 1970)

Throughout the correspondence with LeVann, and in her description of the events to the ombudsman (whose investigation she ultimately found to be very unsatisfactory), this woman seemed convinced that the institution did not want her to be involved in her son's care or to be a regular visitor to the institution. In a similar vein, a series of incidents written up by a worker to the relief manager of the adult section describes an impromptu visit by another inmate's mother, illustrating the institutional ambivalence in parent–staff interactions. The mother, having learned by letter that her daughter was ill, and having become further upset on her arrival when seeing that her daughter's face had been badly scratched, complained that the staff had been neglectful and perhaps even abusive. She refused to be assured that the scratches were self-inflicted and instead accused the staff of "deliberately trying to upset her" (Leithead, 1976). The mother was calmed down and sent off the ward for the evening, but she returned the following afternoon. A nurse described it thus:

> I had Mrs. X again this evening. She is very radical and demanding. She said we are mean to [her daughter]. It was a very upsetting evening again. I had to ask her leave ... She said she will have to move to Red Deer so that [her daughter] is looked after better. I told her if [her daughter] is so good she could take her home and keep her all the time. I told her to come on day shift before 3:30 so she could speak all her complaints to the Charge. She is really cross! (Leithead, 1976)

Parental visits such as the one described above, and even those that were less dramatic, were seemingly viewed with some trepidation; the Unusual Incidents files recurrently mention parental complaints about their children's condition following visits to the wards or following the occasional visits of children to their homes. Although many of these complaints did result in investigations, the complaints were often responded to as if they were misguided or ill-informed. For example, a concerned mother wrote:

Every time we see [our daughter] her teeth are very dirty. And ... all they have is a little paper cup by there [*sic*] bed side with a little bit of water in it enough to wet the brush ... And another thing is, that we seen in there, is very bad is, only one toilet for the children that [our daughter] is with. And there are 24 children in her group. (Anonymous, 1976b)

In response, the assistant director of nursing wrote that she "would feel free in assessing [the daughter's] dental services to be more adequate than the majority of those received by children in the community," going on to note that the mother's "criticism of toilet facilities is really quite unfounded" (Garrett, 1976, p. 1). As can be intuited from the unhappy tone of the letters to the facility, and from the equally tart tone of the institutional response, parent–institution relationships were often adversarial, and visits were less than embraced by staff and administration. It is thus reasonable to speculate that at least some of the social isolation of inmates from their families stemmed from an institutional hope of keeping parents out of the daily management of their children's care.

Finally, the institutional policy of curtailing family visits and loosening the bonds of affection between parents and their children was reflective of overarching attitudes and practice among professionals of the day. Ontario psychiatrist C. B. Farrar, an expert with whom the province consulted to evaluate Alberta's Provincial Training School, illuminated this broader doctrine. In a paper on euthanasia and intellectual disability, he articulated the need for all physicians and professionals to actively work to break down the bonds between children with intellectual disabilities and their parents. He went on to refer to the love of a parent for her or his child with a disability as a "morbid obsession" and to identify "the 'fondness' of the parents of an idiot and the 'want' that he should be kept alive" as a "psychiatric problem" (Farrar, 1942, p. 143).

Loss of Identity

Once family members left their children behind on admission day, isolation and depersonalization seem to have been central and routine parts of the admission process. Almost all the survivors described spending their first few days in the institution in a bare, private room, where they had little contact with anyone outside of the nurses or doctors who occasionally brought them in for psychological testing or for other medical examinations. This experience was often described as a quiet but anxious time of uncertainty, expanding in many ways on Mary's question, "What is it going to be for me?" This period was also one in which vestiges of the children's former lives quickly and efficiently began to be stripped away. Mary Korshevski, who was admitted at 15 years of age, offers a fairly typical description, saying, "When I first came there, I didn't know where to put my purse. They showed me this attic. We put everything in the attic." These newly admitted children had their clothing, their toys, and the few possessions they had brought with them removed, and very often they never saw these things again. This experience was universally shared by all survivors; even though the admission letters to parents did require them to provide a broad range of clothing for their children, the management of these objects was surrendered to institutional control, and, most often, these possessions found their way into the common stock of institutional clothing. Although the removal of personal belongings may have ostensibly streamlined the daily operations of the institution, the net effect was the undermining of personal autonomy and personal identity. Instead of having access to their own things, the children were provided with institutional clothing chosen by staff for them to wear. Michener clothing was sometimes produced by the residents themselves in the institution's sewing room, but more typically clothing came from other inmates, distributed for common use. It is important to also note that some of the survivors did recall receiving new clothing – often sent from home – at different points in their tenure at the institution; however, they were never really able to choose their own clothes on a daily basis or to be sure that their clothing would be safe from loss in the institutional laundries or safe from pilferage by others in the institution.

This inability to direct their own appearance must have had devastating effects on the children's sense of identity and self-image. Thus, it is not surprising that the issue of clothing remains an important memory for survivors. Mary Korshevski told a poignant story of the first time she, as a 36-year-old woman and more than 21 years after her first night in the institution, chose and purchased something of her own to wear:

> I remember when I first come out, we'd go downtown shopping, and I was a little bit leery about looking at things in stores, but this one time we went and [my friend] was looking at something and I decided, "You know, I'm going to start looking around too." And I spotted this yellow dress ... and I showed her this yellow dress. And I asked her, "Can I buy this?" and it was the first thing I ever bought myself, was a yellow eyelet dress, and I felt pretty proud, because we weren't able to go and choose anything we wanted. They did it for us, you know?

Like Mary Korshevski, Harvey Brown also recalled how excited he had been the first time he bought his own clothes as a 19-year-old man on the outside. During the interview, more than 30 years after the fact, he could still recall the name of the store where he made that first purchase.

Erving Goffman, in his foundational ethnography of life inside a total institution, noted that entrance into these institutions is marked through "obedience tests" in which the staff provides new inmates with a clear sense of their new role and place in the world of the institution (Goffman, 1961, p. 16). For Goffman, a foundational and ubiquitous obedience test was the removal of the individuals' "civilian" clothing and identity, both providing a symbolic stripping away of the outside world's hold on the individual and ushering the individuals to an understanding of their new place inside the institution (Goffman, 1961, p. 18). The descriptions these survivors give of their first days in the institution match Goffman's observations; in those first days, the children's identities, their connections to outsiders, and their sense of place in the world was abruptly and unwaveringly stripped away.

Family Life and Social Death

At the same time as these children began to lose their sense of their former selves, their ties with family and their former worlds began to be systematically eroded. Recall that one purported advantage of establishing an institution for "mental defectives" in Alberta was so that children would be closer to their families. However, from the beginning of the children's internment and continuing throughout their entire institutional stays, relations with family members and visits to their homes and communities remained rare events for most of the survivors in this study. It seems that once these children walked through Michener Centre's front doors, they began to experience "social death."

David Sudnow, in his observations of patients terminally ill with cancer, noted that terminally ill individuals often experience social devaluation and exclusion long before they actually pass away; they are often ignored or discounted by their families and loved ones as a form of anticipatory bereavement. For the mourners of those individuals experiencing social death, the process of bereavement preceded the death because the patients' involvement in and contributions to their social world had already ended (Sudnow, 1967). More recently, health researchers have expanded Sudnow's model to include the absence of behaviours, courtesies, and considerations that would normally be extended to someone who is alive; in other words, social death is treatment of someone as though they were dead, despite the fact that the individual is, in fact, still physically alive (Williams, 2004). There are several reasons we can speculate that the Michener Centre's children would have experienced this premature, social death.

As we have learned, the first wedge between the survivors and their social worlds was the Michener practice of discouraging or refusing permission for parents to visit during an initial period of acculturation. Although the official admission documents indicated that this period would last only a month, multiple survivors recalled that parents were not permitted to visit for the first year, so it seems the institution contributed to the inmates' social isolation and lack of social contribution, the hallmarks of social death. One can speculate that the longer such isolation went on, the less involved or connected these survivors became to their families and friends. After that first year of separation, and as time passed, it is likely that social distance made visits increasingly difficult. Indeed, survivor Bonnie Cowan's mother, when writing Bonnie's history of her institutionalization, provided some insight into the various difficulties faced in staying connected to an institutionalized child:

> The institution was some distance from home and due to small children and work schedules, visits require pre-planning and eventually family visits diminished in frequency. Having made that heartbreaking decision, we tried hard to justify it and to believe that it really was best for Bonnie.

In this mother's narrative, we can hear that physical distance made visiting difficult, but we can also hear that the social distance of not seeing a child regularly, and of feeling heartbroken by the child's situation, ultimately made the effort seem to be too much. In this mother's narrative, we can also detect echoes of the broader rhetoric used to argue in favour of institutionalization: that being removed from society was really best for the child.

This mother's response was perhaps understandable; survivors who did have opportunities over the years to visit home or to spend a holiday with family described how wrenching it was for them to be returned to the institution; they repeatedly asked to be allowed to stay at home, and they cried terribly or became angry on their return to the institution. The scenes that accompanied the ends of those visits must have been difficult for the children and for the family members. Not only were children's visits to the family made difficult because of the children's reactions, but when parents visited their children in the institution, they would also have had to face some of the realities of their institutionalized child's life, which must have been unpleasant and unsettling in many cases. As we will see in the next chapter, the institution was, despite efforts made to keep buildings tidy and gardens inviting, a terrible physical environment. To stay away might permit parents, as Bonnie's mother intimated, to avoid the ugly realities of their children's lives and to rationalize the decision to put the children there in the first place. Not seeing the institution would make it possible to, as Bonnie's mother said, "believe that it really was best" for these children.

That visits to the institution were often extremely difficult is further intimated in the following exchange with survivor Jim Molochuk:

JIM: I felt lonely.
INTERVIEWER: Who did you miss?
JIM: I missed my mother.

INTERVIEWER: Did she come and see you at all, Jim?

JIM: Once. And that was once in 1949.

INTERVIEWER: They came up all the way from Lethbridge to Red Deer?

JIM: Yeah.

INTERVIEWER: How old were you then, do you know?

JIM: No. I was quite young, very young then. [This would have been when Jim was 13 years old and had been there for a year].

INTERVIEWER: Tell me about that visit.

JIM: I don't know. We walked around the institution. We walked around.

INTERVIEWER: Did she think it was a good place for you, do you think?

JIM: I don't think so. She was crying.

It is difficult to imagine this visit as anything but painful for both Jim and his mother. For her to see the setting where Jim spent his days must have been very upsetting since she visited only once in all the years Jim lived in Michener. For Jim as well, the much anticipated visit from his mother must have been disappointing – perhaps he had hoped she might take him home or at the very least that he would have more pleasure and comfort from her visit than simply walking aimlessly around the institutional grounds feeling helpless and unhappy.

A final consideration concerning the social death of these children rests not with the parents, or even the institution itself, but instead relates to the general social stigma prevalent during these decades about intellectual disability, one that hearkens back to eugenic ideas about "taint" and "degeneration." In this chapter I have argued that despite claims that after World War II eugenic ideals were no longer commonly held as scientifically legitimate or morally acceptable, we know that these ideas continued to hold sway over admissions to the Michener institution and over the continued practice of legal, involuntary sterilization in Alberta. There is evidence that these ideas persisted beyond the province's borders as well. Nicole Hahn Rafter (1997) discusses the phenomenon of social death in her survey of moral degeneracy. In addition to the obvious arguments that physical distance and limited family resources were impediments to visiting institutionalized children, Rafter reminds us that, because of eugenic moral degeneracy discourse and its assumption that disability occurred as a result of taint in the family, significant shame was attached to having a child who was mentally deficient. James Trent (1994), in his history of mental retardation in America, echoes this claim; he notes that the shame of parenting a defective child kept the plight of institutionalized children out of the public eye until the late 1960s. According to Trent, it was rare for anyone to admit that they had a defective child until deep into the 1950s and 1960s, when several prominent parents of children with developmental disabilities,

including Rose Kennedy and Dale Evans (whose otherwise stellar eugenic credentials as white, upper-class, apparently wholesome women placed them in a
position to debunk some of these ideological holdovers) went public with their
stories (Trent, 1994, p. 187). The persistence of the stigma of producing a child
with intellectual disabilities may have meant that at least some of the parents of
the children in this study felt some relief in placing the child out of sight and
moving on with their lives without having to live with that stigmatizing child.

It is nonetheless unfair to assign the entire responsibility for children's social
death to parents who may have preferred to avoid the pain of visiting. There is
also evidence from Michener documents that parental visits were regarded
with ambivalence and even hostility by Michener staff. From an examination of
Unusual Incidents reports made during the mid-1970s, it is clear that parents
and parental visits were often perceived as disruptive and troublesome. In a
series of reports and letters, among them a report to an officer of Social Services,
Executive Director Dr S. J. Koegler responded to parental complaints. In one
particular instance regarding the scalding of one resident and the "bruises and
scratches" sustained by another, he worried that these situations "could result in
parent action," a concern that seemed to be a recurrent institutional anxiety
(Koegler, 1976a). Because parental visits provided opportunities for parental
surveillance, they seem to have frequently resulted in complaints and struggles over what constituted proper care of the children involved. The Unusual
Incidents reports and letters that were written to parents often discussed post-
visit complaints parents made about the treatment their children were receiving, about the condition of their teeth, about the bruises they saw on their
bodies, about the conditions of the wards themselves, and about their children's
reluctance to return to the institution following occasional family visits. Thus,
it is perhaps not surprising that the institution did little to encourage parental
visits; they were often contentious and required significant institutional investigations and paperwork to satisfy parent complaints. Nevertheless, this dis-
couragement, coupled with social pressures, often applied by family physicians
when advising parents to surrender their children, to forget about the child and
get on with life for the well-being of the rest of the family did result in serious
social isolation and the social death of many of these child inmates.

A poignant example of moving on can be read in a report on the death of a
child in custody. In it, Kathleen Swallow, the director of medical services, noted
that the parents had not contacted the child or the institution for more than
four years before the child's death. The director described contacting both parents' former employers and Social Services to no avail; the family had apparently moved to the United States with no forwarding address (Swallow, 1976).
From this sad tale, we can understand how isolated this child must have been

in the years that preceded her death; long before she physically died, she been socially and psychologically dead to those who were supposedly close to her. It is important to bear this social isolation and the lack of resources in mind as we move into the chapters that follow. The daily depersonalization and neglect that occurred within the institution, the regular violence and discipline that punctuated those endless days, and the routine institutional abuse that occurred in conjunction not only with institutional practices but also with the Eugenics Board activities within Michener was, at least in part, permitted to unfold precisely because these children did not have allies outside to expose the institution and make it accountable for its actions.

Chapter Three

Dehumanization as a Way of Life

By the 1960s and early 1970s, when most of the individuals who participated in this research went to live and work at Michener, the imposing brick building that had housed the institution's first 105 children had become the administrative heart of an enormous complex of multi-storey residences for inmates and staff, service buildings, offices, recreational and physical plant facilities, farm and workshop buildings, and greenhouses, all arrayed on two campuses kitty-corner to each other. The South Campus (located to the south and west) housed the Provincial Training School (PTS), the children's services side of the operation, and the North campus housed Deerhome, the facility for adults. Eventually, both campuses were combined and renamed to the current Michener Centre. According to property maps made during the 1970s, the South Campus had no less than 36 buildings on about 60 hectares (Reid Crowther & Partners Limited, Cartographers, 1977), while the North campus consisted of another 26 buildings on a similarly sized plot (Alberta Government Department of Public Works; Site Development Section, 1971). The buildings included 10 two- or three-storey wards for children, which went under the names of various trees, such as Ash or Pine or Cherry, and another eight multi-storey wards for adults, which carried the names of birds, like Bluebird and Nightingale, for women, and the names of Canadian flora and fauna, such as Juniper and Caribou, for men. On both the South and the North campuses, these wards appear from the outside to be low-rise, 1950s-style brick apartment buildings, spaciously arrayed along walkways or small green spaces punctuated by copses of trees, well-groomed shrubberies, and colourful flower beds.

In addition to these wards, the campuses had many other structures, including similar apartment-sized dormitory buildings for nurses and male staff on each campus, and a private home built for Superintendent LeVann and his family on the South Campus, which perched on a hillside overlooking the town of

Red Deer. Ancillary buildings were also abundant, including a power house, woodshed, three chicken coops, a granary, two greenhouses, a barn, root hous-es, storehouses, breeder houses for livestock, a fire hall, a mechanical shop, a carpentry shop, and a garage. In addition to residential and ancillary buildings, a variety of service buildings existed, including an infirmary, a clinical building, a small school, a vocational training centre, an occupational therapy shop, a summer barracks, a small recreational hall, tennis courts, a curling rink, wad-ing pools, and, in winter, an outdoor skating rink. In sum, the two campuses composed a self-contained and self-sufficient village that accommodated more than 2300 inmates and several hundred resident staff, and serviced an even larger complement of off-campus workers. The two campuses, situated on gen-tly rolling parkland on a hilltop at the outer edge of the small city of Red Deer, were connected by a walking path and a quiet, tree-lined roadway. The cam-puses were edged by farmland on most sides, with residential streets to the west of the children's campus and a tree nursery to south of the adult's campus. In the distance, farmland and forest spread out as far as the eye could see. In all, the campus must have appeared as a place of order and calm; indeed, the campus might have appeared on first impression to be almost bucolic.

Dehumanization and Its Functions

Despite these first impressions, however, it is clear from the descriptions given by residents and ex-workers alike that the inside of these buildings were any-thing but idyllic. Instead, the spatial arrangements, the control of inmates' time, and the personal care that occurred inside these building operated as an inten-tional vehicle for depersonalizing – indeed, dehumanizing – the people who lived there. Dehumanization, the process of attributing less-than-human or non-human attributes to members of a group, facilitates several outcomes. First, it permits those in dominant or in-group positions to explain the actions, behaviours, and attributes of those who are being dehumanized as naturally not belonging in the in-group's social world. For example, in Nazi Germany, Jewish people were constructed as dangerous because they were matter out of place, a people who did not belong to the natural social contract, obfuscating the reality that their position as outsiders resulted from historical and contemporary prac-tices that left them with no choice but to live in ghettos or to interact with others as outsiders (Hughes, 2002). In this aspect of dehumanization, then, in-dividual traits are erased and the person comes to be seen as a member of a group that is not fully human, that has neither the capacity nor the desire to be human, and hence cannot be taken into account as a member of the in-group's own species. Both Hughes (2002) and Savage (2007) argue that the definition of

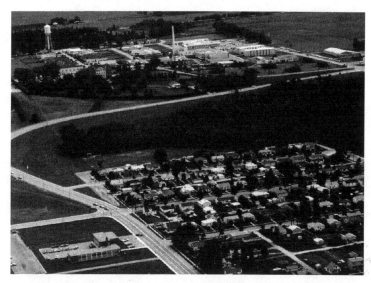

Figure 3.1 Aerial photograph of Red Deer, circa 1975. Michener Centre (top half of photo) sits on the hill, separated from the town of Red Deer by a dark row of trees. Courtesy of Harold Hopp.

out-groups as matter out of place is a particularly modernist obsession; in modernity, order and predictability are synonymous with goodness, while difference or matter out of place is seen as a threat to order and a moral flaw. It is thus perhaps not surprising that people with visible intellectual disabilities during the twentieth century found themselves sequestered in places like the Michener Centre; their unruly minds and bodies did not fit in modern civil societies, and hence removal may have seemed both necessary and proper.

Once inside the institution, order, routine, regimentation, and an erasure of inmates' individuality were major components and goals of daily life at Michener as a means of making their routine isolation seem both natural and necessary. By way of illustration, in a photograph taken in the mid-1950s (admittedly somewhat earlier than most of the inmates' descriptions that will follow), a dorm comprised of a simple room without dividers houses two long rows of metal bedsteads, each with a coverlet patterned with stripes and stylized pine trees. Reportedly, Dr LeVann was very particular that the stripes on these bedcovers should line up perfectly so as to create an atmosphere of precision and order; indeed, LeVann, who seems to have run the institution with an iron hand, showed an obsessive attention to detail and the creation of orderliness in every aspect of institutional life at Michener (Pringle, 1997). However, such obsessions go beyond the simple preferences of an institutional autocrat; they also reflect an overarching institutional precept that the "children"[1] in all their unruly individuality were to be subordinate to institutional regimes.

Another aspect of dehumanization is that it not only naturalizes the outsider status of those it targets, but it justifies the prejudices and abuses of those in the powerful in-group. Again using Nazism as an example, the systematic ill-treatment of Jews by the German authorities resulted in poverty, illness, and lack of dignity for Jewish people, and, in turn, these outcomes were used to legitimatize old abuses and develop new inhumane treatments of these people – after all, so the logic went, they were animals who deserved the ill-treatment they received (Tileaga, 2007). In the case of Michener, with its chronic over-crowding and staff shortages, inmates were treated with little dignity; housed in large warehouse-like spaces; fed, clothed, and showered en masse; and often medicated so heavily[2] as to erase their humanity. In the end, such dehumanization of the inmates was used to justify, or at the very least make less problematic, the careless and neglectful feeding, housing, cleaning, and regarding of inmates because, after all, they seemed to deserve or demand little more. For workers in such situations, dehumanization can lead to the assumption that human feelings of shame, decency, modesty, or entitlement do not apply to inmates; in turn, such assumptions can make it seem reasonable to simply toss people unthinkingly into a wheelchair and leave them for hours or hose them down publicly in a communal shower.

A third outcome of dehumanization draws on medical discourses of infection, contamination, and disease containment so that members of dominant in-groups come to see out-group members as scourges and dangers to the cleanliness, decency, and health of the modern social body. In turn, this enables dominant-group members to see cleansing or the actual removal/disinfection of the polluting group as a desirable goal in terms of protecting the proper or hygienic social body (Hughes, 2002). Thus, Nazi discourse spoke in terms of Jewish contamination and of the "necessity to sweep clean the world [of] sick people, cripples, psychologically immoral people, contaminated by Jewish, Gypsy or other blood" (Lifton as cited in Savage, 2007). Indeed, these types of discourse and practice have become such a normalized part of dehumanization that, although we might be horrified by the Nazis' use of the word "disinfection" to describe their state's genocidal practices, by the 1990s we were able, without irony, to use "ethnic cleansing" as a common descriptor of similar practices in the former Yugoslavia (Savage, 2007). At Michener, this third type of dehumanization directly relates to involuntary sterilizations that occurred routinely and to more passive eugenic processes as well. While I will discuss sterilization or active eugenics later in the book, in this chapter it will become clear that the daily routines and spatial and social arrangements at Michener operated as a form of passive eugenics. In passive eugenics, potential "bad breeders" are removed from society and from the sexual arena to prevent breeding; thus, the segregation of children by sex within Michener acted to prevent inmates from developing healthy and fulfilling relationships with members of the opposite sex,[3] while the campus itself, set apart from the world as it was, also contributed to the social, romantic, and sexual deprivation of inmates in terms of learning about or engaging in partnering or parenting.

In this and the next chapter, I argue that all three outcomes of dehumanization – the naturalization of abject otherness among inmates, the justification of abuse against them, and the rationale for culling them through passive and active eugenics – were facilitated through processes that were routinized in the institution. In the next chapter, I turn to more extraordinary examples of institutional dehumanization, while in this chapter, I focus on how these dehumanizing processes were threaded throughout every aspect of daily institutional life at Michener, occurring along axes of space and its use, time and its management, bodily privacy, and personal property. In deploying these various technologies of dehumanization, the institution, it is also clear, used them to construct hierarchies of humanity; to paraphrase George Orwell, some inmates were more human than others. Further, it is likely that these hierarchies served to create divisions among inmates that were highly disciplining, making the management of all those children's and adult's bodies more controllable for staff.

In the following sections, I draw on inmates' and ex-workers' recollections of their first impressions of the institution and their memories of daily life inside to outline the spatial, temporal, and hierarchical properties of life within the institution. While offering these descriptions, I invite the reader to imagine entering and living in PTS/Michener. How must it have been to be a young child, missing one's family, not understanding why or for how long one would be staying, and beginning to understand that this terrible place and its dehumanizing practices were to become one's new world?

Space and Its Uses

From estimates made by the workers and ex-residents interviewed, and from observations made during a belated tour of the Michener Centre – in which I was able to visit two old wards that had been partially emptied, locked, and left since the early 1980s (see Appendix II) – each floor of the primary, multi-storey residential buildings contained two wards, each designed to house between 35 and 45 children. The layout of the buildings, from an aerial view, was an E shape, and the buildings were entered through the end of the shorter, middle arm of the E. A child walking into these buildings for the first time would enter through a heavy, locked metal door with an adult-height metal panel that, when slid open from the inside, provided a view of the buildings' interiors. Once through this door, the child would be led along a narrow, shiny hallway 12 or 15 metres long. On either side of this hallway, with its terrazzo floors, shiny walls, low ceilings, and overhead lights, were rooms opening onto collective toilets, utility rooms, and small kitchens. At the end of the hall, and through a second, similarly portholed and locked metal door, the space opened up into the ward proper. Directly in front of this entry, along the spine of the E were ranged three large, open rooms, sometimes used as a dining room and two day rooms but more often simply used as three day rooms.

Each room was about 15 metres deep and 12 metres wide, with the expanse broken up by metal pillars. The rooms were tiled with industrial flooring and, similar to all walls in the facility, were painted a shiny white. In these wide, bright spaces, sounds must have reverberated and privacy would be virtually impossible to obtain. In wards with permanent dining areas (many wards did not have these because of overcrowding), trestle tables with long benches or smaller metal tables with chairs would be set out, but in many wards, there was little to break up the expanse of these noisy, hard surfaces. The rooms were lit by large, bright, bare mesh-fortified windows, and in the corner of each room was a television set built into a sturdy wooden, locked, mesh-covered cabinet. As the new child passed by, he or she probably would not yet have been aware that these day rooms would provide the setting where most days were to be spent in the coming years. Even so, the sight of these rooms, filled with inmates, must have been shocking.

The day rooms were generally filled with people, and there were few chairs for people to lounge in so that very often people milled around aimlessly, sat or lay on the floors, leaned against walls, or, in some cases, sat in wheelchairs or on the occasional hard chair in the rooms. In discussing a typical day, Ray Petrenko described the day room in his ward in the following terms:

> We would all go to the Day room there. They would lock the door behind us and we all would be, some of us would sit on the floor, and some of us would sit on the chairs, because they didn't have the ... didn't have very many chairs and we were sitting on floors.

These uncomfortable settings did not serve as simply brief holding areas where people might spend a few minutes waiting to be taken somewhere more hospitable to learn or play. Rather, once they had been toileted and fed, inmates were

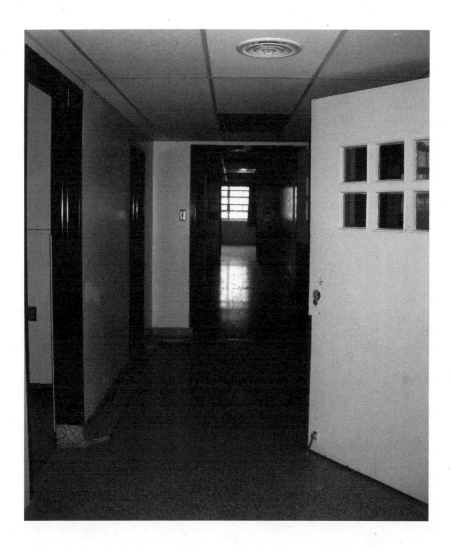

Figure 3.2 The entrance hallway, Nightingale A Ward. Taken in 2005.
Courtesy of the author.

put into the day rooms and spent very long stretches of time there. The lack of furniture or decoration in these rooms, and the resulting lack of comfort they afforded, seems to reflect a belief that inmates were not entitled to, indeed, did not require, a comfortable or pleasant place to sit while whiling away the hours, like any "ordinary" person might. Instead, these rooms were little more than holding tanks or warehouses and could have as easily been used for storing objects as for housing human children and adults.

Segregation and Dehumanization

Not only does it seem that the children's (and later, the adults') comfort was not a consideration, but it also seems to have been assumed that these children would not require interaction and stimulus to grow and develop, perhaps because they were not expected to grow and develop like "normal" human children. In describing her impressions of the day rooms and the activities in them, ex-worker Evelyn Stephens said:

> Most of the people were very drugged up, you know, I can't think of anything more mind-numbing and monotonous and deadening than – and I felt that so often – the routines of the day. Everyone was just walking around, like the walking dead ... people were sitting, pacing, rocking, watching T.V.

Ex-worker Coral James's description of her working life at PTS supports this view; she noted that while nursing staff spent most of their days in the nursing station counting meds and charting, support staff spent their days doing primary care (bed-making, washing, toileting) in the wards. Although Coral was herself such a support worker, she was unable to recall anyone spending their working days in the day rooms; indeed, when I asked her about the day rooms, she was unable to recall much more than that her job was to put those patients who were deemed capable into the day room and leave them there until they needed feeding or toileting again. Jim Sullivan, who worked on several wards in various capacities, concurred, saying that once the primary care was done "you just basically sat there [in the nursing stations] and talked to other staff ... Nothing with the patients or anything like that." In the day rooms, then, there was little to entertain or distract inmates outside of their fellow inmates, or the ubiquitous, droning television set, left on whatever station the staff had chosen.

It is difficult to understand what six- or seven-year-old children might have been feeling when they first saw their future home. Indeed, in most of the interviews, it was not always easy for the survivors to describe their emotional reactions to the day rooms or of entering the ward for the first time. Perhaps they were so young at admission that they have forgotten that first sight, perhaps

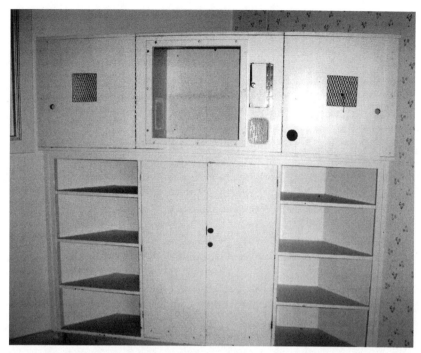

Figure 3.3 Locked television cupboard in day room, Michener Centre.
Taken in 2005. Courtesy of the author.

they spent so long in such rooms that they eventually came to see them as normal, or perhaps they have blocked out their feelings from those early days. However, it is certain that any child's first impression of this space as her or his future home would not have been comforting – instead, it must have been terrifying to see all those people milling around, seemingly without purpose, securely locked away, suspecting that – soon – you would be one of them.

Panopticism on the Wards

To one side as the children passed through the main day room area on their way to the ward would be the nursing station. Raised a foot or so off the floor, and through yet another locked door, the nursing stations overlooked the day areas in front of them and, to the side, the wards where the children slept. Coral, who worked on several such wards, described the layout of these nursing stations:

The office was not unlike the one in *One Flew over the Cuckoo's Nest*. Only I don't remember the glass – there being a total glass front. But there was a lattice glass on three sides. [It was] Not accessible at all. Not at all. I think there was a room, a doorway and a room, to the back of it where the meds were and it was actually raised up a little bit above floor level. That's right, and there was a long counter and there were – so if I was looking out, I could look out into the day room area when I was looking forward from the office. Behind me, there would be charts, lots and lots of charts.

This enclosed space, sitting higher than the rest of the rooms, and open visually onto all the patient spaces, operated as a kind of watchtower from which inmates' every movements were easily observed, their behaviours were readily recorded and charted, and their actions could be speedily responded to by nursing staff.

Michel Foucault (1994, 1995) has shown us convincingly that the spatial arrangements of buildings, public places, and interiors are not simply haphazard or aesthetic but are instead functional and political; from his work, we learn that modernity has been characterized by the development of large public institutions, such as prisons, army drill halls, and institutions like Michener. These facilities are built and organized to offer surveillance of and control over large populations, reducing the need for force in keeping individuals acquiescent. For Foucault, this use of space to monitor large congregations of docile bodies is a hallmark of modern disciplinary societies. Rather than brutally punish transgressors, modern disciplinary organizations work preventively, through the organization of space and surveillance by knowledgeable professionals, to keep individual members of the group submissive and disciplined. As Foucault argued, being able to view inmates, to measure their activities, and respond to their transgressions immediately with modern instruments, such as charts or patient records that track every action, is a powerful tool of preventive discipline. Foucault offered the Panopticon as a metaphor for these modern disciplinary practices, drawing on the ideal prison design devised by Jeremy Bentham, which was a hexagon-shaped, multi-storeyed prison with its cells arranged open to view from a central tower. From that tower, guards could gaze out but inmates could not tell whether the tower was staffed or empty. As a result, not only did inmates behave well to avoid being seen and punished, but they would also come to police themselves *in case* someone might be watching. The Panopticon thus is more than simply a viewing tower or, in this case, a nursing station on a raised platform. Instead, it is a multi-modal set of practices that permit regulation through seeing, knowing, coding, recording, and normalizing the actions of those at the distal end of the

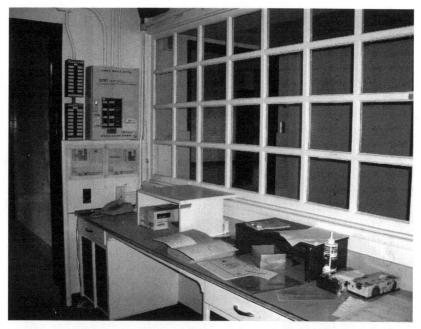

Figure 3.4 Nursing station, Michener Centre. Taken in 2005. Courtesy of the author.

gaze. The point for Foucault and those who build on his work is that even when inmates are not being watched, they come to learn that they must act as if they are being watched or could be caught at any moment because their movements are not only constantly observable but recorded for others – the record stands as an additional layer in the discipline of unruly bodies (Foucault, 1982, 1995; Rose, 1990). Thus, the functions of the disciplinary gaze, in this case emanating from the physical layout of the raised dais and windows of the nursing station, coupled with professional knowledge in the form of the openly visible array of patient charts, would of course have facilitated nursing observations, but these arrangements at the same time offered a visual display of power and knowledge to inmates who could clearly see that they were being observed and charted on an ongoing basis.

After a child passed this nursing station/Panopticon and the day rooms, she or he finally would be led through one last set of locked double doors to enter the ward itself. In the following interview exchange with ex-worker Coral, we gain some insight into how the child's new home would have appeared:

INTERVIEWER: They were in private rooms?

CORAL: Oh no. Oh no, not at all. The ward – the dorm – was a big wide- open area and it ran the width of the building. And there were probably – there were pods. There would be one, two, three, four beds in a pod. And then there would be ... a half wall and a pillar. And then four beds in the next pod with a half wall and a pillar. There was no privacy whatsoever. None whatsoever. So there must have been close to 50 people, I would think.

The wards that I was able to view held nine or ten of these "pods," each housing four beds, all of which would have been fully visible from the nursing station at the entrance to the ward. There were no curtains to separate the beds, no carpets on the floors, no bedside dressers on which to array personal items or photographs, no personal touches, such as playful coloured bedspreads or stuffed toys on the beds, no pictures on the walls – indeed, there were no walls to speak of. In one small room off each ward were clothing storage cupboards, approximately one metre tall and one or one and a half metres wide, filled with cubbyholes with names taped to the front; in these small spaces, no larger than 30 centimetres wide by 30 centimetres high and 45 centimetres deep, each child's clothing would be kept.

Privacy and Hierarchy

These large, open wards were the most common arrangement for housing inmates, but they were not the only kinds of sleeping units on the campus; the size of the wards varied considerably. The ways that personal sleeping space was organized not only conveyed assumptions about the less-than-human status of all inmates and their presumed lack of need for privacy, but they also telegraphed the reality that within the institutions some inmates were seen to be less human than others. The four-bed, nine-pod rooms that many inmates described were fairly common, but some inmates described rooms that had as many as 50 people in one large open space, while others described having rooms with "only" three or four roommates. The large, heavily populated wards would have been primarily allocated for what the institution termed Low Grades, or people deemed to have more severe intellectual disabilities (classed as Idiots or Imbeciles), while High Grades (those identified as Morons or Borderline)[4] were often afforded somewhat more privacy and dignity. Nevertheless, even in High Grade rooms, the paltriness of personal space and personal belongings was ubiquitous. Sean Hoskins was a High Grade who was given some classroom instruction while a child in PTS, entitling him to be called a School Boy, the term for the most advanced inmates on the children's

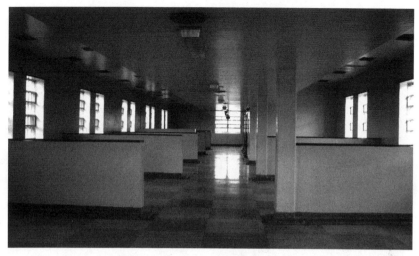

Figure 3.5 Typical Low Grade ward (Nightingale A). Taken in 2005.
Courtesy of the author.

campus. When asked about his first sleeping situation, Sean said, "I slept in a dormitory. There were six beds in a room, six drawers." Sean's description intimates that, even when sleeping rooms were relatively capacious, there still was not a lot of personal space or room for personal belongings: six drawers to accommodate the possessions of six children can hardly be termed private or adequate.

Because most people lived in Michener Centre for long periods that straddled childhood and adulthood, they often lived in a variety of accommodations. In some cases people, depending on their behaviour and institutional classification, were transferred at adulthood from the children's side into some of the better wards for adults on the Deerhome campus, as Ray, Jim, and Michel described. In other instances, the opposite occurred so that an inmate who may have had relatively luxurious housing as a School Boy or School Girl in childhood might then be moved into a wide, dormitory-style setting on the adult side of campus, as happened to Mary Korshevski. Mary described her various rooms as follows:

Oh, when I first went there, I had – I was on a ward for school girls. And it was a bedroom, we shared, three to a room. And I was on one ward for four, and then I went to a ward in Deerhome where I was for 13 years. That was a dormitory, and there was 38, and we slept side by side!

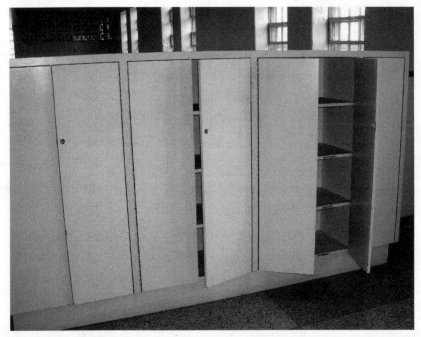

Figure 3.6 Cupboards for storing inmates' possessions. Note the names written on tape
on each shelf of the far right cabinet, and the holes where locks once were.
Taken in 2005. Courtesy of the author.

In Mary's case, this seeming demotion may have been related to her physical
condition. As a child in the institution, she was a valued School Girl because
intellectually she had been identified as a relatively High Grade inmate. However, on reaching adulthood when inmates shifted even more into a worker
role, because Mary had polio and was quite frail, she might not have been seen
as such a desirable or positive kind of resident, and her accommodations reflected that assessment.

Before a child would deposit his or her few remaining personal possessions
into the allotted cubbyhole in the storage room, she or he would have passed
several smaller rooms where daily hygiene took place. In the first areas were the
toilets, followed by shower rooms. As with the sleeping quarters, the lack of
privacy and the routinization of negligence were built right into the architecture of these rooms, which expresses much about the attitudes of those who ran
the institution concerning their charges. The first and most obvious thing that

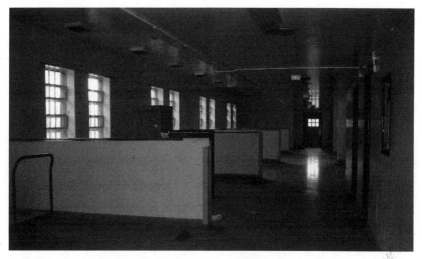

Figure 3.7 A smaller side ward. Each bay held eight beds. Taken in 2005.
Courtesy of the author.

struck me when observing the toilets and showers that I was permitted to see was that they not only did not have doors but that there was no evidence that they had ever had them; the Panopticon even extended into the most private moments of these inmates' lives. In another example of the lack of privacy afforded to inmates, several rooms with elevated bathtubs in them also housed wash racks for equipment and a hopper for cleaning out bedpans. In these arrangements, it would be conceivable that one staff person might be cleaning up urine or feces while another staff person might be bathing a patient who could not use the shower facilities but instead required more personalized care. In the layout of these most intimate spaces, it is clear that the residents of the institution were conceived of as other than human, as not-human, and as undeserving of the most basic human decencies.

Hygiene and Dehumanization

Although the survivors often had difficulties describing their first impressions of the rooms and layout of the buildings, several of them were clearly able to recall their first impressions of the showers when they arrived. Donna Bogdan was able to describe quite compellingly her first experiences of showering during her admission to Michener:

They said I was going to Red Deer, and I was going to Training School, and I thought, oh, that's fantastic. I'm going to really learn something going to school. Well I got quite a big surprise! As soon as I was admitted in, they stripped us and we had to take some showers. They sprayed some stuff onto us ... something to get rid of bugs, to get rid of lice ... so we were sprayed with some stuff and we were all stripped naked and they gave us a bath. I wasn't too happy with what they did, but I guess that's what they did to everybody.

In this description we can link the cleansing of the newly admitted child to dehumanization, to stigma, and even to eugenic discourses about cleansing the gene pool of undesirable stock. These practices illustrate how cleanliness, othering, and dehumanization were intertwined in the institution. Most obviously, because the showers were public and done in groups, it is clear that privacy and modesty were not seen as important, perhaps not even relevant, to Michener inmates. The impersonal, abusive roughness attached to being stripped down, sprayed off, and cleaned up in a public setting not only shows a distinct disdain for the individuals' dignity but is indeed a degradation ritual, a hallmark of total institutions and of depersonalization. Degradation rituals are designed to usher in personality change; in total institutions, such rituals operate to symbolically erase the person who existed before admission, opening the way for a new identity as "inmate" or "prisoner" to be constructed in that previous person's stead. Thus inductees learn through these degradation rituals that the things that people typically can expect in terms of social niceties and human interactions can no longer be counted on; in the institution, their rights to a full identity and human dignity are forfeit (Goffman, 1961). Finally, the routine delousing that Donna experienced on admission reflects eugenic discourses about pollution and cleansing, indicating that staff presumed that these individuals, perhaps because of their family backgrounds, ethnic categories, or socioeconomic status, were naturally unclean and would thus require disinfection before entering into institutional life.

Whether sleeping, toileting, bathing, dining, or spending time in day rooms, privacy was an elusive property; bodies were handled, observed, and processed, always in groups, and always under the watchful eye of someone in a position of power. Survivor Ray Petrenko described a typical shower experience:

And if we went to take a shower, there was no private stalls. All there was were stalls from one wall to the other. We had to stand in a long line in the hallways, and then we were paraded to go inside in the shower. There was no curtains or nothing. Everybody had to go into one stall, all at the same time. We would all line up and you had to parade with your clothes off and walk down the hallway and into the shower.

Former worker Evelyn Stephens confirmed this description, noting that for people like Ray, who was identified as a High Grade, at least the showering itself would have been left to the individual to manage under the watchful eye of staff. However, for Low Grades the experience was even more humiliating, as Evelyn described:

> They'd be standing naked waiting for you. It was awful. Really, I mean all of this is awful ... There was like this long room with shower heads coming out of the wall. And umm, we had, the staff had rubber aprons, we had to get in there and scrub and um (pause) and then, yeah, so they were showered that way and then we hosed them off there as well. I remember that.

Evelyn, who spent much of her time working on an adult ward for Low Grades went on to describe the toilet facilities on that ward, noting that, unlike the usual doorless toilets divided by partial walls that typified many of the institution's facilities, the toilets on the Low Grade ward she worked on were not even partitioned but instead stood in a row in an open, tiled room. Thus, like other architecture on the complex, the different layouts of toilet rooms reflected hierarchical distinctions in the institution between those deemed worthy enough for three walls on their toilets and those less-human inmates whom it was presumed could do quite nicely without. A final aspect of the Low Grade toilets described both by Evelyn and by survivor Donna Bogdan was that at least some of these toilets could be flushed simultaneously by staff who used a pull-cord hanging near the door of the toileting room, thus maximizing workers' efficiency. This last detail conveys a dystopian vision of a mechanized, routinized delivery of human services within the institution that completely denied the individuality, privacy, dignity, or humanity of the people being served: in this scenario, the utility of saving workers a few steps to flush individual toilets was seen as more important than the probability that inmates would be forced to sit in the collective stench until that final, efficient flush.

Time and Its Management

The dehumanizing qualities of the institution not only were embedded in the spatial arrangements of the day rooms, sleeping quarters, and hygiene facilities but were also entrenched in the ways that inmates' days were organized. Days at

Michener were characterized by long, painfully dull stretches of time inter-
rupted by brief, intense bursts of activity. A typical day began early and followed the same numbing routine each day. Harvey Brown, who lived most of
his time in High Grade facilities on both the children's and the adults' sides of
the campus, described how his days unfolded as a relatively prestigious School
Boy during his childhood:

> Got up at 6:30. Had breakfast at 7:00. Made your bed and all that stuff. Had inspec-
> tion. Went to school at 8:30. Came back for lunch at 20 to 12, went back to school
> at 1:10–1:30. Stayed til 3:00. Supper at 5:00 or quarter to 5:00 and then a bath or
> shower at 6:30. And you just sat around and watched TV until 9 o'clock and then
> you went to bed.

These routines were adhered to on weekends and in the summer as well but
without the activity of schooling to break things up. Further, for the vast majority of children who did not attend school, there was even more monotony. As
children, most of the survivors (and indeed, most inmates in general) did not
go to school, a topic that will be discussed more fully in Chapter Five. Those
survivors who did not attend school described days that were, as Jim Molochuk
put it, spent in the day rooms, "walking, day after day, day after day, seeing the
same thing over and over again." Thus, echoing the hierarchical spatial arrangements within the institution, the ways in which time was organized and allocated also reflected internal hierarchies: those High Grade residents who were
deemed to be Morons or Borderline were more likely to spend their days with
at least some stimulation in the form of school time, while those Low Grades
who had been labelled as Idiots or Imbeciles were likely to spend mind-
numbing hours doing virtually nothing, day in and day out.

The fact that inmates had significant stretches of unfilled time every day does
not mean that their time was free, as the following interview exchange with
Guy Tremblay clarifies:

ME: What about shower time and all that kind of stuff? Did they tell you when you
were going to have a bath and when you were going to brush your teeth and
when you were going to go to the bathroom?
GUY: Absolutely – for sure. Mind you, they would unlock the bathroom door for you.
ME: They locked the bathroom door for you? So that was the only time you ever got
to be private?
GUY: They locked and unlocked it for you every time you had to go.
ME: Oh! So you couldn't just go on your own?
GUY: No. Not on the wards I was on anyway.

This exchange shows that because of my own position as a privileged outsider, I failed to understand the point Guy was trying to make – that the bathrooms (and all other rooms in the institution) were locked and that movement – of any kind, really – was not freely granted. Inmates had to gain the attention of busy staff, ask permission to leave the day room or their bedrooms to use the toilets, wait for that staff person to unlock the room for them, and then, finally, be free to use the facilities.

In a similar vein, inmates' food and drink intake was also regimented and determined not by the individual's needs or wants but by the institution's requirements for order and control, and these things followed a highly regimented schedule. Donna Bogdan explained:

> We only ate at certain times. At 7:00 a.m., 12:00 p.m., and at 5:00 p.m. and at 8:00 p.m., night lunch. That was it. There were no other times. And all we did was have water during the day. I wished I would have had tea back then.

Thus, simple human bodily needs – to eat when hungry, to drink when thirsty, and to use a toilet when full – were routinely denied because of the rigidity of the schedule, or delayed because of the necessity of finding an available and willing staff member to unlock the doors that led to bed, food, or toilet.

Although these routines were undoubtedly inhumane, they were not necessarily solely intended as techniques for dehumanizing and disciplining inmates; they were organized in this way because of spatial and staffing constraints in the institution. It is clear that, long after the process of deinstitutionalization had been underway at Michener, overcrowding and understaffing were still putting pressures on the organization of inmates' time. The following excerpt, taken from a series of articles from the mid-1980s in the local newspaper that reported on the new, more humane changes at Michener, describes the routine of "Lyla," an older inmate:

> she rises with the other 61 people on her floor at Robin, a two-storey residence for elderly people who are moderately to severely mentally handicapped.
>
> They file out to the washrooms and bathe before they assemble in the dining room for breakfast. They must leave the dining room when the 64 people who live on the floor above come down for breakfast.
>
> The smooth operation of the institution depends upon adherence to the schedule. Few variations are permitted. (Martindale, 1983a, p. C1)

This excerpt illustrates how spatial limitations, literally written into the design of the institution, meant that inmates' time had to be controlled – to fail to meet the schedule could mean delaying another 60-odd people in getting their food and might mean a disaster in terms of managing the rest of the day. In addition, inhumane routines that operated to control inmates' bodily functions were also established as a way to facilitate staff efficiency and to pre-empt the inconvenience that accidents, emergencies, and inmate demands might place on already burdened workers; the predictability and regimentation of daily routines made the management of all those bodies possible. As Evelyn said, her workdays were characterized by a "routine [that] was based around cleanliness and dressing and feeding and hosing down and putting to bed and giving medications and just – controlling them." This need to control inmate's bodies, while not necessarily intentionally degrading, nevertheless did operate in dehumanizing ways, subordinating inmates' natural bodily functions and needs to institutional efficiency.

Staffing and Time Management

Adequate staffing seems to have been an ongoing preoccupation from Michener's early days, and the difficulties in hiring and keeping trained and compassionate staff are mentioned frequently in the annual reports written by administration to the government and, more informally, in ward reporting for internal use. Staffing was always tight, and the routines for staff, as for inmates, were often characterized by long stretches of dull inactivity or routine impersonal work, such as cleaning or charting, punctuated by intensely demanding activity when dealing with inmates. Evelyn described the night shift on her ward, with 30 to 40 inmates to a side, as follows:

> There'd be two of you – one for each side, basically. You'd come on at 11:00 at night, then of course you'd have all the sort of ... putting things away, tidying things up, making sure the charts were in order, and then, we did bed checks to make sure everyone was in their bed and where they're supposed to be ... it would be times of quiet then times it would be times of howling and screaming, or they moaned and groaned ... you tried really hard to stay awake. Made yourself toast, 'cause there was always food available for staff. So there wasn't a lot to do then, unless there was a disturbance, particularly in the Side Rooms. And your job was really only to tell them to shut up and go to sleep, so to say.

Thus, with the exception of unusual incidents, such as escapes, falls, or disciplinary issues, which will be discussed more fully in the next chapter, much of the night shift consisted of a quiet and often dull routine. However, because the staff-to-inmate ratio was kept low, with two night staff for as many as 70 to

80 inmates, the early morning routine was an entirely different experience, as ex-worker Jim Sullivan, when describing a relatively Low Grade ward for boys, explained:

> By 5:30 you're getting people up and dressed, because you have to have that all done before the day shift comes on. It was a frenzy first thing in the morning, because the night shift is responsible for making sure everybody is up and dressed before the day shift comes on. Then, the breakfast carts would come in and that kind of stuff and you would get it going and start stripping beds. So everything is done around staff scheduling, so that means they get up earlier.

The early morning routine on Jim's and Evelyn's wards that had to be accomplished by night staff before the first day shift arrived at 6:00 a.m. included waking patients, getting them out of bed, stripping wet and soiled linens off the beds, toileting inmates, and cleaning bodies that needed cleaning outside of the regularly scheduled shower times. At 6:00 in the morning, the first members of the day shift would arrive, adding another two or three people to the staff roster, and all three or four staff members would begin moving inmates into day rooms for breakfast, putting out breakfast trays, feeding inmates who might need assistance, putting breakfast trays back on the carts, finishing up the charts, and then taking part in a change-of-shift staff meeting with the incoming day shift. Clearly, in this brief period, with the small staff numbers, there would have been little time for social interaction or even for taking particular care in providing these services to inmates.

By the time the second shift of day staff arrived at 7:00 in the morning, many of the people would already be lined up, as described earlier, naked and waiting to be let into the shower room, and much of the early morning was taken up with showering and bathing people, and then moving them back into the day rooms. In addition to showering inmates, day staff bundled laundry, washed floors, checked bedridden patients to make sure they were still dry, turned them to keep them from getting bedsores, opened up toilets for day room patients needing to use those facilities, put lunch trays out, fed inmates, returned trays to the carts, checked bedridden patients again, peeked in on day rooms, and mopped up messes on floors when people waiting for toilet access failed to contain themselves. In short, the day shift was a constant round of housekeeping and cleaning that kept staff busy for much of the day.

Evenings, with staff arriving at 3:00 or 3:30, began yet another round of moving bodies, feeding them, cleaning up after them, tidying beds, changing linens, putting out trays and returning them to carts, wiping up messes, and putting inmates to bed, typically at a very early hour. Although in the beginning of this section, we heard from Donna Bogdan that her last activity of the day was "night lunch" at 8:00 p.m. in preparation for bedtime at 9:00, Donna was a High Grade inmate, and her experiences were not shared by all inmates. Instead, on Low Grade wards, the schedule was even more grinding than on the relatively privileged upper wards, reflecting the hierarchical thinking that pervaded institutional life. On Evelyn's Low Grade ward, she noted "they were in bed by 4:30 or 5:00 in the afternoon. So you got to be asleep for a long time, which, when you have nothing to do all day and are very drugged up was – well, what else was there?"

The ward where Coral worked seems to have housed people of the Lowest Grade, and although some inmates on this ward were able to go to the day room before being put back to bed by 5:00 p.m. as Evelyn described, many patients were never moved from the world of their own beds. As Coral explained, "Some of them we would get up and put in a wheelchair and wheel them into the day room for their breakfasts and lunch, but the majority on this particular ward were patients who stayed in the dorm all day long. All day, all night." Thus, on Coral's ward, most of these extremely devalued people passed their days without any stimulation at all except for the changing of a bed, being fed, or being turned to avoid bedsores.

The Effects of Time Management – Sensory Deprivation

Although it might be possible to say that this routine did not really matter to inmates who had severe disabilities, we cannot assume that these Low Grade inmates would not have minded the deadening routine because they were not able to cognitively take in the grimness of their situations. Coral told a story about a woman who lived on this ward who was aware of, and perhaps less than happy with, this grim daily schedule but who had no way to resist it:

> And there was one woman, oh my goodness, I don't know why she was there. I will never ever, ever forget her. She was 21 years old and she had very severe – we called it at the time "spastic" – cerebral palsy, I guess. And she was always in a bed. I think her name was Diane. Jeepers I can't believe I can remember that. She was very thin. She was 21, so she wasn't that much older than me. She was always in a bed ... And she – I don't know – I don't know why she was in that hospital and I don't know why she was on that ward, but she was a breath of fresh air, because she could speak. It was very hard work for her, but you could have great conversation with her, you could have a laugh with her.

The kind of interaction Coral described reflects a rare moment of humanity in an otherwise bleak world; that Coral found time to stop and notice that this young woman was aware and capable, and then managed to carve out the time to sit and talk with her, was a precious exception in the institutional routine, probably for both worker and inmate.

We can hope that a person with physical disabilities but no perceivable intellectual disabilities living on a ward for people with severe intellectual disabilities was simply a mistake, a rare instance of inappropriate treatment in the institutional setting. However, this young woman's situation was not unique within the institutional walls. As noted earlier, Leilani Muir, who launched a successful court case against the government for unlawful sterilization and unlawful confinement, was also wrongly diagnosed and spent many years in Michener. Likewise, after leaving the institution, several people who provided interviews, despite years of institutional neglect, had gained literacy skills, sustained friendships, married, and taken up meaningful employment. In short, many of the institutional survivors, despite years of sensory deprivation, managed to prove the institution wrong, going on to reclaim their lives and become integrated and productive citizens. Thus, although they may have been numbed and silenced by their lives within the institution, this was by no means proof that their treatment was appropriate because they were simply too feeble-minded to care about their circumstances. Further, it is important to understand that although mistakes were certainly made in assigning people to wards or in admitting people to the institution itself, the real issue is that the kind of deprivation that occurred every day in both Low Grade and High Grade wards would have been inappropriate for *any* child or adult to experience.

The literature on sensory deprivation is often criminological and focuses on its ill effects, with the research situated primarily in countries where sensory deprivation is a form of torture used by the state to terrorize its people or in total institutions, such as the current "super-max" prisons that house severe and dangerous offenders in the United States (Lippke, 2004; Moisander & Edston, 2003; Richards, 2006; Sarraj, Punamaki, Salmi, & Summerfield, 1996). In this research it is clear that sensory deprivation is implicated in personality breakdown; post-traumatic stress disorder; depression; other serious mental health problems, such as psychosis; and heightened vulnerability to pain and stress. Further, much of this research literature argues that isolation, lack of human interaction, and reduced stimulation are unethical and should not be used in any institutional setting. This criminological and human rights literature focuses on adults who have been isolated or deprived, but there are suspicions that the effects of this sensory deprivation may be even worse for children. Although it is unethical to engage in social experiments that might gauge the effects of lack of stimulation on children's development, studies with children who have been raised in similar institutions to Michener – such as the orphanages of Romania in the mid-1980s and in Haiti currently – indicate that sensory deprivation tied to institutional conditions can lead to similar problems to those identified above for adults. The effects extend to developmental delays, cognitive delays, antisocial behaviour, and reactive attachment disorders, which manifest either in an extreme inability to interact socially or extreme and inappropriate over-friendliness (Schell-Frank, 2000). In other words, it is clear that institutional life as it was organized at Michener would not have helped the children and would instead have caused them to have adjustment, developmental, and attachment problems that would have made reintegration into the community more difficult. In short, situations like those that prevailed inside Michener have been shown to cause the very problems that would have made admission and retention of inmates seem appropriate. Thus, the dehumanizing aspects of institutional life undoubtedly reduced the likelihood that inmates would ever be deemed fit to live in the community.

Sensory Deprivation and Dehumanization

Sometimes, the effects of this numbing, empty daily schedule led to violence. Michel Aubin surprised me when we were discussing Side Rooms. Side Rooms, which will be covered more fully in the next chapter, were solitary confinement cells used to punish misbehaving residents. Michel said:

> I spent a lot of time in the Side Rooms. Sometimes I made sure of that, just to get away from the staff. It was kind of a break to be in isolation like that – just to get away from the staff. So you'd run up and kick one of them or bite their arm, you know, then you knew where you were going to go.

Michel's comments shed light on yet another effect that sensory deprivation, crowding, and low-level brutality can engender – violence. For Michel, the only way to obtain some control over his life and gain some privacy was to lash out at someone, just as a way to change the order of things and get a break from his bleak reality. It is astonishing that Michel found his daily routine so terrible that he preferred to spend time in solitary confinement as a kind of holiday from life on the ward.

Not all the violence on these wards was as intentional or strategic as Michel's was. Instead, all the relationships in the institution, including those between fellow inmates, seem to have been shot through with dehumanization. Almost all the survivors told stories of routine low-level violence – fights over food, or sometimes over nothing, bites and kicks that came seemingly out of the blue, emotional and physical outbursts from fellow inmates that could be neither predicted nor avoided. Indeed, Michel added later in his interview that one of the reasons he would attack a staff member and get into a Side Room was that "it was less violent in there than on the ward, just you on the cold floor."

In addition to engendering violence among inmates, it is also fair to say that these brutal daily schedules were designed to keep staff and inmates from developing positive and meaningful human relationships. As ex-worker Jim Sullivan described:

> You didn't have time. You couldn't sit individually with the kid, you know, when kids are upset, you know the nine-year-old when he's going to bed and he's sort of upset. You couldn't sit and chat with them because most of the other kids were going to sleep. There were only two staff members, remember, so one is with 40 kids. They're all getting into pajamas and getting showered and getting their snack before they go to bed and brushing their teeth and all that, and once that settles down, you might have maybe an hour that you could sit and talk with individual kids but that would be max, and nowhere private because you weren't to bring these kids into the chart room or the staff room. That was sacred territory. So it was tough, and then the supervisors would come around at that time and if you were caught sitting, talking with a kid, you weren't doing your job. You're supposed to be cleaning, or writing your bloody reports.

In Jim's description we hear again evidence about how space, time, and its organization led to dehumanization; certain spaces were only open to "real" humans, while time and its management was purely the domain of those with power inside the institutional walls. Thus, the glass-enclosed, raised-platform nursing station was not only a Panopticon but also an isolation chamber that segregated the clean, orderly world of the staff from the chaotic, smelly, foul world of inmates.

I will be discussing violence by staff against inmates in the chapters that follow, but here it is important to note that the gruelling daily routine, the chronic understaffing, and the hierarchical nature of the institution affected both inmates and staff. This institutional routine actively distanced staff and inmates, causing inmates (and indeed, some staff, as was indicated in the interviews) to experience social isolation and emotional distress. It is not surprising, therefore, that when survivors were asked to speak about a favourite staff person or asked whether, after all their years in the institution, they had kept in touch with former staff members, all but one of the survivors emphatically replied that they had never really had a close relationship with a staff member and that they had no interest in being in touch with staff after they left the institution. The rare exception to this lack of relationships was described by Sam Edwards, a boy who did not live in the main institution but instead lived for six months

in Linden House, a special, small unit for emotionally and behaviourally troubled "normal" kids. Among several harrowing stories about negative interactions with staff, Sam did describe one particularly kind staff member with
whom he felt a personal connection and with whom he developed a bond during his relatively brief stay at Michener:

> There was one guy, Mr Jansen, he was like a, uh, a nurse I guess he would be. Big
> nice old guy. And I really liked him. Even after I got out of there, about a week or
> two later, I phoned Linden House and tried to talk to him. And that really set them
> off. They're, "Why'd you phone here? Don't call again." But I really liked Mr Jansen.

What Sam described is almost a mirror of the way that inmates were cut off
from the outside and their support networks once they were interned. In Sam's
case, once he was gone, he was cut off from and denied a relationship with the
staff member who had been a positive force for him during his time in the institution. In both actions, it is clear that the institution saw itself as separate
from real life, that human relationships were subordinated to institutional regimes, and that the children's need for intimacy were seen as a problem rather
than a natural human need.

Such emotional deprivation would have made it difficult for many survivors
to know how to build and maintain positive interpersonal relationships, either
with their families or with their neighbours and co-workers in community life.
However, the lack of relationships between people who left the institution and
staff, who in many cases had supervised the children from a very young age,
indicates more than just clumsiness in establishing social relationships. Instead,
it indicates that human relationships simply were not a normative part of daily
life inside.

Private Property and the Private Self

Clearly, personal space and personal time were virtually impossible to access or
control for inmates in Michener. In addition, there was little possibility of having
or controlling their clothing, toys, or mementoes from their family, or even their
own body parts or personal pleasures. As with the appropriation and devaluation of personal time and personal space, the institution's obsessive control over
inmates' bodies, pleasures, and possessions was a common and devastating form
of dehumanization for inmates.

As mentioned earlier, on admission the trappings of inmates' former lives
were quickly and relentlessly erased; children were stripped of their clothing
and their personal possessions, ostensibly because in an institution as large and

fully populated as Michener, keeping track of inmates' possessions would be an administrative nightmare. Before admitting their children, parents were advised of how much clothing to provide and how to label these clothes; however, it seems that this clothing rarely made it onto the back of the appropriate child, often disappearing into the common stock of goods that circulated in the institution for all inmates. In daily ward reports of the early 1970s, discussions about missing clothing are common. These discussions, taking place during the last years of Michener's heyday, occurred at a time when the institution was responding to the criticisms of journalists, some family and community advocates, and the government-sponsored and highly critical Blair Report of 1969. In this report the depersonalization of inmates was a central criticism. Among other measures, it seems that the institutional response determined that giving children their own clothing was an important first step in what was then termed *normalization* – the attempt to make institutional life mimic life outside, with an eye to beginning to release inmates. However, the tone of the ward reports during this period concerning clothing and the fact that personal clothing was now being assigned to specific children was quite contentious. Perhaps this conflict occurred because considerable effort would have been required to track clothing processed through central facilities; at the same time the instigation of such personalization also undoubtedly caused concern among workers about the effects of such innovations on their careers.

If it was difficult to track inmates' belongings during the period of normalization and population reductions, it must have been even more challenging when the institutional population sat at more than 2300 inmates, which was the case for much of the time that the survivors in this study lived in the institution. However, the size of the institution was not the only factor in the institutions' problems with clothing. In the winter of 1969, Sam Edwards was placed into Linden House, which was a special unit that operated on the Michener children's campus for a little under a decade. Linden House was a small, purpose-built, and independently run unit, located apart from the regular wards. It accommodated approximately 30 "high-functioning" children with behavioural rather than intellectual challenges, and with its relatively small size, unique population, and separate location, it was theoretically more able to offer access to personal belongings, private space, and control over one's time. In principle, this meant that Sam and his fellow inmates wore their own, regular clothing. Even so, in a setting with only 30 children, none of them requiring physical care, it still seemed to be very difficult for children to hold on to their possessions. Among the institutional documents Sam shared during our interview were numerous contentious exchanges concerning where Sam's clothing had gone. Sam's mother claimed to have sent everything on the list provided to her before Sam's admission and complained about lost items and the costs of replacements; on the other hand, the institution denied that anything had gone amiss yet demanded she send more clothing.

Like Sam, survivors who lived in High Grade wards should have been able to have at least some of their own clothing, but often this proved to be more promise than substance. As Sandra Karnak said, describing her life on a High Grade ward:

> ME: Where did you keep your clothes?
> SANDRA: In a wardrobe, but they kept the good stuff in an attic and wouldn't give it to you. They also took some to the sewing room to put nametags on it, and they were all supposed to come back to the person who owned them. Half of them we never did see. We had good clothes and never did see them.

For High Grades and those in Linden House, the combination of the lack of space for personal possessions, the barring of inmates from storage areas where goods were stored, and the necessity of using the vast central laundry system that, between inmates and staff, served several thousand people, meant that personal possessions, particularly desirable ones, were virtually impossible to keep. Thus, the institution's efficiency in centralizing laundry resulted in a system where all clothing was interchangeable, and hence all children were similarly seen as interchangeable units in the broader population. In addition to loss, several inmates described having clothing stolen by other inmates and having no recourse for getting those items returned to them; it was either too much work or simply viewed as unnecessary by staff to return items to their rightful owners – the clothing, like the children themselves, just didn't matter enough.

Reflecting the highly stratified qualities of life in the institution, people who lived in Low Grade wards had access only to institutional clothing. Jim Sullivan stated that adult inmates who were working while living on one of these wards "basically wore working clothes. You know, bib-overalls for the older men, same with the women." In childhood, inmates who were able to attend school wore what Jim described as "institutional clothing, [that looked] like a regular kid in the community," but this clothing was different from what a regular kid in the community might wear because it came from a central stock of clothing and conferred little individuality on the wearer. Sometimes, the demand for institutional efficiency resulted in a truly bizarre apportioning of resources. Jim went on to note:

> I remember very clearly, on the school boys' ward that would be about 80 young boys from the age of 9 to 16, there were such limited resources that only half those

boys could go out at a time, for example, so they would dress them, send them off to school. They'd come back, change clothes with the other kids and that's how limited the resources were.

This story clearly shows how undifferentiated the children were seen to be by staff members. For that part of the day when the children had to be out of the ward, they warranted "real" clothing; however, for everyday they simply wore nondescript and uniform child-size coveralls or smocks, very often without shoes or socks.

Clothing was, of course, not the only aspect of their personal lives that inmates had no control over. Every single person interviewed – including the ex-workers – mentioned how terrible the institutional food was. The quality of food and the ability to make choices about what kinds of food to eat, the times to eat, and even the size of the portion were not individualized, as is evidenced in the following story, told by Ray Petrenko:

> This attendant put a whole bunch of spaghetti on Keith's plate and Keith told him in a nice way, he couldn't talk very good, but he had a big loud voice and he said, "I'm not hungry, this is too much for me." And they said, "Well, you eat this or else." So this one guy was holding his hands and this other guy was pushing this food down Keith's throat. And Keith was really gagging.

In this incident it is clear that even as rudimentary a decision as how much food a man would eat was not to be determined by his own hunger. Rather, routine portions of food, like routine bathing and toileting, were left to the discretion of staff who seemingly exercised limitless control over inmates' bodies.

For some inmates, the quality of the food was even worse than average, and this difference, as many others, reflected hierarchies of disability within the institution. On Low Grade wards, it was very likely that the food would be puréed, as Evelyn explained:

> In this case, on this ward all the food was puréed. 'Cause most everyone didn't have teeth. And uh, they'd either rotted out or they'd been pulled out because they'd bit somebody. Um, and so we fed everybody.

However, it is important to note that the quality of the food – whether diced, whole, or puréed – was not necessarily tied to how many teeth inmates had. Donna Bogdan, who at the time of her interview had most of her own teeth, complained about her food, saying, "staff thought we should get [our food] mashed up. I didn't like getting treated like that because they thought we were kids and we weren't kids, we were adults. And I didn't like being treated like a kid." Donna's assessment of the food and its rationale is quite insightful; the food, like most other things inside the institution, was designed for people whose individual qualities did not matter and who were not seen as human beings but as perpetual children without rights.

The problem of teeth is mentioned in daily ward meetings, in annual reports, in letters of complaints from parents, and in Unusual Incidents reports. The problem was complicated. First, because of time constraints, it seems that there was little time for already-harried staff to facilitate inmates' looking after their own hygiene or to provide careful and effective dental hygiene to inmates who needed more help. Thus, tooth decay and gum disease were epidemic in the institution. Second, because interpersonal violence was a common outcome of the dehumanizing aspects of institutional life, bites between inmates and from inmates to staff were not uncommon. Finally, because of the mind-numbing qualities of daily life in the institution, many inmates bit themselves regularly as a form of self-stimulation. Removing teeth was simpler and cheaper than providing good care or improving the living conditions in the institution. Thus, inmates' bodies were not only controlled in the institutions but were actually altered – a point we will return to when discussing eugenic sterilization and the use of psychotropic medication – to aid staff and to mitigate against the grim effects of systemic dehumanization. From clothing to haircuts to food choices to dental extractions, routine institutional practices conveyed a clear message about the inhumanity of residents and telegraphed that inmates' bodies were not their own but instead belonged to the institution, which had the right to do to those bodies whatever it deemed necessary or convenient.

Dehumanizing Recreation

A final aspect of institutional dehumanization centres, ironically, on the ways that fun and pleasure were regulated in Michener. We can see an example in the way the institution managed to control even the most human pleasure of knowing that one is loved and cared for: only with the process of normalization or deinstitutionalization was correspondence between family members and inmates considered private. This fact is evidenced in the following passage from a charge nurses' meeting dated 15 November 1973: "Villa charges mentioned that mail for trainees had stamps torn off envelopes. However, the effective date for unopened mail to trainees is December 1, 1973." In other words, a complaint lodged about mail tampering was not seen as legitimate because the regulation against it was not yet in force. Thus, only two weeks before the legislated mandate of permitting inmates to receive unopened mail, the humanization of inmates' lives was subordinated to bureaucratic rules, and the comment reflects the reality that at least some staff were resistant to such changes in the regime. There is, of course, an aspect of surveillance attached to opening private mail between parents and their children, but it also seems as though the institution and its workers believed at some deep level that the inmates really belonged to them and saw the inmates' needs to have a connection to a life outside the institution as unnecessary at best, disloyal at worst.

For many inmates who lived in Michener, other pleasures, such as birthdays, outings, trips to camps or town, or the use of playgrounds and recreational facilities, were simply not on the agenda. These residents were, of course, typically Low Grade residents whose needs were frequently seen as limited to being cleaned and fed. All three of the ex-workers interviewed worked at one point on Low Grade wards, and they all noted that it was seen as "enough" that these children and adults were kept clean, fed, and toileted. However, even High Grade residents had limited access to the on-campus facilities, such as the skating rink, swimming pool, tennis court, or even the playground equipment. For one thing, most of these facilities were built very late in the institution's history, following the 1969 Blair Report and driven by the efforts of a parent group that formed in the late 1960s with the express goal of improving the quality of life at Michener. For another, the facilities were not located close to inmates' residences, as Jim Sullivan described:

> They built a curling rink. That was near the end of my stay [Jim worked at Michener until 1978], and they had playgrounds but the silly thing was, when I think back, the playground was over by the Working Men, which is on the farm, you had to walk like a half a mile to get to this silly playground.

From Jim's description, it is clear that constructing recreational facilities, which occurred at the same time that the institution was coming under significant governmental and lay pressure to close, was little more than window dressing, a belated attempt to at least appear to be offering a favourable environment to child inmates.

That being said, inmates did describe occasional outings, including trips to camps and day trips into the local town to see movies or to attend church. These outings were a part of the informal internal economy in the institution in that they were earned as rewards for good work at school or on the job, or for good behaviour on the ward. Conversely, these experiences were often tainted for those who were privileged enough to earn them because inmates were still controlled during these outings. Sandra Karnak described one such outing, to a local church:

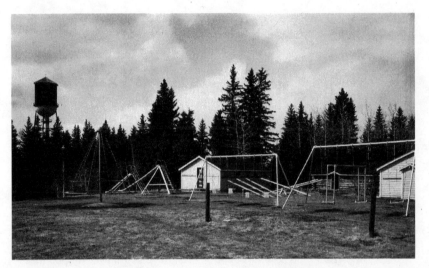

Figure 3.8 The playground, circa 1955. Courtesy Red Deer and District Archives (N2691).

We all went with supervisors. We had nametags on and we all had to be accounted for. You stayed in the line-up and when you went to church, you sat where they told you, and didn't sit with the people.

In Sandra's description, we see how dehumanization can be internalized. Sitting "with the people" was, even in Sandra's own words, not something that the dehumanized members of Michener were qualified to do. Other survivors described similar rare outings to movies or to attend appointments in town, and these were always supervised and almost always done in a group. For the institution, group outings were undoubtedly more manageable and efficient than permitting true freedom of movement to inmates. For inmates like Ray, however, group outing did not provide any real freedom because, "it was embarrassing to be dragged through town like that, in a big group – we always stood out."

Conclusion

Like so many aspects of life in the institution, pleasures and recreation were made impersonal to a level that seems not only thoughtless but cruel and dehumanizing. Inmates, regardless of their age, were treated as though they were children – and not very valued children at that. They were not given choices in their clothing, their personal style, their food preferences, or even their food intake. They were herded around in private spaces, such as showers and toilets, and in public spaces, such as churches and the streets of Red Deer. They were not permitted freedom of movement, freedom of thought, freedom of time, or freedom of choice. In fact, they were not even permitted the normal rights of citizenship: until 1988, Canada limited the right to vote to those deemed to have a requisite level of capacity (Kohn, 2008).[5]

Predictably, the enduring dehumanization and infantilization that these people experienced during their tenure at Michener has had lifelong consequences, particularly for those who were interned in early childhood. After leaving the institution they literally had to learn how to do everything. The effects of this institutionalization have been profound and long-lasting, and some of these effects have been insurmountable.

It is clear that devastating dehumanization occurred for residents who were stripped systematically of the rights to personal space, possessions, and time. These restrictions in turn had profound effects on inmates' abilities, both within and on leaving the institution, to develop interpersonal and sexual relationships, to engage in educational and personal development, to understand appropriate boundaries, to make choices and accept responsibility, to manage money and handle adult responsibilities – in short, how to live as human beings in the world. However, these effects were also profound for those who worked in the institution. The three workers I interviewed all spoke, to varying degrees, about the impact of their experiences on their lives after Michener. All three went on to work in the field of human services, and all three have taken on a political and moral stance of advocacy in that work. One has become a dedicated advocate and educator in community living, another is a leader in special education who offers education not only to children but also to teachers in hopes of increasing "different" children's successes, and the last has been an advocate within the education system for inclusive education. All three attribute their drive, at least in part, to their experiences in Michener.

Not every worker, however, would have been able to use their experiences to gain a broader insight into the human condition or to take on a politicized response later in life as a way of addressing the oppression they observed within the institution. Unlike the three workers interviewed for this project, who spent only a few years in their jobs in the institution, many employees found the work tolerable enough to spend many years doing institutional work, enjoying long-term, well-paid careers that were otherwise not readily available in the small town of Red Deer, a topic we will explore more fully later. The effects of tolerating this kind of daily, routinized inhumanity must have been profound for workers as well as for inmates. Some insight into these effects can intimated from a newspaper article published during the period when Michener was seeing its ranks sharply reduced as a result of deinstitutionalization and normalization (Martindale, [ca. 1984]). The author of this article described conditions on Cedar, a unit for "profoundly retarded and severely disabled" inmates that was similar to some of the wards described in this chapter. The article included an interview with a Mr Larsen, who explained that the lack of doors and curtains, and the public washings, toiletings and feedings, are necessary because of "lack of space, resident safety and staff convenience," reflecting a fairly wholesale acceptance that human rights were to be subordinated to routine and efficiency. The article went on to quote John Runge, a social worker at Michener, who argued that improving the living spaces of these inmates would be a waste of funds and energy, saying instead:

> Use the money for the people where it's going to do the most good. There are a number of them [inmates] that you might as well be talking to a chicken. (Martindale, [ca. 1984]).

From this quotation we are able to see how someone who has worked in a place that treats people like animals can readily make the transition to thinking that these people actually are animals, barely worth the money being spent to keep things at an abusive level, let alone worthy of the expense of treating them with decency. Runge's comments help us understand just how effective dehumanization was not only for inmates but for all who spent time inside Michener. From his comments we are also able to understand how such dehumanization could readily move from systematic neglect to systematic abuse, a subject we will turn to in the next chapter.

Chapter Four

Ordinary and Extraordinary Violence

The previous chapter described how dehumanizing processes were threaded through daily institutional life at Michener in routine and normalized ways. The institutional use of space, its management of time, and the ways it controlled inmates' privacy, relationships, and personal property acted as technologies of dehumanization, making inmates into "others" to their former communities and families and to staff within the institution, and finally giving rise to divisions among inmates. These dehumanizing activities not only separated inmates from their former and potential networks of support but also made the management of inmates' bodies and minds much easier for staff. The dehumanizing aspects also created a culture where violence – spontaneous and institutionally sanctioned, directed from staff to inmates, from inmates to staff, and among inmates themselves – was a normal part of everyday life. This chapter focuses on routine and extraordinary violence in the institution. In addition, it offers insight into resistance to institutional life on the part of inmates, including resistance evidenced by the frequent and sometimes tragic attempts at escape.

Institutional Records on Ordinary Violence

The dehumanizing daily routines of life in the institution facilitated a harsh environment that, in and of itself, was psychologically and physically violent. Indeed, quotidian violence was woven throughout the institutional practices in such wide ranging ways that, as Michel Aubin described in the previous chapter, inmates sometimes would even push for an altercation, just to get away from the grim routine of the day rooms and the constant threat of interpersonal violence. Quotidian violence took many forms, from injuries resulting from routinized neglect to more intentional harms perpetrated by staff on inmates and among inmates themselves.

Unlike Michel, who actively sought violence as a release, many survivors described their experiences with violence as something that they were absolutely unable to control and that came to them without cause. Inmates described being hit or spoken harshly to without provocation as though this was part of the normal interactions within the institution. As survivor Betty Dudnik explained:

> I never did nothing to them, to make them unkind to me. They just pushed me and shoved me and they're not nice to me. Shoved me around and pushed me, and I said I didn't want that anymore, but it didn't matter.

From the tone of Betty's comments, it is clear that neither her actions nor her desire for respect had any effect on her daily life inside and that when violence occurred, it came unexpectedly and often without provocation.

Echoing Betty's description are the institutional records about minor injuries or altercations in which it is difficult to unravel the threads of routine violence, which seems to have occurred randomly and often without warning. The institution's Unusual Incidents files are replete with reports of inmates sustaining minor injuries but without any real sense of how such injuries occurred or could be avoided; indeed, although the violence was depressingly common, it seemed to come from nowhere and no one. For example, in the files, it is "noticed at 0700 in West day room that [X] had 1 inch long laceration over left eye," or individuals are "found in distress, appearing to be choking ... coughing," or "found with a lump on top of spine back of head," and finally "received bump on back of head & reddened area on back." Indeed, throughout the daily ward reports, patients fall, stumble, are found lying on floors, slip out of chairs, and are regularly discovered to be injured or harmed. This kind of description was used even when describing fairly unusual and extensive injuries, as in the following:

> "X" received a stab wound behind right ear – approximately 1 inch in length ... treated with cold compress and application of butterfly bandage – clinical notified – stitches given – returned from doctor 1030 hrs.

The files where evidence of violence was discussed are riddled with passive voice. For example, a resident injured by rough handling was described in language that almost sounds as if she injured herself: "[X] hit right eyebrow on bed rail while being put to bed sustaining a laceration 1½ inches long." In each of these quotes, the use of passive voice, where inmates received or simply sustained injuries, and the finding, discovering, or noticing of these injuries, erases any possibility that such injuries might have occurred as a result of "normal" violence. Instead, harms appeared without incident and without source. This kind of language makes invisible any perpetrator of this violence – unless it was the individual inmate who, through neglect, passivity, or foolishness, does it to herself or himself – and hence there was no way to effect change. In this linguistic representation, not only the perpetrator but the violence itself was made to disappear. Further, although these entries were written in such a way as to protect the worker from recriminations from supervisors, they also speculatively distanced the writer/worker and simultaneously made tolerable to her or him the level of violence that everyone – inmates and staff alike – had to live with inside the institution.

The use of the passive voice and clinical and dispassionate language was also apparent in reporting outside the institution as, for example, in annual reports to the ministry responsible for public health. This language had the effect of minimizing the level of harm incurred and clouding questions of responsibility concerning the causes of these accidents. Reflecting the tone and content of typical reports, an entry under the "Accidents" section of the 1960 Deerhome annual report stated:

> During 1960, a number of patients received injuries through accidents. Many minor contusions and lacerations resulted, which required only first aid treatment. A number of epileptic patients sustained lacerations requiring suturing. As well as these there were 14 fractures [among 867 inmates]. These included three fractured femurs, all three requiring major surgery; three Colles' [wrist] fractures; two ankles and six upper arms. Some were reduced under general anaesthetics, and in the others, plaster casts were applied. (MacLean, 1960, p. 175)

In this report, as with the internal ward records, inmates "received" injuries, damages "resulted," epilepsy appears to naturally lead individuals to have "sustained" their injuries, and fractures simply appeared without cause or explanation. It is important to acknowledge that many inmates living at Michener were diagnosed with epilepsy or cerebral palsy, which would perhaps have made them prone to accidents or falls. However, the way these incidents are reported was singularly detached and uncurious. The causes of such injuries were not speculated on, nor did the record include arguments for increased staffing or suggestions for improved surveillance. Rather, the injuries simply existed and came into being, without remark. This circumspect way of speaking about violence reflects what Michel Foucault has referred to as an authorized vocabulary, where only certain ways of speaking and hence knowing are permissible, indeed, possible (Foucault, 1990). In the discourse of the institution, to recognize violence would have been impossible – recognizing this violence might have meant that things would have had to change or that workers would have had to acknowledge their own complicity in an abusive system. Hence, this way of speaking – the distancing, objectified way of describing violence as though it is not there, forms a discursive framing that not only reinforces the institutional order of things by failing to expose abuse but also protects those complicit in that abuse from having to recognize their own part in it.

Taken collectively, it becomes clear that these recordings of small injuries and spills were reflective of and embedded in systematic problems of over-crowding, understaffing, carelessness, and the numbing dehumanization of daily life in the institution. For example, one daily record entry described how a female inmate "complains of sore toe. Large toe on right foot very bruised – swollen. She states someone shut the day room gate on it." Another entry noted that "[X] fell on floor still tied to commode at 19:15 ... slight swelling of lower leg," while another described how "[X] received a 1 inch laceration to the right side of head while in toilet." In an unusually explicit quote, a staff member de-scribed how "[X] received a 1.5 cm long laceration when he fell in 'B' toilet area while having his pants pulled down." In these descriptions we can comprehend the hurried carelessness that staff might engage in when toileting people en masse or the sustained neglect typified by leaving them unattended for hours in day rooms and hallways, as described in the previous chapter. In turn, we can see how such carelessness might result in injury that was perceived by staff as simply an unremarkable side effect of the normal routine of the institution.

The institutional way of speaking about violence and inmates also reflects the profound level of dehumanization that institutional life effects. Giorgio Agamben, in writing about Auschwitz, described the impossibility of seeing or acknowledging those who were known inside the camps as "Muslims," inmates whose dehumanization and lack of hope brought them literally to the juncture between living and dead, human and inhuman, subject and object. This liminal position ultimately made these inmates invisible to others within the camps (Agamben, 2002, p. 14). In Michener's archival records, inmates seem to have held a similar liminal place; they too were invisible, inhuman, objects. They seem to have been seen or noticed when their injuries were presented or dis-covered, rather than when they occurred. Even on being seen as injured, they were not characterized as victims of violence, or as human actors in the drama of the institution, but instead they were simply marked as recipients of unno-ticed events. Rarely do we read about altercations or accidents as they unfolded; rather, injuries only came to light as part of routine inspections or movements of bodies, or when inmates were occasionally placed outside the institution, and strangers or family members discovered undeniable evidence of violence. In short, like the "Muslims" of the camps, the inmates of Michener were not subjects but barely visible objects on which the marks of institutional life were inscribed and, only when necessary, read.

Ex-workers and Inmates Describe Ordinary Violence

Interviews with ex-workers add flesh to the bones of the skeletal institutional record concerning routine violence and give a clearer sense of how violence occurred. In addition to the violence attendant with neglect, and echoing Agamben's (2002) description of the Muslim and invisibility, ex-worker Evelyn Stephens described daily life within Michener comprising "the kind of violence that has to do with not seeing. I don't mean punching, kicking, beating-up kind of violence, but the day-to-day grinding violence." The violence Evelyn refers to is the kind engendered by not seeing inmates as human and hence not needing to afford them human dignity or decency. She went on to describe the way this kind of routine played out in everyday life:

> pushing, shoving, tying people down, slapping their face ... pushing people with a mop, to corner [them] in a corner in order to tie [them] down, all kinds of bullying and aggressive – people acted pretty aggressively all the time ... Sometimes if someone just made a move that you thought you might get hurt, you'd, you know, hit first. You spoke sharply to people. You weren't comforting. There were lots of threats, verbal threats all the time.

From Evelyn's description, we can gain insight into the varied forms of everyday violence and the lack of respect that characterized life in Michener. We can also get a sense of the fact that not only residents but also staff lived in a state of constant alert, engaging in pre-emptive violence rather than allowing themselves to be vulnerable to the violence inside those walls. Both ex-workers and ex-inmates alike described life in the institution as a mindless and grim routine of low-level violence, punctuated by outbursts that were unanticipated, terrifying, and often unavoidable; Evelyn's description of workers hitting inmates "just in case" is an illustration of this readiness to escalate violence.

Sometimes, violence even performed the function of light relief for staff members, or it acted, as Goffman (1961) might anticipate, as a form of indoctrination for staff members. Evelyn described an early rite of initiation along these lines:

> I remember this woman, Priscilla, who was also part of my early orientation and hazing. She was one of those women who could, um, throw up on command, projectile vomit. So that was one of the little routine tricks, was to get her to puke on you.

Evelyn recalled that this experience was accompanied by tremendous anticipatory laughter and that Priscilla was not really seen as an accomplice in this game but more as a disgusting experience, a thing to be endured as a test of character through which senior colleagues could evaluate and intimidate a junior colleague. Jim Sullivan also recalled a game on the wards played with residents that was particularly cruel and objectifying, in which he as a junior colleague was expected to collude:

> We had an incident there ... where a charge nurse was taking rubber balls [and] making these people line up against the wall and you could throw them [the balls] at them, and if they cried or anything you would put them into lock-up. And this went on for many weeks, and of course, this was a hierarchy there and we were all terrified.

The inmates acted literally as targets in a game of skill for workers and were punished if they acted human rather than simply performing as elements of the game. This account illuminates how dehumanization formed part of institutional life and the role that such dehumanization played in team building among staff. The spectacle of abuse operated not only to dehumanize inmates but also to produce worker solidarity and, it was hoped, silence through intimidation. Despite the climate of worker collusion, after several weeks of this game, Jim's personal values did lead him to complain to his superiors, and he claims he was told to "keep [his] mouth shut – this never happened. This person would never do such a thing," and so the game continued through the remainder of Jim's summer internship, despite his discomfort.

Jim's story illustrates how lack of supervision, a dehumanizing working culture, and lack of staff in the workplace can contribute to an environment wherein workers engage in and encourage others to take on routinized violence. Workers in large institutions are asked to perform alienating and often hopeless work, and their daily routines are numbing and repetitive yet demanding. In addition, workers in institutions serving older residents or people with serious intellectual or mental health challenges may perceive that their work is without value, in part because of the stigmatization of disability and in part because patients or inmates are rarely seen as getting better or moving toward community reintegration. Despite the fact that the institution itself was to blame for these poor outcomes, it is possible to understand how the environment and the inmates shaped by that environment worked to blunt workers' feelings for their charges and moved them to see their work and the residents themselves as without purpose or hope (Schneider, 1996).

The constant culture of low-grade violence, punctuated by spectacles of abuse such as the one Jim describes, operated not only to intimidate workers but also, like the Time-Out Rooms discussed later in this book, to intimidate the inmates who witnessed violence into compliance and passivity. Ironically, inmates and patients in such settings can operate as embodied symbols of the failure and undeniable brutality of the system of care that entraps both inmates and workers, leaving workers feeling not only hopeless but hostile toward their charges for providing living evidence of such brutality. Agamben (2002) discusses this phenomenon in his analysis of German concentration camps. Camp workers, when interrogated by post-war prosecutors, justified their actions by expressing dismay at the passivity and lack of perceived humanity among camp inmates, implying that the lack of resistance equated to acceptance, without any recognition of that these acquiescent behaviours were predictable effects of camp brutality.

Jim's story also illuminates the multiple lines of violence that were ranged, like so much of life within the institution, along hierarchical lines, with a permanent staff member at the top, student interns next, High Grade inmates next, and finally Low Grades at the bottom of the pecking order. This combination of hierarchical relations and the constant dehumanization of inmates intertwined at the Michener Centre to create a climate of brutality characterized by fear, neglect, verbal and psychological degradation, and rough treatment that formed the fabric of everyday life. In turn, this routine, everyday violence facilitated other, more extreme forms of violence, to which I will shortly turn.

The Invisibility of Extraordinary Violence

Similarly to the ways routine and everyday violence is reported, much of the extraordinary violence involving severe injuries appeared in the institutional records in mysterious and disconnected ways, perhaps because the level of tolerance for violence was so strongly inculcated among residents and staff. Even when violence was sustained at levels that made ignoring it an impossibility, it was often difficult for staff to account for how things happened or who caused inmates' injuries, as is evidenced in the following Unusual Incidents report about a child whose everyday injuries were noticed by outsiders when the child was hospitalized for a non-injury-related treatment:

> As requested by Mrs. Vanderhoof [a pseudonym], I am submitting this report as a possible explanation why [the child] appeared physically abused when admitted to the University Hospital on June 29th, 1976 ...
>
> On researching [the child's] medical file, I find that she has had sixteen reported accidents since December 16, 1975. They include a variety of injuries, such as bites, scratches, bruises and minor hemorrhages, which have occurred on various parts of the body; head, arms, back and feet. Four of these accidents were considered

serious enough to be presented to a doctor. Eight of the above mentioned accidents were the direct result of aggression by other residents. The rest with the exception of one, were of unknown causes, but I feel it is fairly safe to assume that the majority of these were caused by self-abuse or abuse from other residents.

It is likely that the original incident reports describing this child's various injuries, and the final report cited above, were written in part with the aim of hiding the possibility that what happened to this child while in care could be attributed to staff abuse. On the other hand, it is possible that none of the staff who wrote these reports really knew how the injuries were sustained. The language of this summary report can be interpreted either way: these reports reflect a cover-up of systematic institutional violence, or they reflect the reality that the institute was so overcrowded, so understaffed, and characterized by such a climate of neglect and low-level violence that it would be easy to find such a series of injuries unremarkable. In either explanation, the violence is unaccounted for – it simply happens, seemingly without explanation, to those unfortunate enough to get in its way.

Indeed it is frequently the case in the institutional records that even quite severe injuries only came to be noted when other incidents or outside witnesses brought these injuries to the attention of authorities. Often, this occurred when children and adult inmates had occasional visits home. The records offer numerous examples of such incidents and convey exasperation on the part of the institution in response to these accusations. The general tone in these reports is one of frustration; parents who made such accusations were seen as overly protective or perhaps even a bit paranoid or problematic, as was mentioned in the earlier discussion about institutional ambivalence toward home visits.

Another way that injuries came to the attention of management in the institution occurred when inmates required hospitalization, sometimes for the injuries themselves and sometimes for unrelated health concerns. For example, an inmate who slid out of her wheelchair and sustained a head injury required admission to the Michener infirmary for observation. Once admitted, the attending staff member wrote:

> Now noted that she has many bruises on her chest, right arm, right side of abdomen, right hip, right and left thigh and both legs from knee downwards, also 2 small bruises on low back and left buttock. They look as if they could have been caused by pinching or nipping.

It is unclear what, if any, kind of investigation followed this discovery, but it is clear that workers in some units on the compound were still able to find the injuries of inmates remarkable enough to report them. The question of how the institution managed investigations of extraordinary violence is one that we can mainly only speculate on; few entries in the records follow the trails of investigation and disciplinary action against staff or other inmates. This lack reflects a culture in which violence was so much a part of everyday life that those responsible showed little inclination to acknowledge or address it within the institutional walls. However, there is evidence of staff covering up for one another when incidents occurred, as in the incident of the game involving throwing balls at residents, mentioned earlier by Jim Sullivan.

Unsurprisingly, inmates themselves were often reluctant to point fingers for fear of reprisals. The following rare investigative report allows us to speculate as to why inmates might be reluctant to disclose issues of violence:

> Mr. Vanderhoof [a pseudonym] was interviewed ... with regard to a statement made by [an inmate] and denied any knowledge ... he stated emphatically that he did not kick [the inmate]. As there was no witness to the incident, I have accepted this statement ... The Unit Charge stated he had never observed Mr. Vanderhoof being rough with the residents, but at times was suspicious that he might have been.

A number of things become clear from this reporting. First, in a hierarchy like the institution, an inmate's word held little weight against the claims of a worker, even when there may have been ongoing suspicions about that worker. Further, because workers at Michener were unionized, without solid evidence, few complaints would end in firing or other significant disciplinary action. This incident report also obliquely illustrates how nepotism may also have contributed to a climate of ignoring or minimizing violence. Mr Vanderhoof, the worker who was questioned in connection to the kicking injury and the resulting incident report was the husband of the worker who, described earlier, investigated the unexplained injuries that were revealed only when an inmate was hospitalized for non-injury-related causes.[1] As married colleagues working in the centre, the Vanderhoofs were not unusual; as will be discussed more fully in the next chapter, although Michener was a huge institution, its host city was quite small, and at times as many as 1 in 25 citizens held the coveted, well-paying unionized positions at the Michener Centre. When community and workers were so intertwined, and further where multiple family members worked together behind the institutional walls, profound negative social fallout would have followed if complaints of abuse, either from inmates or from their family members, were pursued vigorously.

In the above incident report, it is also possible to see how understaffing and overpopulation meant that workers often conducted their business in isolation from one another, providing abusers with opportunities to engage in violence without credible witnesses in the form of co-workers. Finally, we can speculate that individuals who were injured or hurt by staff, and who did report incidents to the authorities in hopes of being protected, would sometimes find themselves at risk of reprisal, which in turn acted as a deterrent to disclosure. This kind of reprisal, it must be added, would not necessarily only come from the individual accused.

An example of the climate of reprisal can be seen in Louise Roy's mention of sexual violence and the repercussions of telling:

> When I was in Michener I was sexually assaulted by this male staff. I reported him and [he] said no he never. And I wasn't lying, and he knew he did it. And I kept telling people about how I felt and they kept saying I was a behaviour problem.

As we will read shortly, to be identified as a "behaviour problem" in the institution was no small matter; it meant more than simply being labelled as troublesome. Rather, being labelled in that way often meant that the individual would be sent for readjustment to the Behaviour Management Unit, a separate, segregated residential unit with much heavier security and regimentation, or it could mean being placed in a Side Room specifically designed to house unruly inmates in solitary confinement. Indeed, in Louise's case, rather than receive a hearing for her complaints, she was stigmatized as a troublemaker, and although it is not absolutely clear that she was directly punished for this transgression, Louise did describe spending time in a Side Room following this incident. In her mind, the two things – telling and punishment – remain firmly linked.

Allegations of abuse were common both against staff and against fellow inmates, with allegations against inmates particularly heightened during the later periods of normalization when sexual desegregation was initiated. The institutional response to these allegations was ambivalent. On the one hand, nursing staff seemed keen to address sexual acting out by separating both same-sex and heterosexual couples and by removing problematic inmates from the general population. On the other hand, reports by parents and by individuals themselves seem to have been treated with dismissal or disavowal. In the Unusual Incidents files, a number of documents compose an investigation into allegations of abuse by fellow inmates made by a female resident living in a mixed-sex unit during the period of normalization. Eventually, because the woman's father was insistent, she was referred to a staff psychiatrist for evaluation. The psychiatrist's report to the executive director after examining the resident included the following comments:

One cannot help wondering if there isn't an element of rather childish, wishful thinking in fantasy about her allegations. I would suspect that her father is a simple man also and he has perhaps become too easily upset by the things she says. (Haigh, 1976)

In this response we can hear echoes of Freud's early assertion that his female patients who complained of sexual assault were merely fantasizing, so it may be that this doctor's comments are simply part of the fabric of psychiatric tradition. However, we can also read in his evaluation that he is willing to dismiss the woman as a gullible and not credible witness, which is an experience common to many victims of sexual violence, particularly when those victims are individuals deemed to be mentally incompetent (McCarthy & Thompson, 1996). Either way, this woman's complaints were not taken seriously despite her and her father's efforts to see justice done. Further, her disability status was used to discredit her; the message is that because she is a woman identified with intellectual disabilities, she and her father (who almost seems to have been diagnosed by association) were not to be believed.

Staff Reporting and Extraordinary Violence

Inmates were not the only people who might have been dissuaded from reporting injuries and ill treatment as a result of the internal culture of the institution. Even though staff was spread thin, it is clear from the incident reports that co-workers observed and occasionally even reported violence. From a lengthy series of entries resulting from a rare enquiry, we can gain some insight into how such incidents unfolded. On 5 June 1975, an inmate was sitting on a chesterfield in a day room tossing pillows onto the floor (this event occurred on a High Grade adult ward during the normalization era so that the day room was quite plush by institutional standards). He was asked to stop by two staff members separately, one a worker on the ward and the other an occupational therapist who was on the ward to pick up a client. He apparently did not stop. According to the report, a junior staff member (Miss Cathy Gordon) observed the following concerning a senior staff member:

[Mr Hildebrandt] kicked him several times, flipped him over on the floor and stood on him with both feet (it should perhaps be noted that Mr. Hildebrandt's weight is approximately 300 lbs, or even more). Miss Gordon also discussed another incident on Thursday, 29th May, when Mr. Hildebrandt kicked [another inmate]. She also mentioned that there had been three witnesses of the two incidents.

Because there were claims about multiple witnesses, the other workers were brought in for questioning. From the questioning, it is clear that Mr Hildebrandt was a routine abuser of inmates. All three staff witnesses confirmed Miss Gordon's story, and added embellishments of their own to the file, including that the man not only stood on the inmate's chest but also jumped up and down on him. They also began to describe other incidents in ways that made it seem as if they were almost relieved to have an opportunity to speak out about this person's behaviour on the job. One member described another incident in the following terms: "Mr. Hildebrandt began to beat [an inmate] ... pull off [the inmate's] helmet, and pull him by the ear onto the floor. He then kicked him in the stomach, then the sides several times." Another noted that "he has also witnessed Hildebrandt kick [another inmate] but at this time, kicking had been the extent of the abuse." A third staff member stated, on further questioning that he had

> seen one or two staff members push residents along by the buttocks, perhaps even giving a slap across the buttocks. He could not decide whether this was a method of moving residents, or whether this was more force than should normally be used, as it is difficult to determine how much force is involved when you are standing a few feet away. Mr. Hildebrandt was one of the people he had seen use this method of moving residents from one place to another.

In this quotation we can see that the institute had a fairly high tolerance for violence; both the investigator and the witness seem to indicate that an acceptable "method of moving residents" could involve pushing them across a floor, aided with the occasional slap. From this report, it is also possible to understand that the everyday brutality of institutional life made things that in other contexts would seem extraordinarily violent instead seem quite ordinary and that, after spending time inside, it might become difficult to see violence precisely because there was so much of it.

We can also see from these passages that although these staff members had often seen Mr Hildebrandt abusing inmates, until the incident was reported by Miss Gordon, none of them had seen fit – or had had the courage – to report those incidents. As one staff member stated, after describing one of the beatings he had witnessed:

> I then walked out of the room, and did not report any of this until today. I am sorry that I cannot give a more detailed report, and I also regret that I did not report this first incident, as it probably would have prevented the abuse of [X] today ... although I am only summer relief, I have seen several such incidents, but this incident last Thursday has been the worst.

This individual, along with Cathy Gordon and the third worker who confirmed her story, all expressed regret at not having told sooner, and all were very junior and hence vulnerable workers compared with the perpetrator. It is easy to understand how difficult it would have been for a summer student and two junior employees to report their superior to disciplinary authorities. As we will see in the next chapter, although work at Michener was in many ways horrifying, it was nevertheless highly coveted employment; these were well-paying jobs in a semi-rural community where such work was hard to obtain. In this particular case, because the evidence was so overwhelming, and because the violence was so extreme, the individual who perpetrated the abuse was relieved from nursing service work. However, he was not fired; he was simply moved to a job involving less contact with inmates.

Another reason that workers may not have reported incidents has to do with the deniability that was engendered within the general culture of violence. This fact is illustrated through a series of reports concerning an incident in which one staff member confessed her inappropriate actions, initiating an internal enquiry. What is particularly telling is the outcome of that confession. The first entry reads, "Miss X confided in me about the 'ducking' of [a resident]. This was to have happened Monday night. From what I heard one of the afternoon staff told Miss X and others (staff) to 'duck' the residents' heads." As the word of this incident spread, an investigation began, and another staff member reported, "Miss X told me that since [this resident] often put her head in the toilet, she held her head down and flushed the toilet." After several such reports, we hear from an interview with the accused staff member that she "insists that she did not flush the toilet while ducking [the resident's] head, but does admit to giving her a push, thinking that this would discourage her [from putting her own head into the toilet]." The report goes on to say, "as there were no witnesses to this incident, I am not making any recommendation at this time." This series of entries indicates that the incident began from a suggestion from one shift of workers to the next that they should engage in some disciplinary or abusive action, perhaps as a challenge, perhaps as a joke, or perhaps even, as was noted in the reports, as a semi-serious way to dissuade a resident from sticking her face in the toilet. This incident is reminiscent of the hazing rituals described by ex-workers Evelyn and Jim, wherein junior or newer workers were induced to be abusive as a part of becoming accepted colleagues. It is hard to know what actually happened, or what the motivations were, but what is clear is that because nobody saw anything, and because certain levels of abuse (i.e., pushing, but not flushing, a person's face into a toilet) were fairly normative, no disciplinary action occurred as the result of this incident. It can be speculated that the strongest lesson this employee took away from the investigation was that it was probably best not to disclose one's violent actions.

A final reason workers failed to report abuse is that they feared reprisals from their colleagues. In one report, an investigation was conducted into an incident in which a worker was showering an inmate, and he "placed the resident's arm behind his back and applied pressure to turn him around, which resulted in a loud snapping noise." According to the report, immediately the worker turned to his colleague and said, "say he fell or else!" As the interviews with colleagues continued, it became clear that this person "had on many occasions been abusive, and that ... the staff were afraid to report incidents because of his threats towards them." In this final incident, where broken bones led to an official intervention initiated by hospital workers outside the institution, staff finally were encouraged to disclose, and it seems they did so with considerable relief. As the evidence mounted, the charge nurse informed this person that he would be relieved of duty pending the outcome of the investigation. Rather than continue as a staff member, the worker requested that he be permitted to resign, which he did. There is no evidence in the record of the investigation continuing further.

In the comfortable distance provided by history, it is possible to judge workers who failed to disclose incidents of extraordinary violence as uncaring brutes who simply ignored what they must have known was wrong. However, given the overall climate of dehumanization and violence within the institution, the conflicts that could arise when the offending staff members were also family members or community friends, and the fears of reprisal or job insecurity for new and arguably less hardened workers, it is perhaps more surprising that some workers did muster the courage to report the violence they saw.

Public Enquiry and Extraordinary Violence

Although workers were reluctant to report on violence of a quotidian or extraordinary basis, it was even more difficult for inmates to make such reports, as will be made clear in the sections that follow. However, occasionally institutional violence was so spectacular that knowledge of it seeped beyond the institution's walls. One such case was the 18 October 1981 strangulation murder of a 22-year-old resident, Brent Keith Stenberg, who was murdered by a former Michener Centre employee (Semanek, 1982). Thirty-six-year-old John Sipos had worked as an institutional aide at Michener for several years, ending in 1975. During this time, he developed a fondness for Mr Stenberg, and on eight occasions over a few years before the incident, he took the younger man for outings on day passes (Lee, 1981).

It seems as though Mr Sipos's murderous actions were in some ways a mis-guided protest against conditions at Michener, in that he made no attempt to cover his tracks, instead strangling Mr Stenberg during a final outing and then delivering his body to a local Royal Canadian Mounted Police station (Lee, 1981). During the pre-trial investigation, Mr Sipos claimed, "I did him a favor. The proper verdict should be not guilty by reason of justifiable homicide" because his intention in committing the murder was to "free the victim from abuse by staff at the Centre" (Zemanek, 1982, p. B2). Mr Sipos's own story gave him reason to understand the conditions in the institution and motivated his decision to take this drastic route. He had himself been hospitalized at a mental institution in Ponoka in the mid-1960s and later again in 1977, and he blamed his personal troubles on those institutionalizations. He said he had killed Brent Stenberg not only to save him from ongoing institutional abuse but also to draw attention to institutional abuse more broadly, saying he wanted to increase awareness, to trigger an investigation into institutional conditions in the province, and to extract revenge against doctors for preventing investigations against the Michener Centre, the Alberta Hospital in Edmonton, and the Alberta Hospital Ponoka, three of the province's largest institutions for people with intellectual disabilities and mental health issues (Zemanek, 1982).

In the end, John Sipos was judged not guilty by reason of insanity for Brent Stenberg's murder; however, much in this incident should give us pause. First, Mr Sipos, who was both an institutional survivor and an ex-worker at Michener, was well acquainted with the atmosphere at the Michener Centre and was clearly so disturbed by it that at one point in his trial he argued he should be awarded a Nobel Prize for Peace for relieving Mr Stenberg of his misery and for bringing institutional abuse to public awareness. Although this may seem to be the argument of a madman, it is also worth noting that euthanasia supporters also use the release-from-suffering argument to maintain that death (albeit death by one's own choice rather than one that is chosen by another) is often a more dignified, even nobler course of action than living in pain and misery. Another consideration in this case is that Mr Sipos's mother claimed to have contacted Michener to express her concerns about the appropriateness of her son taking a relative stranger out for visits. In the court case, the institution denied receiving such notification. However, it is unclear how much screening or supervision occurred when volunteers like Mr Sipos interacted with Michener residents. The question of screening is also relevant to Mr Sipos being hired at Michener; that a young man with a record of repeated institutionalization and mental health problems was hired to work with such a vulnerable population speaks to the difficulties the institution had in finding suitable employees and the compromised hiring practices that arose in the context of such shortfalls.

Problems with screening volunteers for suitability in working with vulnerable people was a problem that extended beyond the Stenberg/Sipos case but that came to public attention only as a result of the few rare cases that ended in criminal charges. Volunteers, from the early 1980s onward, were used to increase inmates' community involvement, working on and off campus with residents. However, screening appears to have been inadequate. For example, volunteer Peter Turton took several residents out on a day trip and fondled one woman and photographed her and another woman in their underwear. The distraught behaviour of and subsequent disclosure by the two women led to a search of his apartment, revealing similar photographs of other inmates. According to statements made at the trial, Mr Turton "had years of volunteer experience, and was a Class Three volunteer [the most trusted and advanced class of volunteer], allowing him to take a resident off grounds" (Monchuk, 1985a). After the trial, Michener increased its screening; however, parents of Michener residents expressed dismay at the small penalty (six months in jail) for Mr Turton's betrayal of a position of trust, and they also expressed concern about the screening process for Michener volunteers more generally (Monchuk, 1985b).

Survivor Stories of Extraordinary Violence

Survivors' narratives help us to understand what it was like to live under a regime such as the one that operated in the Michener Centre, and they also reveal the kinds of behaviour that elicited extraordinary violence. Many of the survivors' descriptions of explosive, unanticipated violence revolve around feeding times or toileting times, the moments in an otherwise isolated and alienated day when staff had no choice but to interact with inmates. The punctuation of the routine violence of everyday care with heightened incidents of brutality added to inmates' insecurity and contributed to a sense that things could go wrong at any time. To complain about treatment or to assert one's humanness, it seems, was to invite a brutal response. As an example of the way violence could escalate over seemingly trivial matters, survivor Donald Graham offered the following description:

> At meal times when we were finished eating we had to stand up behind our chairs facing the wall. We had to cross our arms until we were excused. If you moved or talked we would get knocked on the head.

In this instance, simply moving or speaking to a neighbour is described as grounds for violence. Further, the demands that were placed on residents to behave were frequently impossible to comply with. As Donald went on to say,

"Sometimes I urinated myself because I was waiting for so long. [When that happened] I got sent to the Side Room." In this description we can see how the structure of everyday violence invited mistakes like soiling oneself, which, in turn, would elicit heftier punishment.

Sometimes, even events that were meant to be pleasurable could turn sour without warning. Ray Petrenko described being taken on a walk in the wintertime with a group of people. When he became too tired to go further, "This one attendant pushed my face in a bunch of snow and my face was all red. I got frostbite, because I was tired and I didn't want to go anymore. I fell down." Ray's story illuminates the unpredictability of everyday events in the institution, and the enormity of the power that people working there wielded over inmates. It may indeed have been frustrating to be out on a walk with a number of children and have to deal with a tired child who could not or would not go further, but when staff members at Michener felt frustrated, they had few limits on how they could take those frustrations out on their charges. Thus, the level of violence that could occur truly was extraordinary. Harvey Brown told a harrowing story about an incident that occurred when he was in Deerhome, the adult side of Michener:

> There was a guy by the name of Gregory that was in a wheelchair and ... one of the attendants, he went and he hit Gregory a few times in the chest and Gregory had to be carried out and they wouldn't let us know what had happened.
>
> We asked one of the people, the person that was in charge, what was happening. They said, "never mind, we'll handle this." And they took him away and then the next day we found out on the news that Gregory had passed away. But the people at that time, at Michener, said it was the wrong Gregory – it wasn't the one that we seen, because all we seen was Gregory being carried away on a stretcher.

When pressed, Harvey stated that he did not see Gregory again after the incident. While is it truly sobering to consider the possible killing of an innocent person while in care, it is equally sobering to understand that the effect for those inmates who witnessed these events was perhaps much the same whether Gregory was killed during this incident or not; this incident simply reinforced the reality that these children and adults were living in a setting in which anything could happen to them, over which they had little if any control, and about which it would be prudent to remain silent.

Inmates and the Culture of Violence

It is important to note that the violence that occurred within the institution did not come only from staff members. The Unusual Incidents files list violations between inmates where, for example, "[X] was tipped out of her wheelchair by another one of the residents" or a "resident presents a severe behaviour problem with violent outbursts towards other residents and staff, including attempted strangulation of one of the other residents." An extremely violent incident was reported as follows:

> I found [X's] left arm broken when I went to the dormitory to find why he was crying. Another resident told me [X's] arm was twisted by another resident of the unit by the name of [Y]... I asked him why. He told me [X] was making noise and keeping him awake.

This report shows the effects of a culture in which violence and dehumanization were normalized to the extent that inmates themselves engaged in extreme aggression. We can understand how the overcrowding, lack of privacy, and continual stress of living inside the institution might cause frictions that would contribute to inmates being violent with other inmates. Finally, we can understand how social learning might contribute to the dehumanization of inmates in sobering ways that constructed them not only as victims but also as perpetrators. When we consider the very young ages at admission of many of the people who lived in Michener, and the reality that most would continue to live under this regime for years while growing up, and in some cases, for most of their lives, it is not difficult to understand that the children learned over a long, hard time that violence was something that was neither unusual nor unacceptable. The climate inside Michener was such that acts of kindness and compassion – either from staff or between residents – were rare. Conversely, acts of brutality for seemingly small things, like keeping someone awake or being in their way, became part of the fabric of everyday life. Compassion and solidarity were not encouraged among inmates, and in many ways violence between inmates can be anticipated as a natural outcome of growing up with systematic and pervasive dehumanization.

Institutionalized Violence – The Side Rooms

In addition to routine and extraordinary violence, the culture of the Michener Centre was also characterized by a third, more institutionalized form of violence in the form of the Side Rooms or Quiet Rooms (also sometimes referred to as Time-Out Rooms in the records). Side Rooms were an omnipresent means of exercising both reactive and precautionary control within the institution, and they operated both through routinized violence and the eruption of extraordinary violence. They also represented a built-in kind of violence, one that was an intentional part of the floor plans and procedural protocols of Michener life.

Side Rooms were used to impose seclusion and isolation on unruly patients from the early days at Michener. However, the advent of radical behaviourism developed by psychologist B. F. Skinner in the 1950s and 1960s offered a new scientific legitimacy to the use of segregation in Side Rooms. Skinner argued that understanding why people did things was not important in terms of producing desirable behaviours; rather, he developed operant conditioning, which attempts to shape behaviour through the use of negative reinforcement to extinguish undesired behaviour and positive reinforcement to elicit desired behaviours. The Side Rooms were used as a form of negative reinforcement; undesirable behaviours were to be extinguished by removing the individual from any gains incurred from exhibiting bad behaviours by taking them to an isolated and environmentally sterile place where no positive reinforcement could – even inadvertently – support the undesirable behaviours. Conversely, once inmates began to exhibit desired behaviours, such as being quiet and responding positively to requests, they would be rewarded with release from the isolated environment of the Side Room back into the general population.[2] At least, that was the theory. Thus, in the institutional records, these rooms are consistently described as a benign, clinical form of social control and behaviour modification rather than as a site of punishment. Likewise, they are never referred to as cells for solitary confinement, which in practice is how these rooms operated. Finally, it is worth noting that in 1971, before many of the incidents concerning Side Rooms that inmates described, the Accreditation Council for Facilities for the Mentally Retarded and the American Association on Mental Deficiency issued standards of practice for institutions indicating that "seclusion, defined as the placement of a resident alone in a locked room, *shall not* [emphasis added] be employed" (Joint Commission on Accreditation of Hospitals, 1971).[3]

Despite these professional recommendations, from survivor narratives, it seems that each unit in the Michener Centre had at least one segregation room; Side Rooms were a part of each ward, within the sightlines of warders and other residents in each residential unit. Some wards, and indeed the units that I visited as part of my tour of Michener, had as many as a half dozen Side Rooms for a floor servicing 80 or 90 residents. The Side Rooms were uniformly outfitted: each room had a heavy, locked door with a small aperture through which instructions or food could be passed, and the inside of the room was fitted with a drain in the middle of the floor and little else. A mattress would be dragged in at night for an inmate to sleep on and removed in the morning to facilitate cleaning the cell; for inmates housed in the Side Rooms, cleaning and mealtimes were typically the only times that solitary confinement was broken. According to both survivor and ex-worker reports, stays could last anywhere from a few hours to several days, and in one reported case, for life. Ex-worker Evelyn described how inmates who were housed in the Side Rooms were typically naked, because staff feared that inmates might harm themselves by chewing at torn clothing or perhaps by trying to strangle themselves with strips of cloth. These rooms did have a one-way mirror through which warders (and other inmates) could observe the individual inside and in which the individuals inside could, no doubt, see themselves reflected.

All the individuals interviewed knew about the Side Rooms and spoke consistently about their uses and practices. According to ex-workers and survivors, inmates were housed in Side Rooms as a result of resisting daily practices of the institution; residents could be sent to the Side Room for refusing to eat the food they were given, for refusing to go to bed or wake up at the prescribed times, for aggressive behaviour toward staff or toward other residents, or for refusing to perform work duties as instructed. Finally, survivors noted that people were sent to the Side Rooms in response to attempts to escape the institution. As I will discuss later, the detection of escape was a public event heralded at any time of the day or night by wailing sirens, the chaos of ward searches and calls to other units on the ward, and the striking of search groups to comb the broader campus. The combination of the sirens, the commotion, and the knowledge that those who attempted to escape would inevitably end up in the Side Rooms composed a powerful presence in survivor narratives about institutional life. Hence, Side Rooms were a central form of physical and psychological, reactive, and preventive social control.

Side Rooms as Sites of Foucauldian Discipline

As noted earlier, every survivor in this study knew of and spoke about the Side Rooms and their role as an ever-present means of exercising control within the institution. Jim Molochuk and Ray Petrenko provided descriptions of the procedures for admitting a misbehaving resident into the Side Rooms that introduce us to contradictions between the clinical, measured language of behaviourism and the brutality threaded throughout institutional life. Rather than a detached removal of misbehaving children from the general population, induction into the Side Rooms was frequently accompanied by brute force. Donald described the routine use of a sleep hold, used in martial arts to reduce an individual's oxygen so that he or she passes out. Harvey told me, "They would put you down on the floor in a 'sleeper.' It's like a headlock, and they put you to sleep and throw you in the Side Room ... It was scary, not nice. Had a window and glass, and a mat on the floor, and a drain in the middle." Ray concurred, saying, "They would put you in there in this room. You had no bed. You slept on the floor. They had windows ... people could see you walking back and forth. Some of them, they would put straitjackets on."

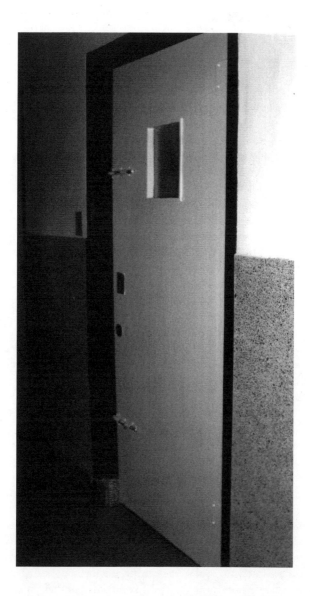

Figure 4.1 Exterior door, Time-Out/Side Room, Michener. This hallway contained several similar rooms along its length. Taken in 2005. Courtesy of the author.

Jim and Ray's descriptions remind us of Michel Foucault's discussion of the Panopticon, with its use of the gaze as a disciplining arm of modern, scientific techniques of power, discussed in the previous chapter. Like a Panopticon, the one-way mirror of the Side Rooms was a window for those who observed from outside and the means through which warders could constantly and easily watch those being isolated. Similarly, because Side Room inmates could not tell when they were being observed or see who was outside, the one-way mirror acted as a visual reminder to inmates of the constant possibility of being observed. Thus, the Side Room could engender compliance and control through what Foucault would term "disciplinary" means – through observations of the self by others and through self-observation to avoid potential punishment.

However, Jim and Ray's comments allow us to see that in the Michener Centre, there was more to social control than the modern disciplinary gaze. Instead, these comments convey that brute power, in the form of the straitjacket and the stranglehold, was a common and publicly displayed accompaniment to the disciplinary control of the Side Room. Thus, rather than the smooth, rational, and impersonal surveillance-based power that Foucault imagined would take place in modern institutional orders, or the detached, clinical effectiveness imagined in the operant conditioning of Skinner's behaviourism, the stories these survivors tell us about the public violence used in routine discipline at the Michener Centre show us a more terrifying and chaotic picture of social control in action. Indeed, we can hear that both discipline-based or modern practices and punishment-based or pre-modern practices operated in concert within the institution.

The Side Room as a Space of Spectacle, Prevention, and Division

Survivors indicated that little secrecy or mystery surrounded the use of the Side Rooms or the ways that individuals came to be incarcerated in them. The highly visible positioning of the rooms themselves, with at least one on each ward, typically part of the regular hallway of resident rooms and within the sightlines of both the nursing stations and the public day rooms, meant that residents of the institution could not avoid knowing about and seeing the Side Rooms. Further, the sirens and flashlight searches that accompanied the internment of runaway residents into Side Rooms, and the struggles and straitjacketing that accompanied the internment of inmates with "bad behaviours" meant that other residents could hardly ignore the violence attached to these spaces.

The public aspect of the Side Rooms' spatial designs is reminiscent of Foucault's descriptions of pre-modern, punishment-based means of social control. Foucault tells us that, in pre-modern societies, punishments unfolded in highly visible public spectacles, which were acted out to symbolically display the brutal power of the sovereign (Foucault, 1995). Although at first glance the Side Rooms, with their locked doors and windowed walls, seem to reflect a more private, disciplinary means of social control, the public positioning of the space, and the often violent and noisy means by which inmates were admitted to the space, in fact offered a spectacle of punishment to other inmates that let them know who was a bad inmate and displayed publicly the might of the institution in response to inmates who resisted. The spectacle of internment to Side Rooms and the public positioning of the space offered all residents a visual reminder of institutional sovereignty, evidenced by swift, brutal, and unforgiving punishment for those who failed to comply with institutional regimes.

Survivors themselves acknowledged the cautionary or preventive qualities of Side Room practices. Sam Edwards, when asked whether there was anyone of whom he had been afraid,[4] described a particularly chilling, regularly occurring event that is instructive regarding the display of raw power embedded in Side Room practices:

> Mr. Wong [a pseudonym]. Because I, I, I could hear him give this kid beatings in this quiet room off the dorm. You could hear. It would happen when we were eating. And I'm sure he did it right at mealtime so everybody's in one spot to hear it. You'd hear the screams. And he, I don't know what he did to him, like I don't think, you know, he punched him and stuff like that, but he'd probably twist his arm and do things to hurt him. Things that wouldn't show.

These violent events, occurring between a staff psychologist and one particular boy, were blatantly public despite being out of sight and behind closed doors. As Sam noted, the choice of a time when all the children were congregated and within earshot seemed purposeful and offered an object lesson for all the boys about what would happen to transgressors and who was to be feared in the institution.

The central locations and ubiquitous presence of the Side Rooms in virtually every ward acted as warnings even when not accompanied by extreme and noisy violence. Jim Molochuk, for example, noted that "some of the kids got put away on the side in this little place. In this dark room with a big window on the door. Sometimes they were there for 2–3 days." When I asked him whether that had ever happened to him, he emphatically noted, "No, I made sure I stayed out of trouble." For Jim, as for others, the architectural, spatial, and physical aspects of the Side Rooms acted as warnings of what could happen to transgressors, prompting preventive self-discipline and conveying an implicit message about the potential for violence that existed for all inmates.

Here, Foucault's concept of technologies of the self is instructive. Technologies of the self extend beyond mere self-policing and are instead forms of self-discipline and self-improvement engaged in by individuals not only so that they can avoid social sanctions but also so that they can come to think of themselves as good, deserving, and worthy citizens (Foucault, 1988a). Drawing on Foucault's work, it is possible to understand from Jim's description of himself as a person who "made sure [he] stayed out of trouble" that more was at stake than simply avoiding punishment. In addition, we can understand that compliance and avoidance of punishment are ways that Jim can see himself as good, smart, and different from those who failed to avoid the stigma and brutality of the Side Rooms. In other words, the use of the Side Rooms within Michener operated to divide inmates and create further hierarchies among them.

Like Jim, most participants in this study were loath to admit to doing time in a Side Room, and they often were remarkably unsympathetic toward those who did end up in them. Donna Bogdan, for example, noted:

> I never went to the Side Rooms, no. I would make sure I wouldn't get in trouble. So I could get out, you know? I thought that with my behaviour that sooner or later, I'd get out of Michener ... I was the kind of person that knew what to do.

As with other inmates' comments, Donna's description permits us again to understand the cautionary value of the Side Rooms, but her description also shows how she was able to distance herself from her surroundings in several ways. First, she was able to assure herself that abuse and violence could be avoided in the institution. In the institution's chaotic and unpredictable environment, in which inmates had virtually no power over their days, their lives, or their futures, the only power Donna was able to grasp was the power she was able to wield over herself. By telling herself that she was the kind of person who exercised positive behaviours, and by believing that these qualities would not only keep her out of Side Rooms but might even provide her with the ability to escape the institution itself, she was able to convince herself that her world was safer and more manageable than it probably was. Beyond Foucault's notion of technologies of the self that are aimed toward constructing a positive social self-concept, Donna's comments allow us to understand that such technologies offer the individual some internal sense power: the power to avoid punishment, the power to imagine oneself as in control, and the power to dream of another, better life. Unfortunately, however, the real power Donna sought, the capacity to get out of the institution by behaving well, was illusory; Donna, like most of the others in this study, escaped institutional life as a result of the deinstitution-alization movement rather than through her own actions.

Ironically, the responses Donna describes not only provided her with a sense of power but also reinforced hierarchical divisions among inmates. Donna's comments show us how institutional orders and self-technologies kept inmates from forming alliances among themselves and potentially against the staff within the institution. For Donna, the unruly inmate was not someone with a sense of justice or an enduring spirit but was instead a person deserving of punishment or an individual who simply was not smart enough to avoid vio-lence and punishment. This framing surely provided residents like Donna with assurances of personal power and safety in a place where both were in short supply, but it also led them to judge others as either pitiful or deserving of the punishments they received. In turn, this skewed sense of institutional justice precluded solidarity among inmates. Side Rooms thus seem to have functioned not only to discipline or punish but also to divide and conquer.

Those purposes of Side Rooms were in keeping with the dehumanizing as-pects of the institution, where inmates were so overcrowded, so understimu-lated, so overmedicated, so much in competition for scant resources, and so constantly on guard for their own safety that friendships, interpersonal alli-ances, and acts of resistance and support were rare indeed. The attitude that this divide and conquer strategy produced is evidenced in the following exchange with Donna:

INTERVIEWER: Did you ever see other people getting punished? Disciplined?
DONNA: Well I know they were put in the Side Room. I know, but I never seemed to pay much attention to things like that.
INTERVIEWER: Why do you think that was, that you weren't noticing things?
DONNA: I don't know, my mind, I don't know. It must have been a shock to my system and I really didn't know. I just seemed to care less, you know, I was very immature and that, so I really didn't know where I stood, and maybe with me be-ing in the Orphanage for 16 years in another Institution you kind of say, well, you get used to it and you just accept it ...
INTERVIEWER: Did you think it was fair though? Did you feel it was all right?
DONNA: No, I didn't seem to know. I didn't seem to care less.

Donna's responses reveal to us how the institution's combination of mind-numbing routine violence, and sporadic extraordinary violence, coupled with the divisive effects of disciplinary technologies like the Side Rooms, could even-tually undermine inmates' own sense of humanity or their imagined member-ship in humankind.

Humiliation and the Gaze

The descriptions provided by those survivors who did admit to spending time in Side Rooms illuminate how the rooms not only acted to demote inmates in the eyes of others but also operated to humiliate inmates in their own eyes. Gene Forzinsky, for example, described the inside of a Side Room as follows:

> The staff could look in from a window in the door, but I couldn't see out of it. There was only a mirror. There was no toilet, and when I had to go, I had to bang on the door with my feet, but most of the time no one would come, so I urinated myself. I had to sit like that sometimes for hours until the staff would come. [Pause] That hurt my feelings.

Gene's description moves our understanding of the functions of Side Rooms beyond discipline, punishment, or the creation of divisions among inmates to their other, central function, which was to humiliate and dehumanize inmates.

What Gene tells us about being watched through the Side Room mirror is reminiscent of Jim and Donald's earlier comments about visibility as a tool of power in the institution. However, he also helps us to move the visual operations of the Side Rooms outside of Foucault's concept of the Panopticon and the disciplining gaze. Rather than a simple description of how the gaze works, Gene's description allows us to understand how such a gaze feels to the individual who is its object. His narrative tells us that being the object of such practices is not only humiliating but that the individual also understands only too well that the purpose of these rooms – despite the clinical language of behaviourism – was to make the inmate feel both violated and degraded. Indeed, it is clear that in addition to fear, a central emotion connected to survivors' stories about the Side Rooms was shame. This revelation helps to explain why only a few of the survivors, with the exception of Michel Aubin, whose story is one of defiance and agency rather than punishment and humiliation, were willing to admit that they had ever been in such a room. It also helps to explain why most inmates spoke unsympathetically about other residents who did get put in the Side Rooms.

Gene's description reminds us that the added visual plane of the one-way mirror operated not only to provide outsiders with a view of the inmate and her or his disgrace, but also to offer a view of the individual that was both sombre and humiliating. Gene's comments permit us to understand that the individuals who are the objects of their own gaze come to be seen not only to others but also to themselves as less than human. Thus, we can see that the Side Rooms existed as more than clinical spaces for the correcting of bad behaviours

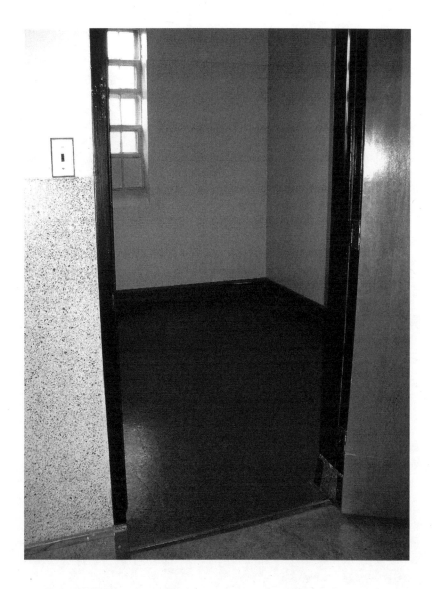

Figure 4.2 Interior view, Time-Out/Side Room. Note the drain in the floor, far corner. Taken in 2005. Courtesy of the author.

through isolationist yet highly visible incarceration. Instead, humiliation and dehumanization lay at the core of Side Room practices.

Nowhere is this function of dehumanization clearer than in a story told by ex-worker Evelyn about a special kind of Side Room resident:

> There were people who lived full-time, all the time, in the Time-Out Rooms, which was a whole other [pause] group of people that weren't there for punishment. They were there because that was the way the institution understood that they could be, uh, controlled and they never left, except to clean out the cells now and then and then they were under strict guard.

Evelyn described these people as incarcerated for the long term because of problems with violent or aggressive behaviour, because their behaviour had been deemed otherwise unmanageable, or because they were simply deemed to be subhuman. Evelyn went on to say:

> So for example, one of the women who lived there was Vicky, who was born in an institution. Her mother had been raped in Ponoka,[5] and she was the child born from that rape, and so had lived her life in an institution and in that locked cell. And Vicky was, she had her head shaved, she was naked all the time, she had a mattress that was pulled in at the end of the day and pulled out in the morning. She spent her whole time smearing her feces over the walls and windows and bars, screaming, and the staff told us that "she'd beat the shit out of you" if we ever let her loose. That was the story. Anyways, everyone was afraid of course.

There are several elements to Evelyn's story. First, we can hear echoes of some of the earlier stories told about senior staff inducting junior workers in to the institutional culture through stories of humiliation and degradation. Vicky's story may have been some sort of terrible tale told to new workers to both frighten them and bond them into the "us" and "them" mentality that seems to have prevailed between staff and inmates. In addition, constructing Vicky and those like her as subhuman may have acted as a way to justify the horrors of the institution and the abjection of its inmates. We must also consider Vicky's life in terms of the earlier discussion about sensory deprivation; this woman, whose entire adult life had been spent in solitary confinement under the most onerous conditions of sensory deprivation, never had a chance. However, instead of understanding Vicky, in Evelyn's words, as "the product of a punishing ... and annihilating institutional life," Vicky instead was treated as a deserving monster, a non-human "other" whose condition literally demanded subhuman treatment. Given her origins, Vicky would have been from birth deemed degenerate –

born in a mental hospital and conceived through rape, her lifelong internment concrete evidence of the horrors of degeneracy and defectiveness, and the appropriateness of the institution for "such people." A final aspect of this story is that Vicky and her life story was known to inmates, and the example of her existence as a lifelong monster, created and sustained through the Side Rooms, could only have added to the Side Rooms' terrifying effects, acting as a powerful cautionary tale about dehumanization within the institution and further galvanizing inmates' resolve to avoid a fate such as hers.

Despite the 1971 standards set by the accrediting body for institutions in North America that prohibited the use of isolation and seclusion, Side or Time-Out Rooms continued to be used well into the 1990s at Michener, as evidenced by an enquiry into the 1997 death of 58-year-old Loreen McPherson, who burned to death in a Time-Out Room. The incident also occurred long after supposed normalization within the institution, where efforts were made to make institutional life more home-like, and residents were given more autonomy and personal freedom than in the years before deinstitutionalization, which may explain why Ms McPherson was placed in seclusion with matches in her possession. According to a newspaper article on the government-mandated fatality enquiry, staff descriptions echo the clinical language of behavioural modification, in that staff "look in every five minutes and if, after 15 minutes, the client appears calm for one minute, they are released" (Michelin, 1999, p. A2). However, in Ms McPherson's case, the staff placed her in the room three times on the day of her death, and the last time left her unattended for long enough that she lit several matches, one of which caught her pyjamas on fire. Even after this death and the subsequent enquiry, the recommendations were not to cease use of isolation as a means of behavioural control but instead to have staff search people before putting them in the isolation room, that staff observe them constantly during their internment, and that it might be desirable to install video surveillance in the rooms (Michelin, 1999, p. A2).

Chapter Five

Resisting the Institutional Order

The impression conveyed thus far through the archival record and survivor and ex-worker stories is that the institution was a terrifying place in which virtually all humanity was ground out of its inhabitants. It is not difficult to speculate on what the effects of these kinds of violence might be for the individual being brutalized and for the individuals who observed such brutality. For staff members who observed or were invited to participate in routine and extraordinary violence, the regimen signalled that to behave violently was permissible and even appropriate in that environment, and often the regimen telegraphed that belonging and collegiality could be built and sustained through abuse. For inmates, observing such events could only convey that individual choices and even very small acts of resistance would not be countenanced. However, despite the overwhelming impression of acquiescence and surrender, there is some evidence in both the archival and the interview data of inmate resistance to the institutional regime, a subject to which I now turn.

The ill effects of institutionalization on children and young adults with intellectual disabilities are well known and long established in academia, with very early researchers finding that children and adolescents who are institutionalized experience depressed mental development, reduced responsiveness, and negative personality effects (Crissey, 1937; Goldfarb, 1943; Skeels & Dye, 1939). Research in the late 1950s through to the early 1970s built on this knowledge concerning the effects of institutionalization on the development and personalities of child inmates. Researchers reported that institutionalized children experienced slower and reduced responses to both positive and negative stimuli, along with a lessened capacity to respond to positive reinforcement (Stevenson & Fahel, 1961); they had decreased language and discrimination skills (Haggerty, 1967); and they developed a marked sense of passivity, acquiescence, and powerlessness (Jaffe, 1967). These research findings contributed to the scientific concept of the *institutionalized personality* in which people incarcerated over long periods were believed to develop dependent and acquiescent personalities that ultimately made them unsuitable to life outside; in a cruel irony, the argument was made that, once institutionalized, children stood little chance of successfully reintegrating into society because they had been "ruined" by their institutionalization experiences (LaJeunesse, 1996). Despite numerous voices who indicated that institutionalized people could and did live full lives (Dybwad, 1961; Wolfensberger, 1970), this pathologizing literature maintained that the personalities of institutionalized people were so fractured that they were virtually incapable of anything but numb surrender to institutional life (LaJeunesse, 1996). Indeed, in the various and recurring debates concerning the closure of the Michener Centre over the years, this argument has been used to claim that it would be cruel to release people from the institution, because they have become used to life inside and would be made anxious by having more freedom and autonomy (Roche, 1994).

However, the stories told by inmates and ex-workers and the institutional records themselves offer up a much more complicated picture of the effects of institutionalization and the inmates' reactions to institutional routines. From these records, it seems that inmates frequently were anything but acquiescent. Instead, they were caught hiding medications, refusing to take their medications, refusing to eat meals, dragging their feet while working, talking back to workers, and even engaging in overt forms of resistance, such as running away or plotting to do so. Indeed, even the architecture of the Michener Centre speaks to resistance; without resistance, locked doors, modes of surveillance, and Quiet Rooms would certainly not have been necessary. In this chapter we encounter evidence of both covert and overt forms of resistance, evidencing that even though many of the individuals involved came into the institution at very young ages and remained inside for many years, they still were able to rally the personal resources to refuse the institutional order of things.

Weapons of the Weak

In many cases, survivors' descriptions of resistance require some imagination on the part of the listener to be understood as such. Resistance was often described as an internal process; for example, Gerta Muller provided a telling example of how, following her sterilization, she developed a bad infection: .

> I thought, "good for you, I'm infected." I thought to myself, "what would happen if I croaked?" Because a girl who had had the operation fell in the bathroom and there was blood all over, and I thought, "What if that happens to me? Wouldn't that

teach them a lesson not to do that anymore? Make them realize they did something wrong?"

It might seem something of a stretch to call this resistance, but Gerta wasn't the
only inmate to offer up descriptions of internal narratives that formed, at least
for the individual, some sense of opposition to the institutional order. Mary
Korshevski also described several incidents in which she was bullied by staff
about her slowness in getting work done:

> She mentioned something to me about being a cripple. And I thought, "Well, one
> of these days, you know, the way people are treated sometimes, maybe the staff will
> be treated the same way. You never know, someday, it will come their turn."

Although the language is passive, and the resistance may have been invisible to
its target, for inmates like Gerta and Mary, these moments stood out as moments of pushing back, and they also provided some sense of self in an environment bent on erasing individuality. As Mary said later, "That was the thing that
I was able to hold on to."

Resistance, as understood by inmates, may not have even been visible as
such to those working in the institution, or it may have been enacted in such
a way as to be ambiguous enough that residents could get away with it. Sandra
Karnak described how she was able to send a message to staff about bodily
control in a way that kept her out of trouble while nevertheless telegraphing
her unhappiness:

> One day I was kind of moody and grumpy and didn't feel good and I told the
> teacher that day, "I'm not feeling good, I have stomach aches." I knew what the
> trouble was, and I told her I have to go back and do some things and she said, "You
> can't go." So I told her, "Can you get the supervisor to bring something down to me
> that I need?" "Nope, nope." So that day you could just see the whole thing and I
> told them, "I hope you're satisfied now."

Although this incident of a bloody accident during a young woman's period
might be read as humiliating, instead Sandra read it as a sort of embodied
"screw you" to authorities that she recalls to this day as an act of resistance.
Other forms of resistance that inmates described included making surrepti-
tious comments (often spoken at such distance that it was not likely that they
would have been audible), covering up or pleading ignorance when being asked
about other inmates or about misdemeanours, or working slower than they
were capable of working. These descriptions of passive and almost invisible

ways of addressing the inequality rampant in the institution are weapons of the weak, which, because overt rebellion is too dangerous to take up for profoundly oppressed people, include things like avoidance, shirking, dishonesty, or failure to respond appropriately and assiduously to superiors (Scott, 1985). In this framing, it becomes possible to see that something as simple as looking away, reacting slowly to a command, failing to understand or agree with directions, or refusing to collude in getting another inmate in trouble are the only tools available to truly subordinated people, and that Gerta, Sandra, and Mary's actions were indeed acts of defiance in the institutional context.

Active Resistance

Given the oppressiveness of life at Michener, it is perhaps unsurprising that passive and covert methods of resistance were common. However, on rare occasions, more overt forms of defiance were also enacted. Mary told a story about a girl who refused the porridge offered her for breakfast, requesting dry cereal instead. The staff responded by trying to "make her stand up and eat" but still she refused:

> So then the charge nurse came, and they told her that Patty would not eat her porridge at breakfast time. So they gave it to her for dinner – they put it in the fridge, and gave it to her for dinner. And she just stood there and wouldn't eat it.

Mary was clearing dishes during both meals, and after the second failed meal, Patty asked her to throw the porridge out when she took the other dishes back to the kitchen. Even though Mary was impressed by Patty's spirit, however, she could not bring herself to match this heroism, instead saying, "Well, I just didn't know if I could do this ... I knew I'd get caught if I did." Eventually, the incident ended with Patty being taken away to a Side Room where she could think about her behaviour, and Mary being left with her own feelings about her role in the event.

On occasion, resistance was enacted simply through witnessing, as Louise Roy described:

> I was feeding [someone] next to them, and they slapped her so hard that she cried. And I kind of thought, "I'm not standing here and watching this." So I fed the person next to them and went and stood by the chart [room], so I asked someone that was giving medication, "Would you come, when you are finished with whatever you are doing, I want to show you something."... And I took her and showed her. And this girl, she had red finger marks on her body, she was helpless, you know?

In this instance, the woman had been hit because she had not been prepared properly for her meal; she was a woman who required some support to help her eat, and this had not been provided, causing her to choke and leaving the workers frustrated. Perhaps because proper procedure had not been observed in the first place, or perhaps because Louise was so polite in her intervention, Louise's complaints were taken seriously, and she described that the two workers involved "had to go and get their walking papers." In this case, and really almost inexplicably in comparison with stories told by other people in this project, there did seem to be some recognition of Louise's and the injured girl's humanity in the institutional response to Louise's disclosure. And it is only fair to acknowledge that "walking papers" did get issued in those rare cases of witnessed, provable, and especially repeated violence. There were a small handful of such records among the many indications of routine and unpunished staff excess. In these rare instances of dismissals, it is clear that the institution was keen to be seen as exercising appropriate protocol, and dismissal letters were copied to several levels of the institution and to the government ministry responsible for the institution.

Escape

As noted earlier, despite the locked rooms and units, the pervasive surveillance in the institution, and the belief of some inmates that good behaviour and hard work were their best hope for leaving the institution, escape attempts were a frequent form of resistance. When people were moved to various training or work placements, when they went on outings for appointments on or off campus, or simply when an opportunity arose and a door was left unlocked or a staff member got distracted or called away, people took their chances and attempted what were referred to in the institutional records as "elopements." It is worth reflecting on the use of this term within institutional discourse. *To elope* has connotations of irresponsibility; an individual who elopes is running away from doing the responsible or proper thing, and elopements, at least in literature, are often followed by tragedy that is more or less deserved. To elope is often to invite shame, to eschew community conventions, and to court disaster. Conversely, *to escape* means that one has a reasonable motivation for running; to escape acknowledges the conditions one is trying to get out from under. Thus, the institutional language of "eloping" accomplishes several outcomes. First, it characterizes the runner as irresponsible and inviting her or his own demise or endangerment as a result of running away. In turn, this reinforces the perceived necessity of paternalism and justifies the draconian level of care embedded in the institution; the subtext is that people in the institution would fall apart if they were not being cared for or protected by the institution. Finally, of course, such language denies the terrible conditions of life in the institution. Thus, to not reinstate such linguistic violence and erasure, and following the language of the survivors and ex-workers who spoke to me about Michener, I use the term *escape* to describe this particular form of resistance.

That escapes were fairly common is made obvious through the institutional documents. Numerous policies, replacement policies, forms, replacement forms, standing orders, revisions to protocols, establishments of levels of alert, and various other official regulations relating to escapes were threaded throughout the institutional records. In a 1972 memo outlining a new procedure to be followed on escapes, for example, instructions were given for intra-institutional levels of notification, and depending on the age of the individual who was missing and the length of time since the he or she was last seen, there were also differing levels of extra-institutional notifications, ranging from notices to family members (where such were still available) and community child welfare services, to the local police and the Royal Canadian Mounted Police (RCMP) (Brown, 1972). The memo included procedures on the appropriate use of RCMP search dogs, the composition of internal search and rescue teams, the proper chain of command for reporting escapes, and the procedures for billing various authorities for costs relating to searches. Wards were to maintain search kits in addition to adhering to appropriate channels for reporting missing inmates; these kits were to include a megaphone, a set of walkie-talkies, eight whistles, a portable first aid kit, and search maps. Whistles were to be used according to a complex code to indicate whether the individual had been located or if assistance was required or if the search was to be upgraded from local to urgent; megaphones were to be used for instructions to move to a new location; no foot searches outdoors were to be made until RCMP dogs first cleared the area, and so on. Other policies gave arcane instructions about who to notify, again depending on the length of the absence and the perceived level of seriousness attached to the escape based on typologies of inmate's impairments (Swallow, 1975). One memorandum indicates that at least some escapees managed to cover considerable ground outside, instating a new policy concerning payments in that "we have no authority to bring a patient back from another Province or the United States and can assume no financial responsibility for [the] same," going on to note that such authorization needed to be referred to the director for a final decision (Brown, 1968). Thus, the various forms and protocols build a picture of fairly regular escapes or attempts and a strong and coordinated institutional response to those attempts.

Inmate stories about escapes also paint a picture of considerable activity following the discovery of a missing person; flashlight searches of wards at night, rushing staff, whistles and alarms going off, and the arrival of police vehicles were reported in most survivors' stories. However, not all escape attempts were accompanied by such draconian or bureaucratic efforts. Guy Tremblay, a man of considerable charm and humour, described several attempted escapes, including this one:

> I ran away one day, the door was open and I just ... headed 'er. Didn't get off the grounds. I remember Mrs Martel, she had a '69 Chevelle and Mr Wong had a 1968 Charger, they were into these muscle cars. And they chased me down with those. Just like the Dukes of Hazard.

Guy told another story about working on a local farmer's fields on a vocational training exercise, when, perceiving an opportunity to make a break for it, he turned his tractor northward, hell bent for Edmonton, a city 90 kilometres away. In that instance, police did apprehend him several hours after he'd abandoned the tractor and hitchhiked up the road. From both of these stories, it is clear that despite having lived much of his life in incredibly demeaning conditions, this man's spirit remained unbowed. Nevertheless, it is also clear from these stories that there was little planning attached to these escape attempts and little chance of success. The lack of planning or preparation for escape attempts is not surprising, given the regimes of institutional life, and the relatively few chances there were for slipping away. Further, inmates had no access to clothing for outdoors or to food or money to sustain them on their journeys. Thus, it is not surprising to hear stories like the one told by Beverly Buszko about two girls escaping during a routine movement from the mess hall to the ward and to learn that the next morning the two girls "came back, on their own, with no shoes."

Some inmates, however, did describe what seemed to be at least minimally planned escape attempts. Mary Korshevski described an incident in which two of her roommates told her they were planning an escape and asked her to come with them. Reminiscent of an earlier comment made by Gerta Muller concerning Side Rooms and being well behaved as a hoped-for means of achieving discharge, Mary declined, saying, "No, I'm not going to. I want to get out of here someday so I'm not going to cause any problems." As planned, the two girls did escape, "in the middle of the night, when people were sleeping, they had a fire chute, and they somehow got the window open and got out down the slide." Nevertheless, the planning did not amount to much, since during one of their routine checks in the night, staff members noticed the absence of the two girls and set a search in motion. When questioned, Mary lied about knowing anything, but covering up for the two girls was not enough. By the next morning, the two girls had been found not far from the campus, and as Mary said, "they took a little walk" for a lengthy stay in the Side Rooms.

Ex-worker Evelyn Stephens also described an incident when she was a young intern in which three female inmates conspired to escape. They hit her over the head during a routine bathroom visit, took her keys, and attempted to lock her in a linen closet. When they attacked her, Evelyn called out, other staff members came to her aid, and as with Mary's two roommates, the women were placed in locked Side Rooms as punishment.

Not all escape attempts were as short-lived or as ill-conceived as those described above. Indeed, it is clear from the institutional record that some inmates escaped and made their way home, and even remained there on rare occasions. In other instances, inmates were gone for a while, living on the streets or staying in shelters, or were picked up and moved into other psychiatric facilities, such as Ponoka Hospital, a few kilometres up the road. Regardless, however, of how long escapees were able to remain at large, in all of these descriptions it is clear how thinly resourced escape attempts were; inmates snuck out of unlocked doors, slid down fire escapes, ran while being transported, and slipped away while working, but they had no access to food, money, warm clothing, or contacts on the outside. Given their typical life story of being incarcerated when very young and living in an institutional culture that gave them absolutely no skills for imagining how to coordinate a plan or manage in the community, it is a small wonder that they failed to stay away for very long. Indeed, we can argue that institutional life made successful escape almost impossible. In addition, the impairments of some inmates added to the unlikely prospects that escape attempts could happen. Jim Molochuk, for example, when asked whether he had ever run away, said, "I was on this medication for my epilepsy and if I ever ran away without it, I would be finished. Otherwise, I would have gone."

Death and Escape

Given the lack of preparation and resources available to inmates who did escape, it is perhaps unsurprising that in the records are several reports of deaths occurring during inmate escapes. Twenty-eight-year-old John Wickstrom was a man with a long history of escape attempts; between December 1971 and December 1975, he escaped no less than 18 times, sometimes for as long as a couple of months and once getting as far as Kamloops, a city 750 kilometres away (Friesen, 1976a). On Sunday, 8 August 1976, staff noticed John's absence while doing a mealtime head count. Mr Wickstrom, like Jim Molochuk, had epilepsy, and his daily medications at the time of the escape included "phenobarbital (130 mgm. twice daily), neuleptil/penothyazine [sic] (20 mgm. three times daily), trilafon/perphenazine (2 mgm. three times daily), dilantin (250 mgm. twice daily), valium (10 mgm. twice daily on a routine basis and an extra dose to be given p.r.n. [as needed] if any seizures occurred), and largactil (when needed, for agitation)" (Friesen, 1976b). These drugs, mainly used to control behaviour and sedate agitated patients, are serious psychotropic medications with severe side effects, such as drowsiness, slowed reaction time, and impaired judgment. Taken together, they compose a cocktail for disaster. It is not surprising then that John Wickstrom's judgment seems to have been clouded somewhat. As he made his way to the edge of campus, he slipped while attempting to ford a river in his bid for escape. By 7:30 that evening, his body was found floating three kilometres downstream from the institution.

A newspaper article reporting Mr Wickstrom's death noted that this was the third death of an escapee in slightly more than a year; in addition to Mr Wickstrom, Marilyn Dewar died of exposure in December of 1974, and Albert Klebe slipped and fell off a culvert into a ravine and died from a combination of his injuries and exposure in March 1975 (Lozeron, 1976). Following this rash of deaths, numerous investigations were initiated, and the results of these investigations were outlined in a memorandum to the director of Social Services and Community Health, a government ministry (Koegler, 1976b). In the memo, the circumstances of each death were outlined, as are the protocols followed and the possible errors made, ending with recommendations for avoiding further incidents. The recommendations focus on tightening security, devising yet more procedures concerning escapes, and hiring additional staff. What the memorandum failed to address is the institutional responsibility for creating a climate that that would lead inmates to risk so much in attempting to escape, nor did it acknowledge that part of the reason that escapees were so vulnerable was because they were underdressed, under-provisioned, unprepared for independent living as a result of their institutionalization, and drugged beyond any reasonably functional level. Instead, the report concluded with a claim that the "real" reason for these deaths while escaping was because of the "recent change in philosophy of care of residents in our Institution," going on to argue that because the institution at this point was moving toward a less restrictive environment and a more residential approach (these specific incidents occurred during the period of deinstitutionalization in the mid-1970s), this meant "new freedoms to the lives of the residents, which in turn introduces additional risks to their lives" (Koegler, 1976b, p. 2). In short, rather than acknowledge that escape was a reasonable enough response to the institution's unreasonable environment, the director took the opportunity to make a covert argument for a return to even more draconian routines, arguing that the little progress that was being made in the institution toward humanization posed a danger to residents that was both inevitable and undesirable.

Chapter Six

Broken Promises: Education in the Institution

The previous chapters have traced the contours of violence, dehumanization, and social isolation that characterized daily life in the institution, examining their effects on the children and adults who lived there. In addition to what life inside was like, we heard how and why people came to live at the Michener Centre. For many, although there may have been eugenic underpinnings to rationalize their admissions, the overt justification to family members and to the children themselves came from a promise of better care. As previous chapters attest, this promise was one on which institutional life clearly failed to deliver, and children instead were subject to brutal conditions while in care. Along with the better care argument, families were convinced to intern their children, and children were in turn enticed by the promise that a stay in a special institution for children with intellectual disabilities would provide them with much-needed education that was unavailable to them in the public school system. In the institution's *Guide and Information for Parents*, this focus was clearly stated:

> First and foremost, we should like to stress that the entire emphasis at our School is one of the residential school (boarding school) where children come to acquire education in conformity with their abilities and in every possible instance teach them some vocational skills so that they may ultimately leave the School and become self-supporting or as near self-supporting as possible. This represents the major portion of the children who take up residence at the School every year. (Alberta School Hospital, 1967, p. 1)

Thus, family members were promised that the services at Michener were geared to education rather than to incarceration, that education would be tailored to individual needs and offered to the majority of the institution's residents, and finally that the educational opportunities at Michener had a strong success rate, as evidenced by independence and, by implication, community reintegration.

In this chapter I discuss the role of education and training in the institution, arguing not only that children were generally not provided with education in any meaningful or personally beneficial ways but that the guise of "training" also laid the foundation for economic abuse by the institution that spilled over into the host community. However, before engaging in a discussion specific to special educational programs at Michener Centre, it will be useful to have a broad picture of the educational options available to Alberta's "special" children during the institution's formative years.

Alberta's Educational Context

In the early decades of the twentieth century in Alberta, public education was characterized primarily by rural school districts with very few towns and urban centres so that schooling took place, for the most part, in one-room school-houses with one teacher delivering instruction to grades one through eight simultaneously (Alberta Teachers' Association, 2002). Children seeking high school instruction typically boarded in larger centres with family or friends when and if such arrangements were possible; however, most children living in rural areas simply did not complete high school. The life of the teacher was difficult, typically involving teaching children of all ages in isolated communities with few resources, compensated by punishing wages. Because of population losses during World War I, further population dispersals during the Depression, volunteerism during World War II, and the generally poor working conditions in the schools, for many decades it was very difficult to recruit teachers in the province. As a result, up until the late 1950s, despite recommended standards to the contrary, the province relaxed its requirements for teacher preparation simply to keep schools open, and teachers were generally not highly educated, let alone educated to accommodate diverse learners (Alberta Teachers' Association, 2002).

The difficult educational conditions for most children in Alberta were compounded for children facing educational challenges. The Province of Alberta School Act was amended in 1915 to make it mandatory for all children between the ages of 7 and 15 to attend school; however, no concomitant legislation required that a child be provided with an education suited to her or his needs (Ballance & Kendall, 1969), and it was only in the late 1960s that Alberta began to establish classes for disabled children, primarily in select, urban schools (Winzer, 2009). In addition, teachers employed in "special" schools or classrooms were not required to have any training in special education. In the 1960s, the government began offering incentives to teachers who took in-service training or summer school in special education, but these incentives were slow in producing results (Ballance & Kendall, 1969). As a result, up until the 1980s, there were very few special education classes available in community schools across the province (let alone inclusive regular class-rooms), even fewer qualified special education teachers, and practically no special education teachers or classes in rural areas. In sum, the possibilities for children with intellectual and learning disabilities to obtain an appropriate community-based education in Alberta remained profoundly circumscribed into the last decades of the twentieth century.

There were, however, options for children whose needs were not being met in the public school system. Under the School Act, children who could not obtain an appropriate education locally were entitled to receive room and board, tuition, and transportation at the expense of the government to attend segregated special day and residential schools, such as the Alberta School for the Deaf in the provincial capital, Edmonton. Children with intellectual disabilities, however, were not treated under the umbrella of the School Act and instead were managed under the 1968 Mental Health Act, which mandated that a child requiring special services because of being "mentally retarded ... or who has any other handicap" could be charged fees for non-residential educational services (Ballance & Kendall, 1969, p. 2). Conversely, the Act also mandated that children between 5 and 15 years of age who could not be schooled publicly were to go to Alberta School Hospital (the children's side of the institution) and ruled that children over 15 years of age deemed "mentally deficient" were to be admitted to Deerhome, the adult side of the institution.[1] This meant that parents seeking appropriate educational services for their children would need to pay for those services unless the child went into residential care, effectively reducing parents' choices concerning institutionalizing their children with intellectual disabilities.

Thus, children with intellectual disabilities in the province were offered virtually no local, cost-free, or appropriate educational services, making them outcasts in their communities. At the same time as it declined to provide community education, the state set laws that funnelled children into the institution and paid for segregated residential education, similarly to the practices in many North American jurisdictions of the time (Amary, 1980). Alberta School Hospital, the children's side of the Michener Centre, promised Albertans a rare opportunity for the appropriate education and training of children with learning or intellectual disabilities, and hence, the claim of education was one that

would have resonated with parents and children alike. Nevertheless, it is important to recall that educational opportunities of any kind were not offered to almost half of Michener's residents simply by right of their age and institutional
location; only children living in the Alberta School Hospital side of the facility
were afforded any educational support, while inmates living in Deerhome, the
adult side of the facility, were not provided with any training except through
work in the institution or the community, as I will discuss later in the chapter.
Finally, even for those children whose age would have qualified them for
schooling, there were few opportunities for real learning, and only 20% of inmates received any formal education.

Sense Training

As occurred with so many aspects of institutional life, educational services at
Michener were divided along hierarchical lines, with "real school" being offered only to an elite few. Low Grade inmates who were deemed educable were
provided with sense training, a form of education based on the theories of mid-
nineteenth-century educational reformer Edouard Seguin. Seguin was a student of pioneering French psychologist Jean Marc Gaspard Itard, who had
worked with an abandoned child known as Victor, the wild boy of Aveyron,
who, when discovered at age 11 or 12 in the woods by local citizens, was unable
to walk, speak, dress, drink from a cup, or engage in other civilized behaviours
(Gearheart, 1972). The method Itard devised, sense perception training, had
moderate success, with young Victor drinking from a cup, dressing himself,
and walking upright after five years of intensive training. The success of Itard's
efforts led to a belief that, with the right educational tools, people deemed to be
"mentally retarded" could be educated. Building on Itard's ideas, Seguin advocated a means of training that involved presenting objects and actions in sensu-
ally rich ways; he believed that people with intellectual disabilities could be
trained to read, write, and conform to societal standards through touching,
tasting, feeling, and hearing the words associated with objects or actions. For
Seguin, sense perception training "emphasized the importance of rapport between the teacher and his pupils," demanding a sustained and individually tailored program for students (Amary, 1980, pp. 4–5). Perhaps this need to engage
children in intimate and continuing learning explains in part why Seguin is
associated not only with sense perception training but also with the movement
toward institutionalizing children with intellectual disabilities; having children
in-house permitted the kind of sustained interactions required by his teaching
methods. Seguin acted as the director of the "school for idiots" at the infamous
Bicêtre (an asylum that at times served as an orphanage, a prison, and a hospital

in Paris), and after emigrating to America, he worked briefly at the Pennsylvania Training School for Idiots before engaging in a career that made him a leading light in the burgeoning field of treatment for children with intellectual disabilities (Gearheart, 1972).

The promise of sense perception training was taken up with enthusiasm in the mid- to late nineteenth century not only for teaching children with intellectual disabilities but also for teaching language to new immigrant children, a growing challenge in North American schools (Lane, 1873). Seguin's methods required long-term relationships between teachers and students, one-on-one sessions that were tailored to individual needs, and a climate of instruction that was gentle and loving. Students were to be housed in small centres with no more than 200 children so that they could be known to educators, and further, they were to learn their lessons within relationships of gentle, individualized care (Gearheart, 1972). Given that the work of Seguin began with such benign intentions, it is difficult to imagine how even the institutions at which Seguin himself worked grew so quickly in population beyond this original vision of small cottage-like settings offering sustained, intimate instruction (Trent, 1994).

From the beginning, the Michener Centre embraced the idea of sense perception training. In 1923, a special Sense Training Room was installed and equipped, and instruction commenced in 1924 for the "lower grade children" (McAlister, 1924, p. 6); by 1938, with a total of 214 children in residence, "14 to 15 children, mental ages ranging from 3 to 6 years, attended the Sense Training classroom" (McCullough, 1938a, p. 131). In 1949, with a total population of 293 patients, four sense training classes were established for an unnamed number of children, but by 1956, new levels of efficiency seemed to be preferred. Although the total institutional population had climbed to 417 residents, the resources apportioned to sense training were reduced; in 1956 only two classrooms were being used, and these were serving some 120 children under a change in policy that limited the attendance of any child to no more than four hours per day and that saw many of them attending only sporadically (LeVann, 1956). In the years subsequent to this policy change, the spatial configurations for sense training remained unchanged; however, the numbers of children being served actually decreased, a striking outcome when the total numbers of residents are taken into account. Between 1957 and 1968 (the last mention of sense training in the annual reports), 71 to 102 children attended each year's classes, while during that same period the total number of children in the institution steadily mounted, reaching 1053 on the children's side in 1967, more than double that of just 10 years earlier (LeVann, 1967–1968). Thus, from the mid-twentieth century onward, the likelihood of receiving this type of training declined at same time that the institutional population grew.

For those children who received sense training at Michener, there was little chance that the training methods were administered adequately or appropriately. As with all schooling in the province, instructors were difficult to obtain, and those who did work in the institution were undertrained and underqualified. The original sense training classroom in 1924 was not staffed by an educator but by "one of our capable attendants assigned to this work as instructress," indicating that teaching was being done by aides rather than educators; elsewhere in the 1924 annual report, it becomes clear that this person's training was accomplished in-house (McAlister, 1924, p. 8). In fact, one survivor, Mary Korshevski, described how she, as an older inmate who had finished her own schooling and was living on the Deerhome adult campus, came to work as a sense training instructor:

> I worked there for two months. I kind of thought, "I wonder why they use the word 'sense' training for these little, little boys and girls. Does it really mean they don't know – maybe they mean they don't know anything. Maybe that's why they use that word." And I – it – it was playschool for them – they used the word Sense Training meaning they probably didn't know much, or they knew very little. But yet, they knew more than they figured. And you know, after I finished working there, after two months, I thought, "You know, that doesn't make sense." Before they go into level I, they've got Sense Training. Those kids know more than the staff do.

Mary's analysis is telling on several fronts. First, it is clear that despite her work in the classroom as an aide, she had little idea what the purpose of sense training was, nor had she received any training of her own specific to the method of sense training or how she could assist in its delivery. As will be discussed later, Mary was provided education only up to the equivalent of grade five during her time at Michener, so her preparation for working with children in an educational setting would have been woefully short by any standards. Her interpretation of the term *sense training* is reasonable enough, given that there was little overt instruction about the philosophy or practice of the program and given the watered-down version of sense training that the institution was able to implement. Finally, Mary's assertion that the children knew more than the instructors gave them credit for is one that came up repeatedly in interviews with survivors and workers and is something that is well documented in the literature on special education. There is ample evidence that in special education generally, children have been thwarted in their learning because of teachers' lowered expectations of them simply because they are identified as having disabilities (Hehir, 2002).

Lack of training and resources were persistent complaints concerning sense training, and ad hoc methods were frequently used, as the 1956 annual report indicated:

It continues to be difficult to find educational materials and aids ... through the research ingenuity of these Instructresses, together with the cooperation of various school departments, many helpful classroom aids have been evolved. (LeVann, 1956).

In addition to spotty teacher training and a lack of appropriate classroom aids, the principle of sustained and individualized instruction that formulated Seguin's original method was also a challenge to achieve in the institution. In 1959–1960, it was noted that the 71 children who attended sense training did so only for one to one and a half hours per day, while in 1961–1962 it was reported that not only were children attending on a part-time basis, but they were also doing so in "nine separate Sense Training Groups ... to cope with the variety of young children who were admitted to the School" (LeVann, 1959–1960, 1961–1962). The use of group instruction, the need to apportion scant classroom time between multiple users, the lack of appropriate training for instructors, and the dearth of materials for classroom aids undoubtedly resulted in a program that bore little resemblance to Seguin's nineteenth-century programs, and it is fair to speculate that the Michener Centre's sense training held little likelihood of success in educating intellectually disabled children. Finally, we must recall that this minimal instruction also took place not within an environment of care and support as Seguin had believed was necessary over a century earlier but as a brief, irregular educational opportunity embedded within the most bleak and dehumanizing of environments, particularly for those children who lived in the institution under the label of "Low Grade."

Given these conditions, it is not surprising that sense training had few successes on the Michener campus. The Michener program laid out its own goals for sense training as teaching children "coordination, socialization, appreciation of rhythm, colour distinction, practical living techniques" and ultimately "being prepared for promotion to the academic school house" (LeVann, 1959–1960, p. 167). However, it is difficult to gauge the success of these programs because most of the annual reports do not indicate student outcomes. The one reporting exception was in 1967–1968, when 99 children attended sense training classes; of these, only 10 were promoted at the end of the year to the intermediate school for more academically oriented programs (LeVann, 1967–1968). In sum, the educational programs that the centre offered to more intellectually challenged or academically unprepared children were inadequate and inappropriate by almost any standard and, unsurprisingly, the outcomes of these scant efforts meant that very few of the children in this group experienced anything near the educational opportunities and hopes for success that had sent them into the institution.

Regular School

For the children who were institutionally designated as "High Grade," the educational prospects were not appreciably better. Although the institution's founding mandate was to provide an education to educable children who were otherwise not receiving education and training in the province, in reality, the Provincial Training School did not start out with any formal classrooms for its High Grade inmates. In the 1923 annual report, a dedicated space for education was requested in the following terms:

> Serious consideration should be given to our need for a building to be used for manual and vocational training purposes ... Certainly we cannot do justice to the higher grade patients without some effort being made to teach them the fundamentals of such vocational work as carpentry, painting, shoe repair, reed work, weaving, knitting, brush making, etc. (McAlister, 1924, p. 10)

Two points are worth noting in these comments. First, despite the promises of education and betterment that were foundational to the institution's existence, from the beginning, the activities of the institution were architecturally prescribed as warehouses rather than as educational facilities. Through its focus on beds and day rooms rather than classrooms and blackboards, it was clear that the main function of the institution was to house rather than educate children. The second point is that the educational facilities requested for the new training institute were not for traditional academic classrooms but for appropriate spaces in which children could be trained for semi-skilled labour. This focus on training children with intellectual disabilities for menial or manual labour has been a founding principle of the vocational rehabilitation industry, resulting in the exploitation of children's labour on the one hand and the undermining of children's intellectual capabilities on the other (Albrecht, 1993). Indeed, the tendency to underestimate the intellectual potential of children in special education is a persistent attribute even in current special education practices (Slee, 2001).

The institutional privileging of vocational over academic learning for children who were seen to be educable had remarkable persistence within Michener. The requested vocational space was added in the late 1920s and was continually augmented throughout the decades, while the first three academic classrooms were created only in 1948, earmarked to accommodate "165 pupil hours daily," triple the previous year's "classes" held in a temporary space on one of the wards (Alberta Department of Public Health, Mental Health Division, 1949, p. 156). In these new classrooms, the children attended academic classes on a part-time basis, instruction was offered only up to the grade-three level, and the focus was less academic than the dedicated classrooms indicate. Not only did none of the students attend classes full time, but "school children in the second or third year of elementary work were assigned, during out-of-school hours, as helpers in the various work departments and thus receive an initial training therein" (Alberta Department of Public Health, Mental Health Division, 1949, p. 158). The report went on to say that, among these children, again reflecting the hierarchical paradigm within the institution, children who were deemed "trainable, but of non-parolable classification" were apprenticed in and assigned to tasks within the institution, while training for more complicated work outside the institution was set aside for those children seen to be of "parolable caliber" (Alberta Department of Public Health, Mental Health Division, 1949, p. 158). In essence, the children's first year of schooling acted as a sorting mechanism for assigning them to a path of training for lifelong work in the institution or for training that might facilitate their eventual release into the community, undoubtedly initiating a self-fulfilling prophecy for those children deemed unfit for the "advanced" training.

It is also important to understand that, in these early years, even the little in-school time and training that was made available to the children was not necessarily academic in focus. The institution's educational goals were "to produce self-controlled, self-confident and at least partially self-supporting citizens" where "character building" was seen as a core focus, and outcomes of "proper social attitudes, good habits of thought and action" were the primary goal of teachers and therapists (Alberta Department of Public Health, Mental Health Division, 1949, p. 158). Thus, subjects such as health, manners, and hygiene formed the core curriculum.

The Schoolhouse

This situation persisted until 1952, with the construction of a six-room schoolhouse, built on the Michener campus with the specific intent of providing more academic training to select Michener children. By 1956, there were 121 children attending classes in the schoolhouse that was "devoted to the teaching of academic work which would correspond to Grades I to VI in the Alberta Educational System" (LeVann, 1956, p. 131). Thus, almost 30 years after opening its doors, Michener/PTS finally offered some of its children curriculum with an emphasis on reading, writing, mathematics, and social studies, and just

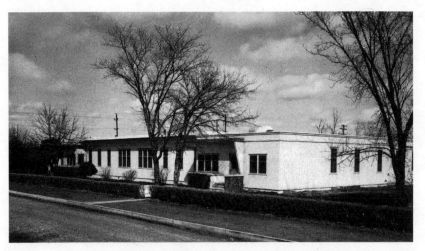

Figure 6.1 Schoolhouse, built in the 1950s, circa 1974.
Courtesy Red Deer and District Archives (N2686).

four years after the construction of the school, some of the children had managed to progress up to grade-six levels, with a couple of children doing some classroom work at the grade-seven level (LeVann, 1956). Clearly, a number of the institution's children had been more than ready for this kind of education, and it is speculatively possible that such training could have been offered to a larger number than this small group of inmates and that the centre could have offered education beyond the grade six and seven ceiling imposed by the number of classrooms available.

Echoing the challenges embedded in the sense training program, scant resources, underqualified instructors, and poor learning conditions also plagued the more advanced educational programs for High Grade children. In terms of numbers, it is fairly clear that a gap existed between the size of the institutional population and the school's capacity to teach the institution's children. From the school's construction in 1952 until the last of the detailed annual reports, the enrolment levels in these academic classes sat between 109 and 153 students (in 1959), despite the fact that the institutional population during the same period more than doubled from 472 children in 1953 to 1055 in 1967 (LeVann, 1954; LeVann, 1967–1968). On the matter of teacher qualifications, ex-worker Jim Sullivan's comments about school staff during the 1970s are illuminating:

The teachers were not certified teachers, because I remember the university students, when they would come, they were Education students, so they would sort of take over ... I was quite shocked because when I left there and went into Education and taught special needs kids here, many of the kids I taught in the integrated settings were much lower functioning than the kids I worked with in Red Deer, so it was sort of shocking to me how things had been done ... There were many kids who never took academic subjects. Literacy? Forget it.

From Jim's commentary we can see that the teaching staff in the institution were perhaps neither well qualified nor particularly competent, in that during field placements, university students ostensibly assigned to the institution for teacher training in actuality "sort of took over." Further, it is clear that this lack of staff education and training played a role in the lengthy institutionalizations of many of these children; because their teachers were trained poorly, they failed to identify the potential of the children, offering only a half-hearted educational program and failing to see that at least some of these children were more than capable of being integrated into mainstream educational settings and ultimately the community more generally. Indeed, several of the survivors gained literacy and numeracy skills through adult education after leaving the institution, indicating that they were capable of learning but simply had not been taught appropriately while in the institution.

Even though the advent of the on-campus schoolhouse heralded a purported new focus on academic learning within the institution, it is also clear from the annual reports that there were challenges to achieving these goals. Reflecting the dismal capacity of the educational system generally, there was little knowledge about and fewer resources specific to teaching children with learning or intellectual challenges. There are repeated entries in annual reports similar to this one, describing the lack of an "authoritative curriculum for the teaching of retarded children on the North American Continent" and the adaptive measures staff were forced to make on "on the basis of teaching experiences during the year" (LeVann, 1956, p. 132). In these entries we can read on the one hand that the institution, despite being in operation as a training facility for more than 30 years, was ill-prepared to deliver appropriate schooling to its charges. On the other hand, there is a tone of self-promotion and a claim to expertise embedded in these complaints about having to forge a new path in special education. In the next year, in an effort to better serve its students, but also as a means to laying claim to a specific level of expertise in teaching special education students, Superintendent Leonard Jan LeVann – a medical doctor rather than an educator or a psychiatrist as he often claimed

(*Muir v. Alberta*, 1996) – and the school's instructors produced and locally printed "primers in Reading and elementary Arithmetic books" which LeVann
claimed would be "suitable for all schools teaching retarded children... carry[ing]
prescriptive techniques necessary to facilitate the teaching of both Reading and
Arithmetic" (LeVann, 1957, p. 130). Despite his hopes that these materials
would find their way into wide distribution, they likely remained in use only
in the Michener classes, as I have been unable to locate any record of their
publication. Nevertheless, despite its slow start in implementing academic
education for its charges, and its limited resources and professional training,
the institution worked quickly to establish itself as an expert in the field of
special education, claiming that there was a dearth of knowledge about such
schooling in the broader context, while setting itself up as the producer of
knowledge about this special educational endeavour. These efforts at building
the academic reputation of the institution were also enhanced, as ex-worker
Jim Sullivan described, by regularly bringing education students from the
University of Calgary and the University of Alberta (each approximately 150
kilometres from Red Deer) into the Michener schoolhouse as part of their
special education practicum placements.[2]

School Curriculum

Despite these ambitions for expert status and the patina of serious academic
education in descriptions of the school program, from speaking with survivors,
and from reading portions of the annual reports, it seems the school days of the
academically focused High Grade children were not entirely literacy or numeracy focused, but instead included significant non-academic work. For example, the 1959–1960 annual report stated:

> The educational program included many field trips to areas in the community
> which included monthly shopping trips by the senior classes. Special efforts were
> made to give the trainees a better understanding of money and its purchases in the
> school canteen.[3] Traffic safety features were taught, such as the recognition of
> street signs, rules for pedestrians and in addition, the constant stress on the need
> for good behaviour, courtesy and consideration of others. (LeVann, 1959–1960,
> p. 158)

Almost a decade later, similar ambitions are outlined as goals for the academic
program, with the educational activities for the institutions' children described
in the following terms: "The academic school program placed emphasis in

relating all academic subjects to practical life experiences. Every effort was made to develop the child to his highest level of academic achievement, combined with vocational training" (LeVann, 1968a, p. 150).

Although this quotation indicates that there was overlap in the academic and vocational work, implying that the vocational or practical aspects of training were used to enhance and make concrete the more academic topics, it is likely that this was not precisely the way things occurred. Rather, non-academic subjects, such as citizenship, comportment, and social skills, were not merely teaching devices but composed a key part of the school's curriculum; ironically, a number of the educational focuses described in the annual reports reflect skills and knowledge that would have been lacking in these children as a direct result of being interned in an institution for their developing years. One could even argue that a great deal of this kind of civic education for advanced students in the institution was in fact remedial work to offset the iatrogenic, negative effects of institutionalization itself.

From survivor Guy Tremblay's description of his educational experiences in the school program, it is clear that even the remedial aspects of this training fell short. When asked about the kinds of subjects that were taught in the Provincial Training School, Guy said, "It wasn't really training. But that's what they called it ... it's not really a school, it's just another name for the institution." He went on to describe the gaps in his learning, noting that when he was discharged, "I didn't even know how to tie my own shoes, because I never wore those kinds of shoes in the institution." From Guy's comments, we get a small insight into the kinds of learning gaps that resulted from years of sensory and cultural deprivation inside the institutional walls, and how inadequate the institution's training programs were in compensating for the numbing qualities of institutional life.

Most of the survivors I spoke with did not have experiences in the academic school, reflecting the rarity of this opportunity for inmates. However, those who did provided a different view of their experiences than the hopeful official narrative. Ray Petrenko attended the school for several years. He described his interactions with teachers as follows:

> I learned some things, but then there were some things that teacher didn't have. She gave up on me. I wasn't going to give up, but she gave up on me, because I guess she figured some people were faster learners than me, so she sent me home, back to the ward, and that's where I stayed ... They were teaching us the things they wanted, like a little bit of adding and subtracting but not much of that. A little bit of reading and writing, and to recognize what our responsibilities were in jobs and stuff like that.

Louise Roy also attended the academic school for a couple years, and when she was asked whether she had learned to read and write in school, she said, "Not at the time. We just printed our names and all that, and what the weather was going to be like. We watched some videos, but mostly we talked a lot in the classrooms." Like Ray Petrenko and Harvey Brown, Louise learned to read and write subsequent to her discharge from the institution; further, she is adamant that the education she was promised in Michener did not occur.

Mary Korshevski, who was described earlier as having worked as an untrained aide in the sense training program for a short stint after graduating, described her education in the Michener academic school as follows:

> When I was 15, I went to Michener Centre and they had what you call levels – Level 1, 2, 3, 4, 5, instead of "grades" ... so when I first went there, they tested me to see what level I would fit in. And I was tested as a Level 5, so just – that's where they left it. I stayed there until I was 18 ... We did some reading and writing ... and then when I was 18 they told me I couldn't learn anymore. And I was even taken out of school at Easter time because of my birthday. You know how school ends in June? But they figured I couldn't learn any more so I had to be taken out at Easter time.

It seems that Mary's three years in the school, spent at the same academic level at which she entered and terminated only when she came of age rather than as a result of any academic milestones achieved, amounted to little more than a way for her to pass the time until she could be moved into the adult side of the institution to begin her working life in earnest. Indeed, it is fair to assume that the academic competence that Mary did have on "graduating" was that which came with her into the institution.

That the institution abrogated its responsibilities to provide an education to its inmates became clear during the lawsuits launched against the provincial government in the 1990s. These lawsuits, focusing primarily on unlawful confinement and sterilization, also included claims for damages not merely because the institution failed to provide inmates with an adequate education but because institutionalization in fact reduced the plaintiffs' likelihood of obtaining an education that would prepare them for the workforce. In the Leilani Muir case, the courts did not award damages for loss of employment income, arguing that it was difficult to assess what exact employment opportunities would have been available to Ms. Muir had she not been interned. However, the judge did acknowledge that it was clear that the "government failed to provide her with the education and training that she might otherwise have achieved" (*Muir v. Alberta*, 1996, p. 4).

Occupational Therapy and Training

Although a great deal of promise was attached to the provision of appropriate academic training for the children who lived in the institution, in keeping with commonly expressed concerns about the productivity and self-sufficiency of people with intellectual disabilities, the institution's key focus appears to have been on the occupational and vocational training of its inmates. As noted earlier, even children attending the academic school had their time divided between academic/school time and vocational time. The blurring of academic and occupational activities following the construction of the academic schoolroom was quite explicit, as the following quote indicates:

> The training program was much like last year's with the greatest emphasis being placed on studying the needs of each individual, his capabilities and how they might best be utilized to prepare him for discharge as a self-sustaining member of the community ... 153 children were enrolled in the academic school program during the year. The stress was placed on practical aspects of education insofar as it was on esoteric studies and more towards properly conditioning the trainees' reactions in society and at work. Proper behaviour, the use of money, shopping and cooking class aspects of training were given wide emphasis. (LeVann, 1959–1960, p. 158)

It is difficult to tell from these descriptions whether this was academic training or simply a more sophisticated form of vocational training. Nevertheless, in addition to this instruction, agricultural instruction, occupational training/therapy (the terms vary from year to year), and vocational training were dutifully reported in each annual report as separate and additional categories.

The number of students engaged in occupational therapy classes was much higher than those engaged in sense training or the academic school; in 1961, for example, approximately 600 students attended occupational therapy classes. Rather than therapy sessions in which remedial aides and approaches were designed to assist inmates with specific impairments and facilitate their learning, these seem to have been "classes" in which inmates produced handiwork and engaged in light industrial work. In the early years, instructors (not educators, but individuals with skills in required areas, such as shoemakers and carpenters) were hired and facilities were built to offer inmates carpentry classes, sewing classes, and classes in reed work, weaving, knitting, and brush-making, the products of which were placed on display at the major Edmonton Exhibition and placed on silent auction sale at the Training School as a fundraiser (McCullough, 1938a).

As the occupational therapy options broadened in scope and grew in capacity over the years, these activities, as always, were assigned in ways that were ordered hierarchically along lines of gender and perceived ability, so that "those workers who were of a somewhat trainable, but non-parolable classification [were] trained to do useful and necessary jobs around the school" while other, more capable students were trained in direct vocational work for placements off campus (Alberta Department of Public Health, Mental Health Division, 1949, p. 157). The school-based training included "contact training in the following departments: Laundry, sewing room, dining room, kitchen, domestic and wards" for the girls, and for the boys, "practical training in general farm work, as gardener's helps, carpenter's helper, and in general janitor and handyman work" (Alberta Department of Public Health, Mental Health Division, 1949, p. 157). Practical classroom instruction was given on a daily basis for boys in "carpentry, painting and varnishing," while the girls received daily classes in "sewing, knitting, embroidery, crocheting, dressmaking and in the use of hand and power sewing machines" (Alberta Department of Public Health, Mental Health Division, 1949, p. 157).

From the very beginning of its operations, the occupational therapy program produced useful and attractive items, and these goods were displayed and regularly won prizes in competitions at local country fairs and at the larger provincial exhibition in Edmonton. By 1961, the offerings included such things as cabinetry, handicrafts, baked goods, soft toys, weaving, knitting and crocheting, basketry, embroidery, leatherwork, and rugs. In addition to being exhibited, these goods were sold through the institution's twice-yearly Sale and Tea, a fundraiser that was attended with great alacrity by members of the local community. At these events, inmates prepared and served community members a luncheon and sold them the goods they had made; however, the proceeds did not go to the inmates themselves. Instead, proceeds went to the Patients' General Comforts Fund, which was used to contribute to the general budget for things like running the small canteen on campus (LeVann, 1961–1962). The number of goods produced by the students was truly impressive; in the 1963 fall sale, students produced "some 200 pounds [90 kilograms] of Christmas cake, plus cookies and chocolates were baked and packaged and found ready consumption" (LeVann, 1963a, p. 182). The amounts generated by the products of the children's labour were not insubstantial; the 1961 pre-Christmas Sale and Tea alone netted $2100, equivalent to approximately $16,452.23 in 2013 dollars (Bank of Canada, 2014; LeVann, 1961–1962). Students also engaged in special projects over the years, including "supplying most of the 20,000 paper flowers for the prize-winning Deerhome float in the Red Deer parade" (LeVann, 1961–1962, p. 170). In addition, during these semi-annual Tea and Sale events, High

Grade children provided entertainment to local officials and community visitors by performing in plays and musicals organized by recreational instructors who were part of the occupational therapy staff (LeVann, 1959–1960, 1967–1968). In sum, the occupational therapy program produced items that not only kept students occupied but also generated income and offered very public proof to the outside world of the productive, educational, and rehabilitative work that went on inside the institution, through these public sales and teas, country fairs, agricultural competitions, concerts, and even parades. In many ways, these activities operated as performances of happiness and productivity for the general public, and reinforced the notion that good things were happening for the children of Michener behind the institution's closed doors.

Vocational and Agricultural Training

In addition to occupational therapy, the institution ran a very active vocational training program, in which male children primarily seem to have participated and which also included an agricultural program. Here, the children engaged mostly in work on the campus, and the vocational training students produced items, including

> many pieces of furniture of solid hardwoods, such as, mahogany, birch, walnut and maple. These included many major projects such as a Children's Playhouse on cement foundation, solid mahogany desks, bedroom suites, lamps and lawn furniture. (LeVann, 1961–1962, p. 162)

As with the occupational therapy products, most of these goods were not produced for use on campus but were sold in conjunction with the twice-yearly Sale and Tea events. These items, too, were displayed and placed in competitions at local and provincial fairs, providing very public evidence of the productivity and skills of Michener's inmates. Not all the work accomplished under the vocational training program was produced for sale, however. In 1957, for example, the carpentry classes were engaged in another special project that involved panelling the institution's boardroom with mahogany panelling and window trim, and the children's playhouse mentioned above was installed in the sole playground on the campus, for inmates' use. In addition, clothing produced by girls in their classes was worn by inmates, and one of the longest-running components of the vocational program was a facility in which children received instruction in making and repairing shoes for use by inmates in the institution.

A final educational avenue offered to children under the occupational or vocational training rubric was the agricultural program in which the boys who attended learned, "the practical background of farm procedures and practices ... what must not be done and dangers to be avoided in relation to working farm equipment" (LeVann, 1959–1960, p. 159). Instruction included occasional field trips to events such as the Red Deer Hatchery and Farm Implement Shows, and daily activities followed a typical farm work pattern, involving not only planting and harvesting, but greenhouse practices and the breeding, raising, and showing of livestock. Again, the products of these efforts were displayed and competed in public shows and fairs in the province. It is not clear from the educational reports what ultimately happened to the food that students produced or the animals they raised; however, it is probable that the produce was consumed in the institution and the animals were either sold to local farmers for use in their operations, sold to local slaughtering facilities for meat, or consumed at PTS/Michener itself.

It should be clear from the above descriptions that the occupational, vocational and agricultural training programs were an important part of daily life for the children's side of the Michener campus. The children's education in the vocational, occupational, and agricultural domains was meant to provide them with marketable skills for self-sufficiency and eventual return to the community. However, these skills were also used to produce high-quality goods in copious amounts for consumption within the institution, for sale to the general public, and as vehicles for the display of the institution's success in teaching children to be productive, happy citizens, despite the reality of what life inside the institution was like and despite the reality that discharge into the community was unlikely for most inmates. Finally, it is important to again note that the educational activities described in this chapter were a focus only on the Provincial Training School or children's side of campus. Once children "graduated" at 18 years of age and were moved to the adult or Deerhome side of campus, their training ended and their labour became simply the medium through which they earned their keep and contributed to the institution and the broader community, as will be discussed in the next chapter.

Conclusion

The promise of education and the goal of returning to the community with new skills and knowledge was in great part what brought inmates into Michener Centre, both as children and as adults. For children, some opportunities for learning, in sense training or regular school, did exist. However, these opportunities were offered to only a small portion of the residents on the children's side of the campus, and even for those children who were fortunate enough to attend these classes, the experiences were inadequate at best. Sense training, offered to Low Grade inmates, was so poorly done that students had little chance of being improved by its methods, let alone graduating into regular school classes; further, it operated within a context that was so cruel that, even had it been run along optimal principles, its chances for success were foreclosed from the outset. Regular school, plagued by problems of inadequate space, inappropriate curriculum, and undertrained instructors, was focused on academics only to a limited extent. Instead, "academic" classes were spent providing remedial civics and comportment instruction, and the curriculum was further blurred between academic instruction and vocational training. Vocational training itself was hierarchically organized, describing its vocational program as training for continuing work inside the institution for children deemed to be Low Grade and as training for work in the community only for those children deemed to be High Grade. In practice, however, it seems that children of any sort rarely found their ways into the community, and their vocational training became a means of funnelling them as children and adults into institutional and community work as an end in itself, a subject that will be explored more fully in the next chapter.

Given that the stated goal of the Provincial Training School was to provide its charges with an education that would prepare them for independence and community reintegration, it should be surprising that few children experienced this outcome. However, the combination of rarely offered, poorly executed education resulted in an environment in which few of the children succeeded. In summing up his impressions of the educational programs at Michener, Jim Sullivan, based on observations during more than six years of working at Michener part and full time in the mid-1970s, provided a chilling assessment of the overall discrepancy between the institution's promise and its actual practices:

> They were told, "They'll be trained," and trained was the operative word. Trained, but for what? To continue living in Michener Centre, basically until they died. I don't recall a person leaving, ever. Not one. Ever. It was a like a life sentence. They never left. Never. Never heard of that. They just grew up and died there.

Although Jim's assessment sounds harsh, it is not unreasonable; the institution's incredible population growth, its expansion to include not only children but its graduating adults in a separate adult facility on the campus, and its persistently low discharge rates confirm Jim's dark view of the rehabilitative functions of the Michener educational system. Further, as I explore in the next chapter, the institution depended on the failure of its academic programs and relied on the continued productivity of its students and its adult graduates.

Chapter Seven

Training, Exploitation, and Community Dependency

In the previous chapter, I argued that vocational training was the most prevalent and valued form of education in the institution, evidenced by the late arrival and relative rarity of education-specific facilities as compared with the early presence and constant growth of vocational training programs within the institution. I also argued vocational training acted as a generator of resources that profited the institution and served as a public symbol of the positive aspects of Michener's educational and treatment programs.

The belief that work can offer a "cure" to children and adults with intellectual disabilities is rooted in the industrial revolution. During the early years of industrialization and urbanization, "mad," "defective," and non-productive people became increasingly visible, and asylums sprang up across Europe and the Americas. Without exception, these were places where people were treated terribly and basically treated as human waste. The only possible economic benefits these individuals accrued was as an attraction for the entertainment of local citizens, as happened regularly at Bedlam (Bethlem Royal Hospital) in England (Porter, 1987). Both in response to the horrors of these early institutions, and in response to the waste of human potential embedded in the early sequestering of mad people and mental defectives, significant reforms occurred during the nineteenth century. In the early decades of the nineteenth century, psychiatric reformer Philippe Pinel, responding to the neglect and abuse he saw in France, instituted a program of moral treatment, based on an assumption that mad or defective people had simply lost their moral core and that providing a rural and gentle environment would facilitate healing and moral reintegration (Porter, 1987). Pinel's followers built on this model, instituting the first uses of active and useful occupational therapies as treatment. A prime example of this was the York Retreat in England, an asylum devised by Quaker Samuel Tukes to house mentally ill people, where pastoral surroundings and a family-cottage model of institutions was coupled with a requirement that inmates perform chores so as to develop a sense of usefulness and propriety. It is interesting to note that Quakerism was highly tied to the notion of increasing productivity through benign, bucolic means and the production of contented workers; the Cadbury family, for example, were Quakers who built their chocolate factory in the English countryside, with fresh air and a corporate village, in an attempt to foster happier workers and to increase productivity. In the York Retreat, and others modelled after it, treatment was focused on productivity as a force of moral regeneration, and weaving, basket-making, carpentry, sewing, and domestic and agricultural work were all part of the rehabilitative program. Typically, we have understood these changes to have been positive and humane advancements over the original asylum system. Michel Foucault takes issue with our historical perception of the "improvement" of the asylums under the regime of moral treatment. Instead of benign kindness, he saw these centres as places for observation, categorization, and the imposition of productivity and docility onto the abject, mad, or defective body (Foucault, 1988b).

Andrew Scull's analysis of social junk as an outcropping of capitalism is also informative to our understanding of the mechanism of work and training in the institution (1984). "Social junk" is a term Scull takes from Marxist interpretations of the production of deviance in which individuals who are unable to participate fully in the demands of the capitalist system are characterized as dependent, useless, and disposable. Although containment satisfies the need to manage this group, it also serves to commodify them, making them into consumer objects and products for the profit of others, in ways similar to what Gary Albrecht (1993) has described as the disability business, in which able-bodied people gain valuable employment and income as a direct result of keeping disabled people dependent. In this model inmates at Michener can be seen as social junk, acting as both burdens and resources.

Foucault's critical perspective on the real purposes of seemingly benign institutional vocational reforms, coupled with Scull's and Albrecht's insights into the utility of maintaining disability as a form of dependency informs my analysis of vocational and occupational "training" at Michener. I extend Foucault's cynicism about the purpose of training programs and Scull's perceptions about commodification to argue that, far from fulfilling its promise of providing its inmates with meaningful training for life outside the institution, the vocational programs instead operated as a training ground for a captive workforce that was used to run the institution and enhance the neighbouring community of Red Deer's economic prosperity. In this sense inmates at Michener provided unacknowledged labour that was used to further the interests of capital outside the institution's doors. In addition, the training programs available for non-inmate workers in the institution provided a privileged and rare opportunity to members of the Red Deer community for well-paid work with rich avenues for advancement, reflecting the commodification role of disabled people as fodder for the profits and careers of others, as outlined by Scull and Albrecht. Before engaging in an analysis of these aspects of work and training, I will situate Michener's practices in the broader context of vocational education and institutionalization.

Utility and the Institution

As noted previously, the Michener Centre saw tremendous growth during its first 50 years, with a particular population surge from the early 1950s forward, following the appointment of Dr LeVann as the institution's superintendent. The town of Red Deer, where Michener was located, also saw phenomenal growth and development between 1923 and the early 1970s. In 1921, the census year closest to the opening of the PTS, the population of Red Deer was 2328, representing only 1.9% of the total population of Alberta. By 1971, Red Deer's population had burgeoned to 27,751, an almost 12-fold increase, and it composed 2.3% of the total provincial population (see Table 7.1). Although this may seem like a small increase in the proportional population of the province, this growth stands in contradiction to general trends between rural and urban populations in the province. Since the early settlement of Alberta in the late nineteenth century, the province's rural areas and small towns have represented an ever-smaller portion of the overall population; in 1921, fully 70% of the provincial population was counted as rural, while by 1971, it was cities that contained 77% of the total population. By way of comparison, the city of Lethbridge, with a 1921 population of 11,907 (five times the size of Red Deer at the time) represented 6.7% of the total Alberta population, yet by 1971, with 41,217 people, it represented only 3.4% of the total population.

Observing the proportional population of Alberta's three comparatively sized second-level cities (Figure 7.1), it is clear that despite a general trend of migration from smaller centres to larger ones in the province, Red Deer was the only town that had increased its proportional share of the Alberta population (MacLachlan, 2005). Medicine Hat, with a population of 9634 (four times that of Red Deer at the time), represented 5.4% of the provincial population in 1921, but by 1971 with 18,773 citizens, it shared only 2.4% of the total provincial population (MacLachlan, 2005). Lethbridge showed a similar decline. Of the three mid-sized cities in the province, only Red Deer managed, albeit slightly, to increase its proportional population over those decades.

Table 7.1 Population Distribution in Alberta, 1901–1971

	1901	1911	1921	1931	1941	1951	1961	1971
Edmonton	2,626	31,064	58,821	79,187	93,817	159,631	281,027	495,702
Calgary	4,398	43,704	63,305	83,761	88,904	129,060	249,641	403,319
Lethbridge	2,072	8,050	11,907	13,489	14,612	22,947	35,454	41,217
Red Deer	323	2,118	2,328	2,344	2,924	7,575	19,612	27,674
Medicine Hat	3,020	5,608	9,634	10,300	10,571	16,364	24,484	28,773
Urban Alberta	12,000	109,936	177,170	227,882	266,000	450,000	851,576	1,196,255
Rural Alberta	61,000	264,359	411,284	503,723	531,000	489,000	480,368	431,620
Urban as %	16	29	30	31	33	48	64	73

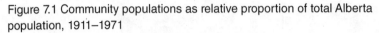

Figure 7.1 Community populations as relative proportion of total Alberta population, 1911–1971

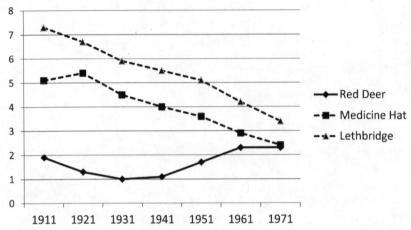

Although there may be more reasons for Red Deer's demographic success than that it hosted a large institution, it is nonetheless clear from survivor narratives and archival data that the Michener institution played an important role in providing employment and educational opportunities for its citizens. In addition, the city drew from the vocationally trained adult institutional population as an available pool of cheap, and often free, labour to assist in the development of local farms and businesses. Thus, I am arguing that in contrast to the institution's own rhetoric, establishing and maintaining an institution for "mental defectives" near the town of Red Deer did little to satisfy humanitarian motives of housing disabled children and adults closer to their Alberta families, nor did it solely accomplish the lofty ideals of educating inmates for independent community living. Instead, establishing the institution on the outskirts of the then very small town of Red Deer contributed to the growth of one Alberta town in ways that spectacularly benefited the economy of, and the non-disabled citizenry in, Red Deer. Indeed, the benefits of the institution to the local economy were a central pillar of the very public and highly charged debates that occurred during deinstitutionalization, where the reliance of community members on the jobs provided by the institution was positioned as a key reason to keep the institution open and operating.

The benefits that flowed from the institution to the community stemmed from three interrelated aspects of the Michener operation. The first benefit

came from financial arrangements that existed within the institution, where inmates were expected to pay their own way through placing their assets in trust to
the institution, through transfer funds from their home municipalities, through
support payments from family members – a practice that only ceased with a major shift in ministry and policy in 1972 (Government of Alberta, Department of
Social Services and Community Health, 1972–1973) – or through contributing
their own labour inside the institution. Thus, although commonplace ideas about
such institutions were that they placed heavy financial burdens on their societies,
in the case of Michener the institution was in many ways dependent on inmates,
their families, and their home communities for its operations.

The second benefit that accrued to the institution came through the blurred
boundaries between education, training, and unpaid labour that characterized
the occupational and vocational programs for the institution's children, whose
training and education was focused on learning skills that would satisfy institutional and community labour demands. These arrangements persisted for the
adult residents of Deerhome, whose work in the institution and the community
was extensive, underpaid, and frequently characterized as continued vocational
training. For children and adults, training in sewing, cooking, farming, and
small machine repair was offered to High Grade inmates who in turn used those
skills in their work in the community, while Low Grade inmates were trained in
skills that would serve the smooth internal running of the institution.

Finally, examining the educational and employment opportunities that the
institution provided to members of the outside community reveals that individuals in Red Deer benefited both educationally and occupationally from having the institution close by. For many years, the Michener Centre was one of the
largest employers in the Red Deer area, and it also operated as a unique postsecondary educational facility for local citizens who participated in training
programs that culminated in a three-year certificate program that credentialed
workers as mental deficiency nurses (MDNs).

Economics, Productivity, and Exploitation

Traditional histories of institutionalization have come from the perspectives of
helpers, authorities, and professionals, resulting in narratives that have been
remarkably devoid of a critique of the motives for establishing and maintaining
such institutions (Digby, 1996; Hubert, 2000). Recently, historians have begun
to take a more critical perspective, arguing that the fates of individuals deemed
to be mentally incompetent have been tied to economic changes in their societies. Thus, in wealthy, mid-nineteenth-century eastern and southern America,
small, cottage-style facilities with a strong focus on education and the goal of

reintegration and communitization sprang up (Bailey, 1997; Trent, 1994, 1995; Jordan, 1993; Rafter, 1997). At the other end of the scale connecting economies to disability services, during the impoverished interwar years in Germany, housing people who were deemed to be burdensome came to be seen as an unaffordable luxury, and institutions emptied their beds, leaving ex-inmates to fend for themselves (Poore, 2007). Similarly, back in North America in the late nineteenth and early twentieth centuries, large-scale institutions became the norm for people deemed to be "unfit," driven in great part by economic concerns about eugenics and race suicide, where it was assumed that immigrants and the poor were overbreeding and placing an undue burden on the state. The growth of the institutions was also connected to an urgency about freeing citizens from the burden of care for their children with disabilities so that they could aid in rebuilding more established states in America after its Civil War and contribute to ambitions of colonizing the west in the United States and Canada (Dowbiggin, 1995; McLaren, 1986; Trent, 1993). The new large institutions, drawing on progressivist rhetoric about individualism and improvement, sought to extract whatever productivity could be had from the "feeble-minded," under the guise of education and training. A focus on productivity was used simultaneously to justify the institutionalization of children who were deemed to be at risk of becoming dependent and non-productive citizens and to validate the institutions themselves as contributors to rather than burdens on the nation's coffers (Jordan, 1993; Rafter, 1997; Scheerenberger, 1983; Trent, 1994).

Productivity within the Institution

These concerns about economy, productivity, and dependency are reflected in early documents relating to the Michener institution. As noted previously, in the inaugural reports to the government, the first medical superintendent of PTS took considerable pains to describe the ways that maintenance costs for inmates were covered through payments from private family members, transfer funds from the residents' home municipalities, the sale of inmates' clothing, and the contributions of inmates to renovations and the running of the facility farm (McAlister, 1924, 1926). Inmates, from the start, were expected to contribute to their own care through communal labour and to pay for their stays in the facility through family, community, or personal funds.

In 1922, at the same time as plans were being made for opening the PTS/ Michener institution, the government implemented the Estates of the Mentally Incompetent Act, which permitted government seizure of goods and properties to cover the costs of maintenance for individuals placed in institutions or asylums in the province. As a result, an entire administrative branch of government, the Estates Branch, was established to administer the assets of inmates of various institutions (asylums, hospitals for veterans, and several smaller institutions for mental defectives, in addition to Michener). Through this office, inmates' possessions were held in trust, rented out, or sold to offset the costs of maintenance. The records from this branch do not provide figures that are broken down in terms of the proportion of the assets that came from Michener residents; however, the assets held by the government to offset aggregate inmate costs were substantial. In 1940, the public trustee "disposed of real and personal property for a total of $342,438.11, of which the Administrator's sale of real property [was] for the amount of $40,000.00" while "assets under administration ... total $5,101,900.16" (Wilson, 1940, pp. 1, 4). In addition to proceeds from sales, the government invested those assets that were liquid into Dominion Bonds, which in 1940 amounted to a total aggregate investment of $1,082,650.68, a princely sum for the times. The branch reported a net revenue of $21,551.95 for the five years ending in 1940 (Wilson, 1940).

It was only in 1972, six years after the establishment of a Canadian national public health care program, that private citizens no longer were required to pay for their internment in the province's asylums and institutions. In the Michener annual report for the following year, this shift in funding is reported with some ambivalence:

> On June 1, 1972 a new policy was implemented, relieving parents of their children under 18 who reside in institutions for the mentally retarded, of the responsibility for payment of mixed maintenance charges. The response from parents has been favorable and some voluntary maintenance payments are continuing, but revenues from this source are down. (Government of Alberta, Department of Social Services and Community Health, 1972–1973)

The loss of this source of income, despite the continuing voluntary payment by some parents, was being missed in the institutional budget. Parents, from the mid-1950s forward, in addition to contributing to their children's maintenance costs, contributed voluntarily to the operation of the institution through fundraising and contributions for special projects. Those projects, although they did not contribute to the institution's bottom line, did produce assets for the institution, and they reflected parents' attempts to improve the quality of life for children in the institution. The children's playhouse, mentioned in the previous chapter, was funded through a donation made by the Parent-School Organization, and over the years the parent group donated "thirteen television sets so that every villa[1] is provided with a T.V. set" (1957), "a wading pool at the School Camp and also continued maintenance of the T.V. sets" (1961a), "necessary materials and equipment for a curling rink with artificial ice" (1963) and a "new commercial electric stove" for the small summer camp that the institution operated for higher grade children at a nearby lake and a "small eight-seater bus" for field trips and medical appointments (1964) (LeVann, 1957, p. 131; 1961–1962, p. 163; 1963a, p. 183; 1964, p. 193).

Despite inmates' families and their estates covering the costs of maintenance and contributing to the enhancement of institutional life through donations, inmates were expected to contribute to institutional life through their labour. I have already discussed the overlap between occupational, agricultural and vocational training, and work provision for children under the age of 18, and it is clear that adults, too, were engaged in these sorts of contributions. The annual reports for Deerhome consistently included a heading of "Occupational Therapy." In the 1960 Occupational Therapy entry, for example, out of a total of 867 adult inmates,

> the number of patients receiving occupational therapy was approximately 200, attended to by a staff of three females and two males ... females occupied their time at embroidery, knitting, weaving, leather and copper work, basketry, rug hooking ... male patients produced some very fine articles in woodwork such as lawn furniture, lamps, bed-side tables and numerous other saleable articles. Approximately 216 male and female patients were profitably employed in departments such as stores, laundry, kitchen and at outside work such as snow-shoveling, field work and gardening. Five female patients were employed in the nurses' residence. Approximately 84 females and 50 male patients assisted with work on the wards. Several women and men patients were permitted to work in the nearby city of Red Deer, either doing housework or assisting with gardening or doing other chores. (LeVann, 1959–1960, p. 176)

In the institutional parlance, "receiving occupational therapy," which sounds as though some sort of constructive and supportive opportunities for rehabilitation were being offered, in actuality meant either producing goods for sale with minimal supervision or simply working – mostly on, but sometimes off, campus – to make a contribution. In the annual reports, there is no mention of payment to inmates for the work done. In their interviews some survivors acknowledged that they occasionally received a small stipend that enabled them to buy the odd treat from the canteen. Most of the interviewees, however, indicated that they received nothing for all their years of work, since work was often characterized as training or education by those who were in charge. Indeed, this was in keeping with the tone of the annual reports, where work accomplished by child and adult inmates was simultaneously characterized as occupational therapy, as vocational training, and as academic instruction.

In their interviews almost all the survivors spoke about working within the institutional walls in a broad array of occupations throughout the years of their internments. Ray Petrenko, who entered the institution in his late childhood and spent more than 20 years there, spoke about his life inside as a set of work experiences that were broad-ranging and ongoing. He said:

> Even as a kid you had to work ... In the Training School, if they figured you were good, they'd find you some kind of workshop job, you know. Shoe shop, cleaning up ... But then, we got a little older, I had some responsibility and that was just working in the kitchen ... where we would get everything ready to put in the dining room ... and eventually later on, the people who were older, they had to work out on the working crew outside. That was even worse because you had to shovel snow and there was always somebody around to watch if you worked out in the garden or something like that.

Both male and female residents engaged in work that contributed to the smooth internal running of the institution, often replacing staff positions with their unpaid labour. Some of this work related to doing their own personal care, making their own beds, and cleaning their own rooms, but often, the work that the survivors described doing involved labour that one might assume would have been done by employees of the institution. Gerta Muller, who spent several years in the institution in her mid-20s, described her work as follows:

> You washed the floor of the day room first, and then let it dry – it builds muscles, you know ... I had kitchen detail. You had to make sure the porridge was good and hot. And then you take it to the ward. Let's say it's like you're wheeling a carriage, only it was heavier.

Some survivors described providing care to others within the institution. Like Ray, Mary Korshevski, who arrived at the institution at the age of 15 and remained for 21 years, experienced a broad range of jobs within the institution. Eventually, she was "promoted" to doing primary care work with other inmates. She described this work in the following terms:

> I ended up working with people that had real bad disabilities, but I went every day and worked on whatever ward I was told. And some of the wards that I worked on, it was some very sad cases. I've seen very sad cases. They had to be fed every meal

and they had to be really taken care of. I went to feed people that couldn't feed themselves. I fed seven of them by the time it was my time to go for my own meal. And I can remember one time, I fed a girl that was very, very hard to feed, and I would ask them to wrap her up in a sheet, in a bed sheet, and she would eat.

The situation that Mary described reflects persistent systemic hierarchies within the institution based on notions of productivity; Mary, who had contracted polio as a child but was highly mobile and capable, was considered to be a High Grade inmate in great part because of her ability to contribute to the productivity of the institution. Note that a focus on productivity within institutions was not limited to Michener Centre. James Trent (1994), in his excellent history of the social and professional treatment of intellectual difference in the United States, has argued that the very foundations of the institution rest on determinations of productivity; individuals were admitted because of concerns about their potential productivity, and those who were released were "given" their freedom as a result of proving themselves self-sufficient. Given these foundations, it is not surprising that hierarchical rankings based on productivity within Michener characterized almost every aspect of the daily operations.

We can also not assume that this kind of work was simply a therapeutic regime designed to rehabilitate inmates into a productive life outside the institution or that work inside the institution was organized simply to keep inmates occupied or entertained. Rather, high productivity levels were important in these working arrangements, and several inmates described being disciplined or having privileges withdrawn if work was not accomplished satisfactorily. Gerta, for example, described missing a movie night on the campus because she had to re-wash dirty dishes until late into the night, while Mary described the tensions of working for a charge nurse who repeatedly watched her work and dressed her down in front of others for being a "slow cripple." The need for a productive inmate population was also not particularly unique to the Michener Centre; disciplines such as occupational therapy and vocational rehabilitation throughout the twentieth century drew heavily on progressivist and pragmatic theory, and hence had as core functions the discerning of the useless[2] from the productive, sometimes, as in the case of Nazi Germany, with horrifying outcomes (Burleigh, 1994, 1997).

The institution's annual reports lend credence to the probability that inmate's labour within the institutional walls was critical. Although no detailed reporting of actual inmate work hours is provided, the annual reports from the very early days of the institution provided lists of assets in the form of produce harvested from the gardens and revenues received from inmates' families and estates. As well, each report described increases or decreases in production and acknowledged the labour of inmates in indirect and direct ways. The scope of this labour was substantial. In 1957, for example, the garden and grounds sections of the annual reports indicated the following:

> An estimated total of some 25 acres [10 hectares] have been seeded to lawn, 53,000 bedding-out plants were set out last Spring, all of which were started from seed in the School's greenhouse. Twelve hundred yards [nearly 1100 metres] of black dirt were leveled in various areas [and] approximately 1,000 shrubs and trees were set out. (LeVann, 1957, p. 133)

Although residents may not have accomplished all this work singlehandedly, as part of the children's vocational training, and of the adults' preparation for life in the community, inmates regularly formed an important part of the workforce.

Inmates' contributions were often justified in indirect ways in the annual reports. For example, under the heading "Agricultural Activities" it was noted that, "in a Province where one of the major industries is agriculture, the need to prepare boys ready for discharge for this work cannot be over-emphasized" (LeVann, 1964, p. 192). And the boys were prepared well for agricultural work while incarcerated. In 1963, the garden produced 290 metric tons of vegetables, while in 1956, it produced 4700 bushels of grain, 105 metric tons of hay, 6800 kilograms of pork, 6700 dozen eggs, and 145,000 kilograms of milk, "which was pasteurized and delivered to the Kitchen" (LeVann, 1956, p. 136; 1963a). In some years, there were even surpluses, and goods were either sold in the market or sent to other institutions, such as the Ponoka Mental Hospital several kilometres away, thus contributing to the bottom line of institutions outside Michener (Alberta Department of Public Health, Mental Health Division, 1946). As usual, despite acknowledgement of the volume of goods produced, the magnitude of inmates' agricultural contributions were hidden in the institutional records because the work was often reported as an "educational opportunity for residents" rather than as a direct accounting of hours worked *as* work. The inmate hours also remained hidden, of course, because inmates were not paid for their contributions.

Despite the lack of detailed figures relating to inmates' labour, narrative entries in the institutional records can give us some insight into inmates' working lives. In the 1964 report, the director indicated that the shoemaker was able to service the entire campus through the assistance of "some of the higher grade boys" who were deemed unable to accomplish heavier labour (LeVann, 1964). Occasionally, the record did directly acknowledge inmates' contributions to daily operations, as in the 1962 annual report that credited the labour of

approximately 330 male and female patients (out of a total adult population of
population of 718) in accomplishing routine work in the adult portion of the
campus (LeVann, 1962a). This work included inmates' labour in the laundry,
kitchen, storehouse, seasonal occupations, and male and female staff residences, where they were used as cleaners. It also, as Mary Korshevski's descriptions of caring for children in sense training and in residential wards indicated,
figured into work performed by High Grade inmates in the care, feeding, and
cleaning of Low Grade inmates. This broad array of worker skills no doubt
helped to offset the difficulties that the superintendents of the institution had in
finding competent and long-standing staff, a common complaint right up until
the last years of the institutional reports. Inmates who could cook, clean, do
laundry, and provide primary patient care could work under the supervision of
fewer employees and could be made to accomplish the least desirable aspects of
institutional work.

Finally, inmate labour figured into the institution's bottom line through sell-
ing the products of inmates' occupational therapy and vocational training, as
noted in the previous chapter. This included "lawn furniture, bedside tables,
sewing cabinets, gun cabinets and china cabinets" made by the boys and "embroidery, knitting, weaving, leather and copper work, basketry, rug-hooking
and other crafts" by the girls (1962a, p. 172). Indeed, the 1962 annual November
sale includes 2157 articles for sale that were contributed by the female occupational therapy department alongside 433 items produced by the male occupational therapy department (LeVann, 1962a). Again, the proceeds of these sales
did not go to the individuals who made the items, or even to a collective fund
over which inmates had some control; instead, they went into the general operating budget to pay for recreational activities and the canteen. As when discussing other sources of income, survivors were consistent in saying that they did
not receive any direct benefit for their handiwork, nor were they able to say
what those funds were used for. In short, inmate labour and the capital it generated belonged not the individual but to the institution.

In the above sections, I have outlined some of the ways that inmates contributed to the internal economy of the institution. From the early record of establishing Michener as an institution, it is clear that officials were anxious about
the children's and adults' ability to contribute to the economy. Further, from the
grounds given in the admission records about indigence and marginal family
status, poverty and dependency were often used to justify public officials' efforts to institutionalize the children. Ironically, however, it is also apparent that
once inmates were inside the institution, they were clearly expected to contribute to its bottom line and its daily operations. Further, we can see that vocational training and occupational education programs were used to rationalize

the economic exploitation of residents by having inmates produce goods for consumption within the institution, for occasional transfer to other institutions within the broader mental health system, and for sale to the general public. Further, whether their labour was routine institutional work or involved producing goods for sale, the survivors interviewed consistently asserted that they did not receive financial compensation for their labour. Thus, far from being burdens on the state, inmates' unpaid labour and their family-based assets operated to offset institutional operating costs.

Contributing to the Community

Residents were expected to contribute to the financial well-being of the institution through their unpaid in-house labour, but they were also expected to cover the costs of their own upkeep from monies obtained from their families or estates and from their home municipalities. Records filed annually by the Public Guardian indicated that until the repeal of statute in 1972, properties belonging to inmates were held in trust, leased out, and actively farmed, with the resulting income used to offset institutional costs (Low, 1939; Wilson, 1940). Although the annual reports do not list the funds received from specific families, it was a policy that public funds would be provided for inmates' upkeep only after other financial resources, such as private incomes and assets, were exhausted (Manning, 1958). Indeed, in its own unofficial history, the Michener Centre indicated that even after the change in legislation in 1972, the institution continued to expect payment from wealthy families to provide maintenance support to their family members:

> Residents and/or families having sufficient incomes are expected to assume maintenance charges. Otherwise, the Centre's operation is funded almost entirely by the provincial government. (Alberta Social Services and Community Health, 1985, p. 3)

In addition to private funds, public funds from outside the Red Deer area were also funnelled in to the institution: where private shortfalls occurred, inmates' home municipalities were responsible for local children who were sent to Michener, so that Red Deer itself would not have to support the institution. Because Michener was the only institution in the province for individuals deemed to be mentally defective, its inmates came from across Alberta, bringing their own, their families', and their municipalities' resources with them, and undoubtedly, Red Deer indirectly benefited from this funnelling of assets into its local economy.

In addition to supporting the internal economy of the institution, inmates who were deemed capable were also expected to contribute their labour to the economy outside the institutional walls. Under the guise of educational and vocational training, inmates were regularly placed in unpaid jobs in the town of Red Deer and its surrounding area. Guy Tremblay came into the institution as a child, moved to the adult facility Deerhome at 18, and left the institution at 39 years of age. He described some of the work he and others did while living as adults in Deerhome:

> I worked for a couple of farmers, and some of them [inmates] worked at Jubilee Beverages in Red Deer. Some of them worked at a car wash ... and at a place called "Stellar" Enterprises ... but they weren't getting paid, they were just working, making stuff, and I worked there for a while ... We would go out there on a bus. There was a guy by the name of John X, who used to work at Michener, and he started the whole thing, and we would make things for trailers, for oil wells, too.

Guy thus described a mix of financial arrangements between the institution and community entrepreneurs, such as local farmers and other businesses. Some of the local businesses were designed exclusively for the "vocational rehabilitation" of Michener inmates. The arrangement was that these rehabilitation-centred businesses, some of which continue to operate today,[3] made contributions to the inmates' training while at the same time operating as independent businesses that benefited from a convenient pool of cheap, compliant labour; in some cases, these non-profit organizations even subsidized their training costs by receiving government grants for their supervision of inmates. Not only did inmates' labour in these businesses contribute to the local Red Deer economy, but some of the products, such as instruments and machinery relating to oil and gas development, also benefited locations even further afield, since the oil patch in Alberta is located several hundred kilometres north of Red Deer.

Adult female inmates also worked for businesses outside the Michener Centre. Mary Korshevski, Beverly Buszko, Gerta Muller, and Louise Roy all described working at outside businesses, at restaurants and nursing homes, and as housekeepers and nannies, and each in turn volunteered that they "didn't get very much money, not very much" (Betty Dudnik). Mary even described a meeting in which the matter of pay came up in negotiation with Dr LeVann, the director of the institution:

> When we first started there, we got – we didn't get paid – nothing. And then one time we had a meeting with a fellow by the name of Dr. LeVann ... Just all of the workers ... And he decided that we should get paid, you know. So we told him, you

know, that that would be very nice. (laughing) But you would not believe how much we got paid! (laughing) Twenty-five cents for starters! [I got a cheque] every two weeks, but there for a while it was twenty-five cents, but the more work we did, then they'd add to it.

Louise Roy also described this event and shed some light on why payment may have typically been withheld from workers, saying she was told she should not be paid "because they said that I can't make money when I'd be going to school." As occurred within many aspects of the institution, the ambiguous boundary between education and employment was, in this case, used to justify labour practices that were highly exploitive.

The practice of paying inmates who worked off-site came into place in the late 1960s and early 1970s, concomitant with increasing rhetoric about the closure of Michener and the need to prepare inmates for community reintegration. These shifts toward deinstitutionalization gave rise to new vocational programs that nevertheless continued the tradition of blurring the lines between training and labour. As part of a series of 1983 articles in the Red Deer *Advocate* on deinstitu-tionalization, one article describes the working lives of Dorothy and Roland, who are among the "privileged few" from the Michener Centre who were able to participate in these workfare programs. According to this article, despite the fact that they were being paid significantly below minimum wages, "Dorothy and Roland don't care. They would work for free." In the same article, Bob Greif, director of vocational services, who coordinated work placements for more than 400 residents, is quoted as defending the substandard payment rates be-cause "it is a training allowance and not payment for work. However ... residents are encouraged to believe it is pay" (Martindale, 1983b, p. B3).

Paul Anjou echoed other interviewees when he noted that his work at a voca-tional centre during his time at Michener was poorly paid, although he indicated that he was paid between 15 and 36 dollars a month for his work. Others simply noted that they did not get paid very much, while some, like Jim Molochuk were not really sure whether they were paid or not, because even though they were told that they were being paid for their work, the money was deposited directly into a trust account managed by the guardian who had legal responsibility for him while he was in Michener (as was the case for many Michener inmates, in-cluding Jim, and in a significant conflict of interest, Michener itself acted as trustee for many of these inmates). Several survivors described similar situations in which their money went to a trust fund or to an account from which they might withdraw "pin money" for use in the weekly canteen, but they also pro-fessed to have had little knowledge of or control over the actual accounts. Mary Korshevski, who worked as a nanny and housekeeper for a family in Red Deer for many years, acknowledged that she was paid for her work but noted that "then I had to take it, when I got paid, I had to take it up to the office and they took care of it from there." In Mary's quote, it is clear that she had little understanding where her money went and no ability to use her money as she saw fit. It is ironic to consider that Mary, like many other women in the institution, provided domestic and child-related care as a nanny and a housekeeper to the citizens of Red Deer for many years, particularly in light of the fact that she was sterilized by the Alberta Eugenics Board presumably because she was deemed to be unfit for precisely these kinds of maternal tasks.

In sum, there seem to have been a variety of arrangements made for wages for inmates' outside employment, from not receiving any money at all for work performed, to receiving a small stipend in the form of a cheque, to simply having "something" put into a campus account or trust fund for limited personal use. In any case, it is clear from the survivors' accounts that work performed in the community was undervalued, and it also follows that employers, the local families, local farmers, and local businesses enjoyed significant benefits from using Michener's cheap labour to subsidize their activities. It is also worth noting that in 1971, many years earlier than the stories provided here, the *Standards for Residential Facilities for the Mentally Retarded*, a set of guidelines produced by a coalition of the American Psychiatric Association, the Council for Exceptional Children, the United Cerebral Palsy Association, the American Association on Mental Deficiency, and the National Association for Retarded Children, clearly recommended that residents in institutions should be paid reasonable wages for their vocational labour and be permitted access to and responsibility for their own money as part of their training programs (Joint Commission on Accreditation of Hospitals, 1971).

Education and Employment for Non-inmates

Inexpensive farm labour, household help, and semi-skilled employees must have offered a tremendous boon to the families and small businesses of Red Deer as the town developed, but the city benefited through numerous avenues from its relationship with the institution. In many ways, the town of Red Deer and the institution located on its outskirts grew up together. That being said, even by the mid-1960s Red Deer remained a small, agricultural centre an hour and half in either direction from any real urban locale, and it enjoyed little industry outside of farming, ranching, and the Michener Centre; thus, the institution offered local citizens a rare opportunity for well-paid, stable indoor work. Regarding educational opportunities, Red Deer only opened the doors of its small community college in 1963, so that until that time, citizens seeking advanced education were forced to leave for the big city. In contrast, the Michener Centre was able to offer at least a perfunctory kind of postsecondary training from 1937 forward in a three-year program for mental deficiency nurses (MDNs). I describe this program as perfunctory because although the program did involve some training, these workers were never examined by any outside boards or registered with any outside professional associations. Nevertheless, at least superficially, the centre could offer local citizens some opportunities for study and career advancement, permitting them to avoid moving to the university and technical schools located in the cities of Calgary or Edmonton, both about 150 kilometres distant.

Recurring comments in the annual reports and in the official history of the Michener Centre indicated that obtaining qualified and appropriate staff was a challenge from the institution's beginning (Alberta Social Services and Community Health, 1985). In an attempt to mediate this problem, the provincial government granted Michener/Provincial Training School the mandate to offer a three-year residency program that would train people as MDNs. Between 1935 and 1973, when the program ended, Michener produced 453 graduates, averaging 21 graduates annually between 1955 and 1973. The mid-50s increase in graduates was due to a 1954 decision that new primary-care employees would be required to take the three-year MDN program as part of their contracts. Opportunities for career advancement resulted from these decisions; in the revamping of the MDN program, it was also determined that "all courses should be given by personnel at the PTS, rather than by a number of external lecturers" so that senior staff had opportunities for lecturing and teaching that would rarely be available to graduates without a university degree (Alberta Social Services and Community Health, 1985, p. 13). This teaching was encouraged because the Michener Centre at the time thought of itself as a leading institution for the training, treatment, and therapy of people with developmental disabilities, and it was thought that Michener employees would thus be leaders in the field of "mental retardation" treatment. Of course, the reality behind that reputation remained shaky at best; in the institution's annual reports, MDNs are unevenly referred to as *qualified nursing assistants* or *child care workers*, and the only external review of the institution found the standard of training among MDNs to be woefully inadequate (Blair, 1969).

Regardless of the quality of the program, however, Michener was ostensibly the only place in Canada where young people could obtain credentials for the "specialized education in care and training of the mentally handicapped" (Alberta Social Services and Community Health, 1985, p. 13), so it is possible that students came not only from Red Deer, or even Alberta, but from across the country to receive this training. However, not all students who entered the

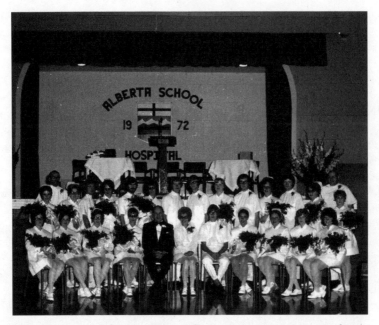

Figure 7.2 Mental deficiency nurse graduates, circa 1972. Courtesy Red Deer
and District Archives (N5475).

program at Michener did so because they understood the training to be worthy
or because they saw working with mentally deficient people as a calling. Instead,
the training opportunities offered through the Michener Centre were attractive
to local people seeking reliable and well-remunerated skilled employment in a
market where farming was the typical, and limited, career path. In a farewell
article written on his retirement, one former MDN had the following to say:

> When I first came to work in January of 1962 at what was then the Provincial
> Training School, I had no idea 41 years later I would still be here when it came time
> to retire. I needed a job at the time and was told they were hiring at the PTS. I ap-
> plied not knowing what I was getting myself into. (St. Denys, 2003, p. 12)

In this man's case, the training came only after he signed on for a job that he had
few expectations of but that, to his apparent surprise, gave him a lifelong career.
Many of the people trained at the Michener Centre came from the Red Deer
area, and many of them enjoyed lifelong careers and a professional status that

would not have been locally possible without Michener's educational opportunities. The role of the MDN program was a boon for the recruitment of workers seeking meaningful, well-paid employment, and it helped to keep staff turnover down. Although it was theoretically possible for people trained as MDNs to obtain work in other psychiatric centres, the training was not as readily transferrable as other, more mainstream designations, such as registered nurse or psychiatric nurse, and the specificity of the MDN credential acted as a deterrent to leaving the institution. Thus, is it not surprising that the constant complaints about hiring and retaining qualified staff seem to subside somewhat in the annual reports after the late 1950s, when the MDN requirement came into force, producing a more or less dedicated and trained workforce.

A number of people who worked at the Michener Centre were not drawn from the local population. Two of the three ex-workers interviewed for this research came to their jobs at Michener as summer students, through arrangements with the University of Calgary and the University of Alberta. Jim Sullivan, who eventually worked at the institution full time as a "psychologist" (with a BA as his sole qualification), described his work over four summers as a fairly common summer job for psychology majors from both Calgary and Edmonton, referring to his summer work as an "internship" and noting that the dorms were filled each summer with young people doing this kind of work. Evelyn, the other university-based ex-worker interviewed for this project, also came to the Michener Centre as a young summer "intern." Similarly to the roles filled by faculty of education students described earlier, who came to Michener for their practicum placements, these training opportunities worked on several levels: they provided a perhaps questionable education to psychology, education, and rehabilitation students in the province; they operated as relatively inexpensive ways to staff classes and wards with university students; and they acted to enhance the academic reputation of the institution because of its role as a site for the advanced professional training of human service workers.

Professional mental health workers, such as MDNs and psychology interns, were not the only workers who came to the Michener Centre. Beyond using inmates to keep things running, the institution required a virtual army of unskilled and skilled workers to maintain its operations, from laundry and grounds workers to physiotherapists, occupational therapists, and cooks. Although the annual reports unfortunately do not provide the numbers of employees for each year, the official history of Michener does give an idea of the scale of employment at the institution. In 1983, when the inmate population had been cut by more than a third (falling from 2300 to only 1500 inmates), the centre employed almost 2000 people (Alberta Social Services and Community Health, 1985). Considering that the entire population of Red Deer in 1983 was only slightly more than 50,000, even as the institution was winding its operations down by moving inmates into community living, 1 in 25 people living in the Red Deer area was directly employed by the institution. Indeed, the institution had a major impact on the local economy, since "the institution is, after all, the largest employer in Red Deer. Thousands of local people have worked at the institution over the years, including in some cases two or three generations" (Alberta Social Services and Community Health, 1985, p. 17).

In addition to working within the institution, there were undoubtedly other opportunities for jobs that the institution brought to the community of Red Deer. Community businesses served the institution indirectly through service contracts, landlords benefited from the influx of workers who came to work at the institution, and local shops and services developed because of the increased markets that the institution created through its very existence. Finally, workers were needed to build the institution over the years. As noted earlier, when the institution first opened its doors in 1923, it was situated in one narrow, three-storey brick building on an undeveloped plot of farmland, but by the time it reached its pinnacle during the 1970s, it comprised 66 buildings on 130 hectares of land. These buildings included vocational training centres; workshops; laundry facilities; light manufacturing facilities; school rooms for inmates and for MDN students; residences for inmates, staff, and MDN students (the residences for staff alone consisted of two large three-storey dormitories); a swimming pool; a recreation centre, a curling rink; a house for the superintendent; industrial kitchens; administrative buildings; several group homes; storage facilities; a power plant; and greenhouses – in short, the workings of a small city were located on the 130 hectare campus. This infrastructure came into being as a result of an investment of significant money into the community; it required construction workers and engineers to build the institution, and it demanded materials and supplies to support that construction. Inevitably the jobs and supply contracts that accompanied the construction of the Michener Centre, in addition to its every day operations, benefited the local Red Deer economy tremendously over the years.

Conclusion

In the late 1960s a number of events combined to initiate a deinstitutionalization process for Michener. First, the formation of a number of parent groups led to citizen advocacy for more community options for children with developmental disabilities. Second, a series of highly critical newspaper exposés on conditions in Alberta's mental health institutions caused a public outcry that ultimately led the government to commission an enquiry into provincial mental health services. The resulting report, referred to as the Blair Report, called for a redistribution of services for children with intellectual and neurological disabilities to smaller training units that would be located close to the children's homes. It also called for a reduction in residential services. In short, it called for the closing of the Michener Centre and a move to communitization (Blair, 1969). In light, however, of the contributions that the Michener Centre and its inmates made to the local economy, it is not surprising that many members of the Red Deer community were vehemently opposed to the deinstitutionalization movement. In 1976, seven years after the deinstitutionalization process began, an editorial in a newspaper expressed concerns regarding the planned closure of the institution. In response to a government decision to maintain the Michener Centre "at 1975 staffing and patient population levels," the editor wrote:

> It's important for Alberta not to waste the facilities. It's important to Red Deer and district to maintain what is still the biggest employer in the area ... We're gratified with the assurance, as we are sure most people in this community will be ... having regard for the waiting lists for this kind of care, the investment in the plant [building, grounds, etc.] and the role the institution has assumed in the region's social fabric and economy, we aren't prepared to see ASH-Deerhome dismantled on some current sociological whim. ("Stability at Last," 1976)

The Red Deer citizenry was not alone in its opposition to winding down the institution; the Michener Centre employees, with the exception of its professional staff (physicians, psychiatrists, and nurses) were bargaining members of the Alberta Union of Provincial Employees (AUPE), so their working conditions and wages were reasonably good compared with those of many local workers. Loath to lose these good jobs, Michener workers, backed by AUPE, also consistently lobbied to keep Michener's doors open and staffing and admission levels high. In 1994, the local Red Deer paper quotes union chairman Jeff Ruder as saying that "the home is losing nearly 100 patients a year and hardly any being admitted," (Roche, 1994, p. B1) and further claiming that the union was seeking to have the Michener Centre run by an independent board of directors, composed of residents' family members who would favour keeping the Michener Centre open. The article described the union's lobbying efforts:

> To gather public support for the Red Deer home for the mentally handicapped AUPE printed about 5,000 brochures which it has been handing out at shopping malls and other high-traffic areas ... AUPE represents nearly 1,500 full-time, part-time and casual employees at Michener Centre. (Roche, 1994, p. B1)

It is also clear that efforts on the part of union workers to keep Michener afloat and vibrant have not ceased. In 2004, the monthly AUPE bulletin called for its membership to keep the public aware of the "threats against Red Deer's Michener Centre" and encouraged its membership to call their local politicians to remind them of the "importance of this facility to this community" ("More Than 260," 2004). As recently as 2013, the union was called to take up the battle for keeping jobs at the Michener Centre. As will be discussed in the final chapter, in March of that year, the provincial government announced plans to close the centre by April 2014. The union responded by asking AUPE employees across the province to sign petitions to keep Michener open, inviting them to attend protests organized in the provincial capital and in Red Deer, distributing 1000 lawn signs to its membership with the demand "Keep Michener Open," and launching a series of television and radio spots (Alberta Union of Public Employees, 2013). This campaign was effective and the threatened closure was postponed until December 2014. Around the same time, Michener supporters issued a court challenge, to be heard in November 2014. In June 2014, the reigning Conservative Party undertook a leadership race that saw the Michener Centre as a central issue of contention, with candidates arguing that closure may not be in the best interests of the community (Henton, 2014). Likewise, Opposition Leader Danielle Smith made her party's commitment to keeping Michener open a central part of her platform (van Rassel, 2014). On September 19, 2014, the newly elected Conservative party leader and provincial premier, Jim Prentice, announced that the Michener Centre would remain open and that former residents could be readmitted to the institution.

Thus the struggle continues; while the Michener Centre no longer provides its inmates as a standing army of unpaid semi-skilled workers for the local farms, homes, and businesses of Red Deer, it remains a key employer in the area, and this function remains a lynchpin in the argument of whether it should stay open, or whether, as the Blair Report recommended more than 40 years ago, it should close its doors forever. Ironically, the economic value of people with disabilities as inmates and residents has meant that community members are strongly committed to perpetuating the institutional system.

Michener's inmates have either been historically excluded because of presumptions about their economic dependencies, or their dependency status has justified exploiting their unskilled labour while at the same time providing rich employment opportunities to those on whom they supposedly were dependent. Further, it is safe to say that Red Deer itself has historically been dependent on its inmates. Without the Michener Centre, the city of Red Deer and its surrounding community would certainly have developed differently than it has over the past 85 years, and further, it is unlikely that it would have enjoyed the quality of life, prosperity, and growth that it has experienced without having had the institution's inmates to exploit and rely on.

Chapter Eight

Bad Medicine: Drugs, Research, and Ethics

The previous chapters focused on the institution's educational and rehabilitative programs, painting a picture of exploitive and abusive practices that belied the institution's mandate as a training facility and its promise of educating its charges for release to a fuller, more productive life in the community. In this chapter, I examine medical and eugenic practices to expose the dishonesty embedded in the institution's promise of care and proper treatment for children whose health needs were purportedly not being adequately met in the community. Despite family physicians and social workers routinely using this rationale to convince parents that institutionalizing their disabled children was the best option, and despite the medical expertise promised at Michener, the quality of medical care in the institution was deeply problematic.

The medical mandate of the institution was reflected in multiple ways. Until the mid-1940s, inmates were referred to as "patients," and following addition in the late 1950s of the adult Deerhome facility on the campus, in 1965 the children's side was renamed the Alberta School Hospital. From the beginning, the institution was directed by a medical superintendent who oversaw the administration but who also was charged with providing health care to the inmates. Dr William J. McAlister, a graduate of McGill with degrees in both medicine and surgery, served in this capacity from 1923 to 1931, followed by Dr D. L. MCullough, whose wife, Dr Mary McCullough, also a physician, provided medical services to the growing inmate population; together, these two headed the institution for 18 years, until retiring in 1949. The arrival in 1949 of Dr Leonard J. LeVann heralded the beginning of a new era; in his first nine years as medical superintendent at Michener, the number of inmates grew from 293 to 1433 (Alberta Social Services and Community Health, 1985). As well, Dr LeVann's medical ambitions extended well beyond providing medical attention to the children and adults in his care to include a sustained program of medical research in conjunction with staff from the University of Alberta's medical faculty (*Muir v. Alberta*, 1996). Finally, the institutional governance did not operate under the umbrella of the ministries of education or labour but instead reported to the Department of Public Health until a major overhaul of government portfolios in the 1980s brought it under the umbrella of Social Services. Thus, despite its stated – but false – mandate as an educational and training facility, the institution was also engaged in and committed to care and health-related activities. A brochure provided to survivor Sam Edwards's mother on his admission explicitly conveyed that medical care would be comprehensive and of a high calibre:

> There is always a Physician on duty to look after our children should any sudden illness occur and in addition we have a Consultant Surgical Staff from one of the clinics in town. A School Dentist ensures that a child's teeth will be examined twice a year or more often if necessary and carry out any required dental procedures ... Immunizations are carried out for Polio, Diphtheria, Whooping Cough and Typhoid Fever on any child coming to the School who has not had this done or who requires booster shots. (Alberta School Hospital, 1967, p. 2)

In the same document, parents of prospective inmates were assured that psychological care would be delivered by professionally qualified personnel and that children requiring more intense nursing care would be attended to by "specially selected nursing personnel who are either student nurses working towards their diploma in Mental Deficiency Nursing or graduates in Mental Deficiency Nursing as well as Registered Nurses" (Alberta School Hospital, 1967, p. 1). This promise of comprehensive, expert, and appropriate care was also delivered verbally to parents, as Carl's mother, Mavis Semkow, described, saying, "Oh, I was told he would get the best care, he'd get everything that he needed. He'd get medical help, and everything would be fine."

As with other promises made to parents and children, however, it is clear that the care provided at Michener was inadequate at best, and the medical aspects of the institution in fact contributed to the climate of neglect and abuse. In this chapter, although I will briefly discuss the institution's medical responses to illnesses and injuries, many of which resulted from violence by staff or between residents, the core of my focus will be the routinized and multiple ways that medicine was used inappropriately to violate and exploit the children and adults at Michener.

Medical Treatment and Care

The annual reports made each year to the government indicate the importance of the health of the children and adults of Michener, and indeed of the staff as

well. For the most part, routine health issues, such as fevers, illnesses, or accidents, were not reported; however, tallies of surgeries performed (excluding
eugenic surgeries, which were reported separately) and epidemics (including
lost work time among staff) are dutifully provided. The extent of medical work
was impressive. In a typical year on the Deerhome (adult) campus alone, "in all
7,592 examinations were made. The consultant surgeon made nine visits and
112 patients were presented for surgical consultation" (LeVann, 1967–1968,
p. 156). The annual reports also provided an account of routine preventive
medicine and screening, indicating that medical surveillance was a significant
part of institutional operations. For example, in 1960 the entire inmate and staff
population was screened by X-ray for tuberculosis, and each year thereafter,

> Upon admission or employment all patients and staff were x-rayed, rectal swabs
> were taken to exclude infection or carrier state of any of the gastrointestinal dis-
> eases. Throat and nose swabs were taken to detect carriers of diphtheria. (LeVann,
> 1967–1968, p. 149)

As well, a regular and comprehensive program of immunization, dental check-
ups, blood screening for medication toxicity, stool screening for gastrointestinal disorder, and blood screening for parasites for all patients and staff was
maintained and reported. In 1968, on the children's side alone,

> 2,474 X-rays were carried out ... 6 E.E.G tracings were carried out ... 9,276 labora-
> tory procedures were carried out at Alberta School Hospital ... 776 laboratory re-
> quests were referred to a commercial laboratory ... [and] two thousand, one hun-
> dred and forty-six bacteriological specimens were sent to the provincial laboratory
> for diagnosis and classification. (LeVann, 1967–1968, p. 144)

Despite the regularity of health reporting, these accounts, using virtually
the same wording from year to year, offer little insight into the physical condition of individuals or the actual quality of their medical care. Rather, they read
as statements of inventory, providing information on numbers admitted, numbers transferred within the campus and to other facilities in the province,
numbers of surgeries and dental extractions performed on and off the campus,
and numbers of deaths in custody. There is little sense in these tallies of why
these events occurred, or who they occurred to in particular, and instead we
are presented with a portrait of the inmate population as just that; a faceless
herd of bodies that were counted, processed, and tracked, but not really cared
for or about in a compassionate sense. Even quite grave experiences were reduced to matter-of-fact numerical reporting, as in these entries from the 1967–
1968 annual report:

Thirty-eight fractures resulted from accidents ... eugenics surgery was carried out
on 59 patients ... [and] six patients were admitted to the Alberta Hospital, Ponoka,
for lobotomy, following which they were returned to Deerhome. (LeVann, 1967–
1968, pp. 149, 143, 157)

In this, and all other annual reports, significant injuries and illnesses, altera-
tions in personality and intellectual capacity, or reductions in reproductive capacity were treated as dry facts provided to satisfy reporting requirements but
providing little insight into the lives shattered or improved by these events.

As we might expect, the daily ward records offer a different picture concerning medical care, much of which seems to have been offered in response to accidents, injuries, and infections that occurred as a result of violence and neglect,
as discussed in an earlier chapter. Thus, the daily records frequently described
staff cleansing and dressing lacerations, applying compresses to bruises and
swollen areas, or giving pain medications for tenderness and injury, very frequently without indicating how these conditions arose. Likewise, the records
described applying restraints to inmates to keep them from falling or getting
out of bed and harming themselves, without acknowledging that more engaged
care might be a more desirable form of treatment. Occasionally, we read descriptions of enemas given for impaction or medications given for nausea and
diarrhea, without much expressed curiosity about why these gastric upsets
might occur. Another frequently reported activity was painting inmates' skin
with Betadine for skin deterioration or packing gauze into the bedsores that
often developed from prolonged inactivity in beds or wheelchairs, without attendant suggestions for increasing the mobility of these patients. A final recurring description was of dealing with the effects of skin breakdown or fungal
infections as a result of inmates lying too long in moisture, presumably due to
incontinence. For example, we read:

> Both groins markedly reddened with pustular eruption at left side. Washed with
> soap and water, dried, and betadine applied. Slight bleeding from bedsore at right
> buttock and lower abdomen bedsore. Thighs kept apart with restraints on each
> side of bedrails and kept as dry as possible. (Nightingale Ward Record, 1982a)

At the end of this entry, there was no discussion that this individual should be
turned frequently, massaged often, gotten out of bed, or toileted more often, or
that other less invasive or preventive measures be used; rather, she is simply tied
down, legs spread, in hopes of keeping the skin dry. Like most of the treatments
described, the action is reactive rather than proactive. Indeed, what was not
mentioned at all – either in the annual reports or in the ward records – was the

provision of treatments that might improve inmates' health or physical conditions pre-emptively. There was no mention, for example, of physiotherapy or passive movement exercises to help bedridden inmates or inmates with limited mobility to avoid contractures, nor do we read of fittings being applied to beds to assist people with movement in bed or in getting out of bed, nor do we hear of testing for hearing difficulties that might help inmates to communicate better, or eye tests so that they could better navigate the hallways and learn to read, or of hydrotherapy to assist in strengthening people's sense of balance and range of motion. In sum, there was no mention of the kind of basic care one might reasonably expect in a residential rehabilitative setting for disabled children and adults.

The long-term effects of this level of care were described by Mary Korshevski's friend Edna, who sat in on my interview with Mary. Mary, after spending 21 years in the institution, went to live with Edna, who was a member of a church community involved in supporting people who left the institution in 1976, during the height of the deinstitutionalization process. Edna described her first impressions of Mary:

> I looked at her, and she was hanging like a monkey and had two teeth and she would walk around the corner and she'd fall. And they told me that she had no – no problems, no nothing like that. So I started on her teeth and on her glasses. You should have heard the doctor that did her glasses. He called the institute – I've never heard anybody swear so bad in my life! Her glasses weren't even near – that's why she was falling all the time. She couldn't see. It was the wrong prescription. So that's how we started.

While listening to this description, Mary pitched in, saying, "It was somebody else's [prescription]! And one other time I remember I had the same glasses for 11 or 12 years."

On a similar note, Mavis Semkow, who brought her son out of the institution during the same era as Mary's departure, described the galvanizing incident that made her decide to contact an advocacy group to help her bring her son home. Carl had experienced an episode in which he aspirated some food, and this eventually turned into pneumonia, requiring his hospitalization in the Red Deer General Hospital. On visiting, she noted,

> When we went to the hospital in Red Deer, when Carl had choked on the food and had that pneumonia, [his brother] said, "I can't stand this Mom, he's so skinny. They're starving him to death, that's why he's going to die; they're starving him to death." And he's got to be 5'11" if he's an inch. We tried to stretch him out, we got

5′11″. So he could maybe even be closer to 6′, because he's contractured a bit. But he was only, at that time, he only weighed 67 pounds [30 kilograms]. So that was skin pulled over bone. He really was starving to death.

Given this description, coupled with our understanding of the conditions under which care work was accomplished – short staffing, overcrowding, high staff turnover, and primary care that was frequently provided by inmates – it is fair to speculate that Carl's malnourishment and the food in his lungs that led to his pneumonia were caused at least in part by chronically inadequate, rushed, or unqualified caregiving. In other words, we can surmise that his medical problems were not improved by the expert medical care the institution promised but in fact were caused by persistent institutional neglect.

In addition to malnourishment, chronic illness also plagued those who lived at Michener. In 1980, for example, the local newspaper reported on an outbreak of Legionnaires' disease that killed 1 resident and made another 20 residents and 6 staff extremely ill. Bacterial cultures and viral checks on tissue samples taken from the victims failed to identify the actual illness, and investigators acknowledged that because of the nature of institutional populations, "the outbreak could have been due to a whole host of respiratory viruses or several bacterial strains" (Lee, 1980, p. B1). Later, in 1989, a sustained outbreak of hepatitis A was identified through routine blood work. This disease, which is usually transmitted when passed from the bowel to hands and mouths, seems to have been endemic to the institution. As Dr Lorne Tyrrell, the medical investigator from the University of Alberta hospital, said at the time, "a number of the clients in the institution are lifelong carriers" of both hepatitis A and hepatitis B, which is "very common in institutions for the mentally handicapped" (Donaldson, 1989).

In the various institutional records (ward reports, Unusual Incidents reports, annual reports, and nursing records), the rare acknowledgments of poor health and inadequate care were mentioned primarily when a crisis arose. Occasionally, these were revealed when staff members discovered broken bones, severe bruising, staph infections or cellulitis, deep lacerations, ulcerations, head injuries, scalds, or abrasions so severe that they required the visit of an outside doctor. Other times, these events were mentioned because of parental complaints during visits to their children at Michener or during home visits by their children. The nursing records included several exchanges between questioning parents and the nursing director or one of her numerous assistant directors. The tone of the institutional response was typically both grudging and dismissive; parents were assured that their children were receiving excellent care, their concerns were responded to as trivial or uninformed, and the general tone was adversarial rather than conciliatory. The following letter, the final in a series of exchanges from a mother expressing concern over her daughter's recurring dental infections and continuing episodes of bowel impaction, provides insight into the tone of these correspondences. The assistant director writes,

> I have done extensive investigation into your many complaints regarding the care given to [your daughter]. She has her teeth brushed three times daily. She had dental appointments in May and June, 1976 and one December 15th, 1976, at which time the dentist ordered peroxide mouth wash four times daily for two months. I would feel free in assessing her dental services to be more adequate than the majority of those received by children in the community. Your criticism of toilet facilities is really quite unfounded in view of the fact that there are five toilets and three commodes available to the children to whom you refer ... I regret that you are so dissatisfied with the care that [your daughter] is receiving. We have excellent staff on [the unit] and I do not think that more care could be given to her than she is receiving. (Garrett, 1976, p. 1)

The letter also included an indication that the child would soon be transferred to a different facility closer to the family home in Edmonton. In tone, this was a letter of dismissal, both of the charges and, literally, of the child and her troublesome mother.

Dental Care

Dental care seems to have been a topic of much importance in the institution; however, despite having an in-house dentist, along with contracted arrangements for regular services at Michener by local community dentists, as the above mother's letter indicates, dental care seems to have been persistently problematic. Dental care provision was dutifully conveyed in the annual reports, and the extent of dental work accomplished is notable. In 1961, "516 patients were examined, 40 fillings were done ... and there were 323 extractions with local anaesthetics, and twelve patients had general anaesthetics for multiple extractions" (LeVann, 1961a, p. 170). In 1963, with an inmate population of 1802, there were 333 fillings, 289 extractions, 8 X-rays, and a number of other lesser procedures; in 1967–1968, 1602 patients were seen in regularly held dental clinics, with 220 fillings and 621 extractions carried out, some under general anaesthetic (LeVann, 1963a, 1967–1968; Alberta Social Services and Community Health, 1985).

These descriptions of dental care provision are remarkable in particular because, although children and adults were provided with regular dental check-ups, dental extractions were far more common than fillings or preventive work. From interviews with ex-workers and family members, it is clear that many inmates were left without teeth, not necessarily for reasons of hygiene or decay but to facilitate care and reduce staff and inmate injuries from bites. Janice Holmes, whose sister wrote her story, lived at Michener for 26 years, leaving at the age of 37. Janice's sister wrote that, "At the age of 24 all of Janice's teeth were pulled to prevent her from biting herself."[1] Ex-worker Evelyn confirmed these descriptions while outlining the daily routines on her ward, saying, "on this ward all the food was puréed. 'Cuz most everyone didn't have teeth – uh, they'd either rotted out or they'd been pulled out because they'd bit themselves or somebody else." However, while reducing violence and self-harm were often reasons for these extractions, it is likely that neglect and poor care also contributed to the poor dental profiles of Michener inmates. Both Evelyn and Coral James indicated that in their daily care work, they provided patients neither with routine dental care, such as tooth-brushing, nor with oral care in the form of swabbing gums and cleaning out mouths for inmates whose teeth had been removed.

Teeth that had been extracted were not always replaced with a denture or partial plate. Janice Holmes's sister noted that after her extractions, Janice was not provided with dentures "as the doctor did not feel Janice could cope with them." Mary Korshevski, despite having had all but her two front teeth removed when she was in her early 20s, only obtained dentures after her release at 36 years of age, because, "sometimes when people had their teeth pulled they didn't bother doing anything else for them. They just left it as is."

Extracting inmates' teeth as a means of reducing interpersonal violence or harmful self-stimulation, or to avoid the work attached to maintaining proper dental hygiene, seems to have been quite common and reflects again an overarching ethos that the convenience of workers, the reduction of labour, and the management of the population was more important than the health of individual inmates. And removing teeth, particularly when coupled with a failure to provide well-fitting dentures or plates to replace them, does have serious health implications. On a prosaic level, lacking teeth causes difficulty in speaking and communicating, resulting in challenges in expressing needs for care with staff or in interacting with others in the institution more generally. On a health-specific level, lacking a full set of teeth has cumulative effects resulting from avoiding important food groups, like fruits and vegetables, and a continuing inability to process most foods properly. These effects include an increased risk of mortality from choking; increased likelihood of respiratory disease and death from aspiration (food in lungs); nutritional deficits in fibre, protein, calcium, iron, and vitamins C and B; weight loss because of poor nutrition; stroke; stomach and bowel cancers; and shortened life expectancy (Abnet et al., 2005; Geissler & Bates, 1984; Sheiham et al., 2001). A newspaper article reporting on a new innovative tooth gel being used at Michener noted that although some 25% of inmates did not have teeth, "some residents cannot be fitted with dentures" and thus they were at high risk for choking (Proby, 1991). In this light, Carl Semkow's hospitalization as a result of aspirating food and contracting pneumonia, as well as his profoundly malnourished state, not only can be understood as the result of poor caregiving but also can be attributed to the long-term effects of having had all of his teeth extracted shortly after admission, as his mother confirmed.

In addition to health concerns, a series of exchanges between Sam Edwards's mother, the provincial ombudsman, and Superintendent LeVann highlights the more draconian aspects of dental routines, particularly as they related to questions of consent. I introduced Sam's story in Chapter One, noting that when he was an 11-year-old child, he ran afoul of his teachers for behavioural and attentional issues. Sam's mother, a school principal herself, was pressured by the family physician and then the members of a visiting Guidance Clinic to admit Sam into a residential program for children with behavioural problems that operated for a decade at Linden House on the Michener campus. Sam spent less than a year there, but his mother left him a cache of Michener-related documents, including an exchange of letters with the provincial ombudsman, George McLellan, and Superintendent LeVann. In both exchanges, Ms. Edwards complained about the lack of psychological support and assessment her son received, the difficulties she faced in communicating with Sam or having him home for visits, the loss of his clothing and possessions in the institution, and, of relevance to this discussion, his dental care. In a letter to the ombudsman, she wrote:

> While at Linden House, Sam was examined by a dentist, a Dr. X of Red Deer. Dr. X wanted to put Sam under general anesthetic and remove eight to nine teeth. I was asked to sign a release for his operation. I refused and Dr. LeVann was furious that I dared to question their opinion. I took Sam to another dentist who pulled two baby teeth and patched two permanent teeth. Sam has always had his teeth attended to regularly and I fail to understand this type of thing. I suggest the dentist was out to make money on my child.

This passage raises the question of appropriate treatment; it is clear from Mrs Edwards's follow-up with an outside dentist that, at least in this case, unnecessary dental work was being advocated by the institution. A more chilling concern is that of consent. On 20 January 1970, Dr LeVann wrote to Mrs Edwards indicating that Sam had been seen by the "School Dentist, who advises that he requires nine dental extractions to be carried out under general anaesthetic" (LeVann, 1970b) and requesting that she sign a document on Department of Health letterhead that read as follows:

The Mental Health Act – 1964

Form Va – Consent to Operation

(Section 13)
I, "Sam Edwards", of Alberta School Hospital hereby consent to undergo the operation of nine dental extractions, the effect and nature of which has been explained to me.

I also consent to such further or alternative operative measures as may be found necessary during the course of such operation and to the administration of a local or other anesthetic for the purpose of the same.

I understand an assurance has not been given that the operation will be performed by a particular surgeon.

Dated at Ponoka, Alberta this _____ day of January A.D., 19 70.

At first read, this may seem like a reasonable document, although it also fairly unlikely that the "effect and nature" of nine dental extractions was explained to 11-year-old Sam. However, given the institution's and the provincial government's unusual approach to issues of consent for eugenic surgeries, the extension of consent in this form to include "such further or alternative operative measures as may be found necessary" is truly alarming. Is it possible that this kind of consent acted as a wedge for eugenic operations? Did Sam, because of his mother's refusal, dodge a eugenic bullet? While such questions might seem alarmist, we will see later that consent protocols in medical research and eugenic surgeries routinely included similar deceitful actions so that, given the context, my questions are reasonable.

(Over)Medication

Although preventive medicine, daily care, routine treatments, and corrective devices for daily living, such as glasses and dentures, were in short supply in the institution, psychoactive drugs were seemingly ubiquitous as a form of preventive and reactive treatment. In the daily institutional records, each shift included an indication that medications were distributed but with no detail on the types or amounts of drugs people were being administered on a regular basis. However, when an inmate was visited by the doctor for medication adjustments, injuries, or uncontrollable behaviour, the physicians' entries into the Unusual Incidents files are telling. For example, in a follow-up examination of an inmate who had been experiencing severe hiccups, the physician made the following observations:

> Appetite seems to be good ... Present weight: 148 lbs. Meds: Zarontin 250 gr. t.i.d., Dilantin 1 ½ gr. t.i.d., Phenobarb [illegible amount] t.i.d., Chloral hydrate 1 oz. [sic] p.r.n. if ineffective. Sodium Luminal gr.iii I/M for muscle spasms. Largactil 50 mg. I/M q.6.h. x 24 hrs. for hiccoughs. Sodium Luminal gr iv I/M after 1st grand mal. (Deerhome Ward Progress Notes, 1974)

From the above, we can extract that this young man was given three Zarontin doses (a sedative and anticonvulsant), three Dilantin doses (another anticonvulsant medication) and three phenobarbitol pills (a barbiturate/sedative and anticonvulsant) each day. In addition, he was given a daily injection of another barbiturate/sedative in the form of Sodium Luminal for muscle spasms that incidentally may have been a side effect of the Zarontin and phenobarbitol regime, since both drugs carry the side effect of severe, spasmodic, and involuntary muscle movements. Finally, he was to receive an additional injection of the barbiturate Sodium Luminal following any seizure activity, and if he showed any agitation, he received chloral hydrate (a sedative/hypnotic/antipsychotic drug that is no longer in common use). It is worth noting that this last drug (chloral hydrate) was charted at a level that would probably be quite harmful; this dosage, noted on a typewritten report dictated by the physician called in to examine the young man's progress, might reflect slipshod charting practices rather than an actual dosage that this young man received.[2] Nevertheless, according to the ward progress notes, these are the inmate's regular medications; the additional medication in this list for the complaint of hiccups is a short-term (24 hour) prescription for Largactil, which does indeed treat nausea, vomiting, and gastric upsets but is also yet another antipsychotic drug that is used to calm people experiencing psychotic symptoms (Schizophrenia Society of Ontario, 2014a).

I am not qualified to speculate on the appropriateness of dosages or the interactive effects of these psychotropic medications; however, it is clear that at the very least, most of them are strong sedatives, and this helps us to understand the trance-like state of inmates in the day rooms that Evelyn described earlier. Survivors also spoke about the effects of the role of medication in their institutional lives, noting that "they kept me drugged. Lots of pills to make sure you didn't know what you were doing" (Sandra Karnak), or "I was on a lot more medication then. We were all walking around like zombies" (Guy Tremblay). The effects of these high levels of medication were more than subjectively experienced, however. For example, Donna Bogdan described the effects of medication on how she was perceived and treated in the institution:

> I was so doped up on pills ... like I was drooling because I was on so many pills. The staff came up to me and yelled at me because she goes, "Are you a Low Grade?" and I said no, because I was drooling all over and I couldn't help it.

In this exchange we can read how the side effects of the most typically used medications (barbiturates and anti-psychotics), which included drooling, tremors, tics, muscle spasms, lolling tongues, and dry mouths, made inmates appear to be in worse psychological shape than they actually were. Further, given the hierarchical nature of the institution, to be heavily medicated could mean being demoted to a Low Grade. In a sense, these drugs not only sedated people but also made them appear to be less functional than they were, which in turn meant they were seen as hopeless and unworthy of the kind of training and care that a more hopeful case might deserve.

The iatrogenic aspects of hypermedication went beyond unattractive side effects; Michel Aubin's high levels of medication seem to have caused behaviours that the drugs were meant to eradicate. He noted that "they had drugged me up so much my brain was fried. They tried to control me, but I was so violent they couldn't." Michel, in keeping with the interviews of all survivors, did not know what medications he was given while in the institution, so it is difficult to know precisely whether or not his particular medication had iatrogenic behavioural effects. However, many of the typically prescribed medications for behavioural problems do carry side effects that include irritability, excitement, and confusion. Michel is clear that during his stay at Michener, he never received any counselling or anger management assistance and received only drug therapy to deal with his anger. After his release, he was able to live without taking medication while simultaneously experiencing significantly less anger and conflict in his life. It is possible to take from Michel's story that at least some of his anger may have come from the iatrogenic effects of inappropriate medication. It is just as likely that his anger stemmed from the alienating and threatening aspects of life in Michener itself, and that at least part of reasons the drugs did not help to reduce his violence and anger was not because as Michel speculated, "they used the wrong drugs," but because those drugs were unable to remedy the institutional regime that lay at the base of his problems. When Michel no longer had to deal with life in Michener, it seems, he was also able to live without the aid of so many mind-numbing medications.

Finally, the administration of heavy sedatives on a routine basis played a speculative role in at least one death described in the records I was able to access. John Wickstrom's attempted escape and subsequent drowning in the river bounding the Michener campus was described earlier, in the chapter on violence. During the investigation of his death, it was noted that his daily medications included an astonishing regime of phenobarbital (twice daily), Neuleptil/penothiazine (three times daily), Trilafon/perphenazine (three times daily), Dilantin (twice daily), Valium (twice daily), and Largactil (p.r.n.) (Friesen, 1976b).

The use of inappropriate or unnecessary drugs was also cited in the decision of Justice Veit on the unlawful confinement aspects of a lawsuit brought against the government by Leilani Muir in 1996. She stated that a particularly problematic aspect of Ms Muir's confinement at Michener was the "administration of drugs to control behaviour: many antipsychotic drugs were administered to Ms. Muir despite the fact that she was not psychotic" (*Muir v. Alberta*, 1996, p. 43). Thus, the judicial records make clear that, in this instance at the very least, an inmate who did not need psychotropic drugs for any medical reason nevertheless regularly received them as a way of keeping her docile.

The overuse of serious psychotropic medication began to be addressed with a new program instated by Dr Robert Lampard, the centre's medical director, who began a systematic review of medication use in 1990. A newspaper article discussing the early changes occurring during this reassessment noted that one resident, who had only communicated through gestures for several years, finally began to speak after having his medication lowered (Proby, 1991). Dr Lampard said that in some instances, he had been able to gradually reduce patients' medication "to as low as one-twentieth of their previous dosage" (Proby, 1991). The article went on to note that, in response to these changes, some staff had expressed concerns, with one staff member writing an anonymous letter to *The Advocate* complaining that behavioural problems had compromised staff safety on the job since the new reductions in medications had been initiated. This complaint tacitly acknowledged that hypermedication was being used as a form of social control on inmates, a subject to which I now turn.

Medications as Means of Social Control

From the archival record, it seems the heavy use of sedatives as a form of social and behavioural control was quite common. In an entry in the Unusual Incidents files, we read a physician's response to an inmate's unmanageable behaviour on the ward. On examination, the doctor made a decision to change the inmate's medications in the following way:

Phenobarb 100 mgm. q. 8 h. is discontinued, given Phenobarb 160 mgm. q. 12 h.
and...Largactil 1000 mgm I/M p.r.n. for severe behaviour outbursts and Neuleptil
20 mgm. t.i.d. x 2/52 and re-assess. (Cookson, 1974)

What this tells us is that before the incident, this inmate had been receiving
300 mg of phenobarbitol in three pills over 24 hours, and that the dosage was
then raised to 320 mg in two pills over the same period of time. In addition,
the doctor prescribed a thrice-daily dose of Neuleptil, an antipsychotic drug
that is also used to control symptoms of hostility, impulsiveness, and aggres-
siveness (Schizophrenia Society of Ontario, 2014b). Finally, a directive is made
that, should any "severe behaviour outbursts" occur, an injection of the antipsychotic and sedative drug Largactil is to be given as needed (Cookson,
1974). In this response we can see that inmates whose behaviours were deemed
problematic were sedated quite heavily, both prophylactically and in response
to perceived inappropriateness. As with much of the clinical reporting, however, we are never really told whether these incidents *were* inappropriate or
threatening to the health of the individual or other inmates. However, the daily
ward reports do give us some insight into the reasons for medicating, particularly in terms of how "p.r.n." (as required) dosages were used.

Standing orders for p.r.n. medications, such as Valium (a sedative), chloral
hydrate (a barbiturate), Mellaril (an antipsychotic and sedative), and Sparine (an
antipsychotic drug) were ubiquitous. The following entries indicate how these
"as needed" medications were administered:

- Given chloral hydrate 1 gm p.r.n. for loud and aggressive behaviour.
  (Juniper Ward Record, 1983a)
- Up banging his head and screaming. Given 1.5 mg. Chloral hydrate p.r.n.
  and settled. (Juniper Ward Record, 1983b)
- Very noisy and agitated. Chloral hydrate 1.0 gm @ 1815 given. Appears to
  settle down @ time of report. (Juniper Ward Record, 1982)
- At 1830 he started to be physically and verbally aggressive. Valium
  10 mg p.o. and chloral hydrate 0.5 gm given. CN [charge nurse] informed.
  Settled down on his own after having 2 cigarettes @ 30 minute interval.
  (Nightingale Ward Record, 1982b)
- Throwing dishes in the dining room and induced vomiting following
  breakfast. Given Sparine 50 mg. I.M. @ 0740. Effective (Nightingale Ward
  Record, 1983a)
- Put in dining room. Did not settle. Chloral hydrate 1.0 gm given. Prior to
  supper, she was given her p.r.n. per Mrs. X. Did not appear to help, as she
  still refused to get dressed and as a result did not go. (Nightingale Ward
  Record, 1983b)

- Very agitated for no reason ... Chloral hydrate given. Appears to settle down @ time of report. (Nightingale Ward Record, 1982c)
- Was asked by staff member to come for a bath. Flatly refused and immediately became extremely self-abusive – uncontrollable. Given Valium 10 mg for severe behavioural outburst. Effective. (Juniper Ward Record, 1983c)
- In spite of increase in Mellaril in April he is still needing p.r.n.'s very frequently. Increase Mellaril further to 100 mg. t.i.d and review in 1/12 (Unusual Incidents Report, 1975).

The p.r.n. medications, which were routinely placed as standing orders on inmates' files, were used by staff as a means of reducing inmate resistance. Indeed, the use of p.r.n. medications was common enough that several people interviewed, when asked about the drugs they were on while in the institutions, while knowing little about the type of medications they were given, referred to this term to explain how their medications were given. Even those who described not being on any medications while at Michener frequently added the phrase, "only my p.r.n." (Sandra Karnak, Mary Korshevski, and Harvey Brown).

Institutional descriptions of p.r.n. medication use were frequently couched as a response to inmates' inexplicable behaviour. The individuals who refused dinner, complained on being roused from bed, disliked their food, or refused their regular medications were not responded to as reasoned social actors who were not hungry, who disliked institutional food, who did not want to get out of bed or go to work, or who wanted to be less heavily drugged. Rather, they were reacted to as a crazed person, to be tranquilized and neutralized medically. Finally, the use of p.r.n. medication was routinely combined with institutional violence; doses were described both in the institutional record and by survivors as accompanied by informal restraint in the form of holding someone down while administering injections, or more formally by tying someone down to a bed or chair, or they are coupled with sessions in Time-Out Rooms, where drugged inmates were placed to cool down following outbursts or behaviours deemed to be inappropriate.

Medical Research

In addition to the inappropriate use of antipsychotic medications on inmates to control unruliness and resistance, there were other ethical concerns regarding medications, particularly the use of inmates as non-consenting subjects in medical research. In her 1996 judgment on the Leilani Muir case, the judge noted, "it appears from his publications in professional journals that Dr. LeVann used Ms. Muir and others as a means of testing the success of different drug treatments" (*Muir v. Alberta*, 1996). The use of non-consenting subjects in medical or social research, even in the early years of LeVann's 1949–1972 tenure as medical superintendent, would not have been seen as ethical methodologically. Although it was only in 1970 that the Medical Research Council of Canada laid down its first formal internal regulations for research (Canadian Medical Association, 1970), the Canadian Medical Association adhered to several international accords and declarations before that date that made obtaining consent normative. In 1946–1947 in Nuremberg, Germany, several high-profile war trials exposed crimes against humanity perpetuated by Nazi physicians and administrators in the form of medical experimentation on unwilling victims during World War II. These trials culminated in the 1948 Codes of Nuremburg, which set standards of practice for physicians engaging in medical research. The Codes outlined that informed consent must be a mainstay of medical research and that there must be a benefit to participation in research to override any potential harms or risks to research subjects (Young, 1998). Although the Codes were not mandatory, in 1948 the World Medical Association (of which Canada was a member) drew on them to construct its Declaration of Geneva, which stated that physicians should hold the health and welfare of their patients foremost, regardless of race, ethnicity, disability status, and other marginalizing categories, and that physicians must never use their medical knowledge to violate civil liberties or human rights (World Medical Association, 1948/2006). The World Medical Association further codified its regulation of research protocols for member states through the 1964 Helsinki Declaration, clarifying risk–benefit guidelines in human subject research and outlining stringent research safeguards (particularly the use of animal testing before human testing for drugs and prohibitions against using unnecessary or inappropriate medications), particularly for clinical settings and drug trials, while at the same time broadening consent protocols somewhat to include consent by proxy for vulnerable and institutional populations (Young, 1998). This last part would have been relevant for individuals at Michener, who often were under the protection of legal guardians or the institution itself. In addition, Canadian physicians' ethical guidelines from as early as 1961 required physicians to be cautious in publishing discoveries, presumably so as not to overstate their findings or mislead researchers, physicians, or the general public (Canadian Medical Association, 1961). Finally, in addition to the international and national guidelines, the Canadian Medical Association issued its own research regulations in 1970, requiring physicians to obtain informed consent, to ensure that no harm or deceit be involved in the research, and to ensure that any research be passed under the lens of an external review board (Canadian Medical Association, 1970).

Although the norms and regulations governing medical research should have resulted in protections of some kinds for the inmates of Michener, the research

Dr LeVann conducted on inmates would not have passed muster on methodological or ethical dimensions, as will be made clear in the following sections. It is also worth stating that LeVann's methods and use of inmates as research subjects were a matter of public record, recorded not only by LeVann's publications but also in his regular annual reporting to the minister of health as the institutional superintendent.

Leonard Jan LeVann was an ambitious man. As noted earlier, during his 1949–1972 administration, the population of the institution grew rapidly, suggesting a more aggressive approach to inmate admissions. His ambition is also evident in the expansion of the facility itself during his tenure, including the construction of significant, multi-storey residential spaces on the children's side of the campus and the establishment of an entire institution (Deerhome) to house adult inmates on the north side of the campus. The population, by way of reminder, grew from 293 children in 1949, the year of LeVann's arrival, to 2400 children and adults at its apex in 1969. In addition to growing the institution numerically and structurally, he also appeared to have been keen to build the institution's reputation. His were the only annual reports that included entries about research projects conducted in the institution. These research entries were also presented with significant pride as compared with the other, more routinized entries regarding health, staffing, and other statistics and accomplishments that composed the annual reports. In the annual reports, he listed the full titles of the articles he published and the names of the journals that published them, as well as the societies, locations, and sponsors of conferences that published his work. In addition, he instituted a new heading in the annual reports, "Visitors," that reported on "honourable visitors" who came to the institution for observation or knowledge exchange. These included the Provincial Hospital Visiting Board, the Eugenics Board (which will be discussed in the next chapter), the chief of the provincial government's Mental Health Division, the chief of the federal government's Mental Health Division, the minister of health, the provincial deputy minister of health, and the province's premier, Ernest Manning, whose son was a resident[3] in the institution for many years. In his reporting on these august visitors, LeVann mentioned them by name, title, honorific where appropriate, and frequency of visits. He also regularly described educational "visits and rounds completed" by nursing students from several hospitals in Alberta and by university students in psychology, public health, and medicine from the University of Alberta and the University of Calgary (LeVann, 1961–1962, p. 165). Finally, he noted that "the Alberta Psychiatric Association Convention was held at Deerhome in October" (LeVann, 1961–1962, p. 172). Clearly, LeVann sought to establish and sustain Michener as a leader in the field of institutionalization and treatment for "mental defectives." As part of this campaign for legitimation, it is worth noting that he also misrepresented himself; despite his degree being in general medicine, he described himself consistently as a qualified psychiatrist (*Muir v. Alberta*, 1996), and he listed himself as either a "psychiatrist" or an "honorary lecturer in psychiatry" on his publications. In addition to hosting a psychiatric conference, conducting psychiatric and nursing rounds for students and faculty, and inviting political leaders at the provincial and federal levels to observe his work, LeVann published his original research in learned journals. The quality of the work he published, however, reads as significantly flawed to modern eyes.

In one article, he reported on the experimental use of thioridazine (Mellaril) on 89 non-schizophrenic children, to measure its effects on unruliness and undesirable behaviours. This drug, used in the treatment of schizophrenia, carries warnings about its use even on individuals *diagnosed* with schizophrenia, because it can cause cardiac arrhythmias as a side effect and even death, indicating that it "should be reserved for use in the treatment of schizophrenic patients who fail to show an acceptable response to adequate courses of treatment with other antipsychotic drugs"[4] (RXList Inc., 2012). Given that the children in this experiment did not require this drug to control any illness but were instead given it to see if it would affect their activity levels, one must question the research's adherence to extant requirements that drug trials, particularly with clinical participants, should involve benefits that outweigh potential risks (Young, 1998). In his article, LeVann (1961b, p. 144) seemed to get around this dilemma by claiming that administering this drug had revolutionized "psychiatric care ... by diminishing the need for more hazardous types of physical therapies such as electro-shock and insulin-shock" and that using it on children was not simply an attempt to reduce staff labour and inmate unruliness by sedating children. Instead, he argued for the benefits of Mellaril for behavioural issues because it "rendered the patient more accessible to his therapist and nursing attendants" (LeVann, 1961b, p. 144). Using methodologies that even for the time would have been questionable (Gould, 1981), he described administering a double-blind trial to three groups of non-schizophrenic children, who did not require such a dangerous drug for medical reasons but instead for social and behavioural ones. The three groups were "Idiots & Imbeciles, High-Grade children, Including Morons and Borderline Cases and Emotionally Disturbed children [who had normal or above-normal intelligence and lived in the Behavioral Unit, Linden House]" (LeVann, 1961b, p. 146). The test drug was given at dosages ranging widely, from 10 mg b.i.d. (totalling 20 mg/day) to 200 mg q.i.d. (totalling 800 mg/day) without any justification given for the differing dosages nor any description of differential outcomes based on them. As well, the article had no baseline information on those patients, which would have been an ordinary expectation even in the 1960s for experimental research (Gould, 1981).

The research report also offered no indication of how "improvement" or "side effects" were measured and no indication of the duration of the "experiment." It provided a note that the drowsiness seen in only one child was so "in keeping with this particular child's attitudes that one would not clearly regard it as a side-effect per se," despite this child being included in a study supposedly seeking to measure the "improved" uncontrollable behaviour of the participants (LeVann, 1961b, p. 146). LeVann nevertheless confidently recommended that the drug could be given for the "control of a wide variety of behavioral or thinking patterns in children" without side effects and that this treatment was so effective as to be recommended for out-patient and institutional use because compliance would be high, because of purported lack of side effects. This final recommendation clearly stands in opposition to Canadian Medical Association (1961) regulations concerning overly enthusiastic research reporting. In short, using a flawed methodology, he showed little fear in making extravagant claims about a drug that is recommended today only for use with schizophrenics who cannot take anything else to alleviate their symptoms. He did have the honesty – in this publication alone – to report his gratitude to the Sandoz Pharmaceutical Company for providing the drugs and placebos used for the experiment, but this last nod to ethical protocols stood in contrast to the balance of the research reports (LeVann, 1961b).

In another experiment, LeVann administered the tranquilizer chlordiazepoxide (Librium) for a duration that "ranged from 4 to 54 days" to 47 children identified as having behavioural problems, 35 of whom also had epilepsy (LeVann, 1962b, p. 124). In this study – again without any baseline indicating medications taken before the study or behavioural patterns before the intervention, nor with any indication why "treatment" was stopped after 4 days for some and continued for 54 days for others, nor any explanation of how "improvement" was measured – LeVann nevertheless claimed that half of the children experienced behavioural "improvement." Conversely, of the 35 children with epilepsy included in the study, 20% experienced the negative side effect of increased seizures. Even so, LeVann concluded that, despite the side effect of increased seizure activity for one in five of the epileptic children in his study, the drug was "of value in treating epileptic and mentally retarded patients with behaviour problems" (LeVann, 1962b, p. 25). In this study, given the lack of baselines for behaviour, the lack of markers for what constituted improvement, the ignoring of harm incurred for 7 of 35 research subjects, Dr LeVann's enthusiastic endorsement of the treatment seems ill-founded.

In addition to the two experiments outlined in detail above, LeVann also published similar articles, with similarly enthusiastic claims, on experiments using trifluoperazine, dihydrochloride, Tarasan and thioridazine, trifluperidol, and haloperidol, all of which would be considered heavy-handed or inappropriate for psychotic or seizure-disordered children, let alone for the otherwise healthy children who were simply emotionally disturbed or intellectually disabled on whom these medications were trialled (LeVann, 1959, 1961b, 1962b, 1968b, 1969, 1970b). Finally, in retrospect, it is evident that LeVann's confidence and enthusiasm for the "less hazardous" (1961b, p. 147) use of serious antipsychotic drugs on children, many of whom did not have a mental illness, was not borne out. During the court cases against the government's involuntary sterilization program, the over-prescribing on a daily basis and the misuse of medication in medical research at Michener were exposed and decried (*Muir v. Alberta*, 1996). When interviewed by media following the final court case, 47-year-old litigant George Boucher described having lived in a fugue state while being a "human guinea pig" to "doctors [who] were like demons from hell" and stated that he still suffered from "flashbacks" decades later (Wittmeier, 1999, p. 13).

Beyond his studies on the effects of varying antipsychotic drugs on children's unruly behaviour, LeVann also engaged in ethically questionable research in which 100 Michener children deemed to be underweight for their ages were administered norbolethone, an anabolic steroid, to induce weight gain. Norbolethene was discovered in 1966 but was never made available commercially because of early concerns about its toxicity (Catlin, Ahrens, & Kucherova, 2002). Although the medicated children did gain weight, the children on a placebo drug for this study also gained, indicating perhaps that simply paying attention to children and their nutritional needs in the institution might have had an effect on the children's ability to thrive and grow. In his report, LeVann did acknowledge the controversial nature of using anabolic steroids of any sort (let alone this particular brand) on children, but he dismissed these concerns as trivial, instead claiming that the gains in weight and height made by the children in his study meant that the drug "was entirely satisfactory" causing "little in the way of untoward reactions" among his research subjects (LeVann & Cohn, 1972, p. 58), an endorsement that again seemed to contravene the Canadian Medical Association's 1961 admonition to avoid excessively eager research reporting.

An unpublished aspect of LeVann's medical research revolved around the collection of testicular tissues obtained during eugenic operations. In particular, a group of 15 males with Down syndrome were castrated under the aegis of the Eugenics Board in the 1950s and their removed testicles were collected for examination by Dr LeVann and his erstwhile Eugenics Board colleague Dr Margaret Thompson (*Muir v. Alberta*, 1996; Wahlsten, 1997). During the sterilization court cases, the presiding judge stated that, because the record showed Dr Thompson had provided LeVann with detailed instructions about removing and preserving testicular tissues, "this constituted encouragement to Dr LeVann to use the trainees as medical guinea pigs" (*Muir v. Alberta*, 1996, p. 32). During the trial, when Dr Thompson was asked about the sterilization and tissue removal from males with Down syndrome, she responded "that *there was nothing lost* by sterilizing the male mongol; she thought everyone would agree with her approach" (*Muir v. Alberta*, 1996, p. 16). In fact, there was nothing to be *gained* by sterilizing these young men either, since males with Down syndrome have historically been understood to be sterile.[5] Further, as will be explained in the chapter on eugenics, sterilization operations were routinely performed on Michener residents without consent, and nothing in the record indicates that these particular operations were handled differently. Thus, several years after the world's horrified response to medical experimentation in World War II and the subsequent production of the Nuremberg Codes, an unnecessary and undoubtedly non-consented operation was performed on at least 15 young men in Canada, simply because "there was nothing lost" by doing so, according to one of the surgeons involved.

Although LeVann never published the results of his experimentation on tissues removed from sterilized males with Down syndrome, Dr Thompson did publish on fertility issues for females with Down syndrome during the time she worked with LeVann on the Eugenics Board. However, the first of these publications is a simple case history and did not describe tissue use in the article (Thompson, 1961). The second did acknowledge the use of tissues; in this case, Dr Thompson described a 22-year-old woman with Down syndrome who was given a hysterectomy while 20 weeks pregnant.[6] Following the abortion/hysterectomy, tissues were removed from the fetus in an attempt to establish the presence of Down syndrome, presumably to bolster a genetic argument for the sterilization of females with Down syndrome. Unfortunately for Dr Thompson, the kidney samples from the male fetus were not adequate for establishing his chromosomal make-up, so the article was only able to conclude speculatively on Down syndrome mothers and the heritability of the syndrome for their offspring (Thompson, 1962). Given the history of involuntary sterilization in the institution and the province, and the lack of reference in the research report to ethical and consent protocols, it is not unreasonable to assume that this research was also conducted unethically.

Consent

It is important to note that although these experiments involved powerful and often dangerous drugs or surgeries, nowhere in the journal articles or in the annual reports where this research was reported, was there ever any mention of efforts to obtain consent from inmates or their guardians. In her judgment of the Muir case, and drawing on more detailed archival documentation than I have been able to access in my research, Justice Veit was clear that consent for such experimentation was not obtained either from inmates or their guardians; rather, residency in the institution seems to have been taken as de facto consent to such experimentation (*Muir v. Alberta,* 1996). Conducting drug research without obtaining consent would certainly have been in keeping with Dr LeVann's disdainful attitudes toward children under his "care." In an article published the year following his arrival at Michener, on the putative improbability that people with intellectual disabilities could also have "true" schizophrenia, he describes intellectually disabled people as subhuman:

> Indeed the picture of comparison between the normal child and the idiot might almost be a comparison between two separate species. On the one hand, the graceful, intelligently curious, active young homo sapiens, and on the other the gross, retarded, animalistic, early primate type individual. It is on this clinical basis that we find it difficult to associate schizophrenia as a regressive disease of the mind, if we may postulate a schizophrenic state in these idiot types. It is rather that the mind has acquired an archaic form of thinking, which in the adult is admixed with his cultural experiences and in the idiot shows itself uncomplicated and primitive with little distortion. (LeVann, 1950, p. 470)

In effect, he argued that schizophrenia could not possibly be a proper diagnosis for children with lower IQ scores because they lack a "regular" human type of psyche from which to develop this "regressive" psychological disorder; they were, to him, already too deeply "regressed" to go any further.

LeVann's ideas about the more social aspects of intellectual difference were not limited to medical experimentation or even to topics directly related to his institutional work. He also published on such diverse topics as the connection between rates of mental retardation and nuclear testing (LeVann, 1963b, 1965), and the causes of alcoholism. In the alcoholism paper, he described the qualities of what he believed to be two types of alcoholics, exploring such attributes as their response to a variety of psychometric and psychiatric tests, including Rorschach's, MMPI and IQ tests, and personality inventories. Based on a sample of 32 people, he speculated that alcoholics fail to accept the Freudian myth of the father figure, going on to note that this probably explained why there are so few Jewish or Chinese alcoholics, because both these cultures consider the father figure as paramount, perhaps even sacred (LeVann, 1953). Clearly, the good doctor did not shy away from sweeping and inappropriate generalizations in his research, regardless of how methodologically or ethically unsound that work was.

It must be acknowledged that, despite the ethical protocols I have outlined earlier in this chapter, invasive and even harmful research on captive or marginal populations could and did continue in North America into the 1960s and early 1970s. The goals of science and progress, often woven together with less progressivist doctrines, such as racism, ableism, and sexism, gave rise to research excesses that rightfully shock current sensibilities.[7] However, the use of captive or marginal populations as research subjects became significantly regulated following the 1947 Nuremburg Codes, and cases of research misconduct were not normative. The medical research described in this chapter was conducted in the two decades following the pronouncement and subsequent broad adoption of the Nuremburg Codes concerning human subject research. Nevertheless, the research projects conducted by Leonard Jan LeVann at Michener contravened several aspects of the Codes, in that they did not involve voluntarism or informed consent because they were conducted on individuals who were incapable of refusing or withdrawing from the projects. Finally, it is important to remember that none of this extravagant, frequently unethical, and consent-free research was accomplished in secrecy. Rather, as noted earlier, through his regular annual reporting, LeVann assiduously highlighted these activities as accomplishments to the ministry that oversaw and regulated institutional activities. We can assume that he was allowed to continue this work not because the government to which he reported was unaware of the ethical quandaries involved in his research, but because the people to whom LeVann reported were not particularly worried about ethical safeguards for these specific research subjects. In the following chapter on eugenic activities at Michener, we will see that issues of consent and unethical medical protocols were endemic to the institution and were, in fact, central to the way the province's sterilization program was implemented on Michener inmates.

Chapter Nine

Eugenics and Sexuality

In 1995, Leilani Muir, a former inmate of Michener, launched the first successful lawsuit against the provincial Government of Alberta as the entity responsible for the abuses of passive eugenics in the form of institutional confinement
and for the abuses of active eugenics in the form of involuntary sterilization.
The question of informed and ethical consent lay at the base of Muir's and subsequent lawsuits. In early 1996, the judge presiding over the Muir case began
her summary with the following statement:

> The circumstances of Ms. Muir's sterilization were so high-handed and so con-
> temptuous of the statutory authority to effect sterilization, and were undertaken in
> an atmosphere that so little respected Ms. Muir's human dignity that the commu-
> nity's, and the court's, sense of decency is offended. (*Muir v. Alberta*, 1996, p. 3)

Justice Veit's judgment represents the closing chapter on the eugenic history
of Michener and provides a sense of how unrestrained and unethical the actions
of the Eugenics Board had become by the end of its reign, acting virtually without oversight or due process. In an earlier chapter I outlined the history, structure, and philosophy of the eugenics movements that flourished in the early part
of the twentieth century in the West. In this chapter, drawing on the official record, I outline the context for and mechanics of active eugenic programs in
Alberta and at Michener. Then, drawing on interviews with survivors, I explore
the experiences and impacts of the eugenics program for Michener survivors.

The Context of the Sexual Sterilization Act in Alberta

Alberta instituted its passive eugenics program in the form of institutionalization for "mental defectives" alongside a more active and formal eugenics

program implemented and sustained through public legislation. Both these programs began in a social context where science, racism, imperialism, and sexual prudishness converged to produce moral panics about the proliferation of undesirables. In Alberta, the movement to instate eugenic legislation comprised people for whom these scientific, racist, and imperialist aspects converged in specific ways. In many nations, the science of eugenics, built on a faulty understanding of genetic traits as simply like begetting like, was taken up with enthusiasm by social reformers of the time. However, because of Alberta's rural and agricultural economy, these ideas were taken up with a particular enthusiasm for and experience with agricultural selective breeding programs. For example, when the Sexual Sterilization Act came into force in 1928, Mr George Hoadley was the minister of agriculture and health – even the name of the ministry belies a naturalized association between animal, plant, and human health in the construction of civic leadership and governance. Hoadley, a keen supporter of eugenics and of the Sexual Sterilization Act, was interviewed shortly after its passage by the secretary of the Canadian Eugenics Society about his support for the legislation (Wahlsten, 1997). Hoadley's response was telling; he noted that in his life as a farmer and stock breeder he had seen firsthand the effects of positive eugenics through good breeding and the improvements made possible through negative eugenics to breed out undesirable traits (Wahlsten, 1997). Hoadley was neither a physician nor a scientist and had received no education in the fields of biology, agricultural science, or psychology; nevertheless, because of his enthusiastic early support of the eugenic program, he was appointed the minister in charge of health, mental health, and the eugenics program (Wahlsten, 1997).

Like many other eugenic reformers in Alberta, Hoadley was a member of the United Farmers of Alberta (UFA), the party that governed Alberta from 1921 to 1935 (Rennie, 2000). In the late nineteenth century, several non-partisan organizations had formed in the territory (this was before Alberta joined Canada in 1905), seeking to protect farmers from corporate excesses and political neglect and to promote the interests of local agriculture. In 1909, these groups merged to form the more politicized UFA, an organization based on cooperative values that retained its original commitment to agricultural reform and family issues. The UFA became the governing party and played a key role in supporting and implementing the Sexual Sterilization Act. Ironically, the UFA held highly progressive values, including a commitment to suffrage and farm women's property rights, collective bargaining for market values on grain prices, state-run medical care, and fairer taxation (Rennie, 2000). By 1918, the United Farm Women of Alberta (UFWA) had become an important and well-organized sister organization; many of its members were instrumental in the struggle for women's suffrage in Canada and held political posts in the province (Langford, 1997). The UFWA was a maternal feminist organization, taking on the work of improving social welfare by maintaining a focus on health, education, young people's labour inclusion, child protection, women's sexual reproduction, and women's rights (Langford, 1997). In turn, many of these issues and experiences directly informed UFWA members' strong support for eugenic legislation.

The women of the UFWA were in a position to exercise influence from within government because when the UFA won a majority government in 1921, it included UFWA women as members of the assembly and as party leaders. In 1919, Irene Parlby, a founding mother in the UFWA, became the British Empire's first female cabinet minister. Echoing the established gendered lines of responsibility drawn between the UFA and the UFWA, Parlby's appointment was as minister without portfolio, with the mandate of advising the government on issues of particular concern to women and children, a position she held until her retirement in 1934 (Cavanaugh, 2012). However, Parlby was not alone in advising the government on family issues. Through her work lobbying for women's suffrage, Parlby worked intimately with other UFWA members who shared her keen interest in women, children, family, and health. These members included Louise McKinney, a member of the legislative assembly who maintained an interest in the establishment of PTS and who expressed enthusiasm for the self-sufficiency of inmates (McKinney, 1919). Another UFWA affiliate was fellow suffragist Emily Murphy, who had achieved the august position of being the first female magistrate in the British Empire.

Similar to Parlby, Murphy's 1916 appointment as chief police magistrate and judge of the juvenile courts in the capital city of Edmonton was a gendered responsibility that brought her into contact with family violence and dissolution, family problems arising from addiction and alcoholism, and criminality relating to family and youth. This work impressed Murphy deeply and she spoke and published widely on the social problems she encountered as a magistrate. Her addiction writings placed a critique of the inadequate or degenerate family alongside racist anti-immigrant sentiment, intimating that addiction was related to the rampant immorality of Chinese immigrants, combined with lax or inadequate parenting that left children particularly vulnerable to predatory Chinese drug dealers (Murphy, 1922). Her strong belief in the social benefits that could be obtained from the scientific control of breeding was coupled with a strong conviction that the founding (White) population of Canada was under threat by overbreeding and morally bankrupt immigrants (McLaren, 1990; Sharpe & McMahon, 2008). She also argued that mentally defective children were "a menace to society, and an enormous cost to the state" that must be curtailed through positive eugenics, such as improved health and welfare programs, and through negative eugenics, such as sterilization (as cited in Wahlsten, 1997). To Murphy, "feeble-mindedness" was at the root of many social ills, and her experience with families and youth led her to argue for numerous maternal feminist reforms, including prohibiting alcohol and drugs, and providing women with access to permanent birth control in the form of sterilization. Murphy lobbied Minister Hoadley assiduously during the debates leading up to the implementation of the 1928 Sexual Sterilization Act, arguing that much social upheaval had been proven to be caused by "mental defect," as Henry Herbert Goddard – whose work by this time was already being discredited – had shown (Grekul, 2008; Wahlsten, 1997).

Another prominent UFWA member who shared the maternal feminist goals of McKinney and Murphy was fellow suffragist Margaret Gunn. She argued that the lofty goals of universal enfranchisement, a strong social safety net, and the cooperative values promoted by the UFA government were not applicable for "mental defectives" because "democracy was never intended for degenerates" (as cited in Grekul, 2008). These women – like other UFA and UFWA members – were convinced of the benefits of positive eugenics in the form of family-supportive policy and programs, coupled with negative eugenics in the form of a voluntary sterilization program and educational programs that would "assist" undesirables in "choosing" sterilization. Further, the rural roots of most of the UFA and UFWA members fostered an overly enthusiastic acceptance, based on their personal experiences as farmers and breeders, of the eugenic argument. Indeed, UFA Minister of Health George Hoadley attributed his experiences on the farm and his observations of the benefits of selective stock breeding as instrumental to his support for the Sterilization Act (Wahlsten, 1997).

The enthusiasm of these local politicians was fuelled by a study commissioned by the Canadian National Committee on Mental Hygiene, an association formed in 1919 of self-appointed but nevertheless highly influential physicians and psychiatrists. Part of the success of this group undoubtedly came from its inclusion of a number of high-ranking military psychiatrists concerned about the state of the nation's soldiers following their World War I experiences, at a time when dealing with "shell shock" was a national problem and priority. In addition, the committee made strong connections with financial leaders who shared its concerns over what was perceived to be a nation-wide increase in mental illness and lack of productivity. The committee was also concerned from its inception with what its director perceived to be an additional burden on the nation state posed by the "inadequate medical examination of immigrants ... deplor[ing] the fact that through loose methods at our ports we have been allowing thousands of insane and feeble-minded aliens to enter the Dominion" (Hincks, 1927, p. 553). The committee, like other individuals and groups involved in the eugenics movement, was also highly concerned about questions of sexuality, arguing for laws that would limit marriage for "individuals with psychopathic tendencies," expressing concerns about the heightened vulnerability that adolescence, menarche, and menopause produced in terms of mental illness and further arguing that clear connections existed between criminality, mental illness, and these dangerous sexual moments (Porteous, 1918, p. 634).

The committee, highly successful in procuring the support of local, provincial, and national elites, was able to secure funding to conduct a survey of western Canada's mental hygiene under the leadership of Dr Clarence Hincks (McLaren, 1990). In 1919 the committee turned its attention to the province of Alberta, publishing the results of its survey of mental health services, mental defectives, the feeble-minded, and the insane in 1921 (Canadian National Committee for Mental Hygiene, 1921). The findings were alarming; the scale of the problem was seen to be larger than anticipated and growing in magnitude and severity, in great part because of "the mentally unfit are breeding faster than the fit" and also because of the problems created by lax immigration standards (Hincks as cited in Park & Radford, 1998). These survey results, expressing values already espoused by the local UFA and UFWA political elite, found a receptive and enthusiastic audience and helped legitimate the eugenic ambitions of Alberta reformers. .

The Sexual Sterilization Act and Its Amendments

The Sexual Sterilization Act was first proposed in the legislature in March 1927. However, because of an extremely busy legislative session it was tabled, reintroduced by Minister George Hoadley in February of the next year, and passed into law just one month later on March 21. The Act is a surprisingly brief document, given its scope. At less than one and a half pages, it established that the Alberta Eugenics Board was to be composed of two medical practitioners nominated by the senate of the University of Alberta and the Council of the College of Physicians, alongside two non-medical practitioners, appointed by the lieutenant governor as a representative of the province. Presumably, the use of two appointing bodies was meant to provide some checks and balances in the Board membership, but in practice, the composition of the Board remained remarkably stable over its decades of operation, which critics have argued contributed to its slipshod practices (Grekul et al., 2004; Wahlsten, 1997). In keeping with the construction of people with mental illness as dangerous breeders, the Act included a provision that "when it is proposed to discharge any inmate of a mental hospital, the discharging institution's Superintendent could refer the inmate to the Board." If, in turn, the Board was "unanimously of the opinion that the patient might safely be discharged if the danger of procreation with its attend risk of multiplication of the evil by transmission of the disability to progeny were eliminated," then the Board should "appoint some competent surgeon to perform the operation" (Government of Alberta, 1928). Thus, from its inception, the Sterilization Act was meant to be a vehicle for freeing people from the institutions and perhaps simultaneously freeing the province from paying for inmates' upkeep. Such operations were to be performed only after obtaining the consent of the inmate, if competent. However, given the choice between sterilization and internment in an asylum, even the original "voluntary" Act posed a slippery ethical slope in terms of voluntary consent. Finally, the Act provided assurances to surgeons performing eugenic surgeries that they would not be "liable to any civil action whatsoever by reason of the performance thereof" (Government of Alberta, 1928).

Despite what to modern eyes seem like extremely broad powers, the Eugenics Board found it difficult to find willing participants. The UFA Party, which had been so instrumental in lobbying for and implementing the original Act, had in 1935 lost their majority in the provincial legislature. However, the Social Credit Party, elected in 1935 and holding power in the province unopposed until 1971, had little difficulty sustaining the eugenic impetus initiated by the UFA. In 1937 an amendment to the Act was proposed by Dr W. W. Cross, the newly elected Social Credit Party's minister of health, seeking broader scope and less restrictive guidelines. Arguing that the benefits of eugenic sterilization for the general population outweighed the imposition on personal liberty of those deemed defective, proponents of the amendment proposed that the Eugenics Board, given unanimous agreement on specific cases, need not always obtain consent to pass candidates for surgery (Grekul et al., 2004; McLaren, 1990). The 1937 Amended Act opened with a section that discerned between "psychotic persons," which it failed to define in any specific way and "mentally defective persons," which it defined very loosely as "arrested or incomplete development before the age of 18 whether arising from inherent causes, disease or injury" (Government of Alberta, 1937). Based on these vague discernments, the Act implemented substantial changes that broadened the reach of the Eugenics Board and lessened its potential liabilities:

- *A shift from the language of heritability to the language of behaviour and risk.* Here, the reasons for deeming a psychotic or mentally defective person unfit for procreation included the transmission of heritable disorders but also extended to the "risk of mental injury, either to such person or his progeny." In these broadened clauses, the notion of risk and the assessment of appropriateness moved into the realm of speculation rather than science.

- *A significant loosening of the parameters of consent.* Now, only psychotic people who were deemed capable by their assessors were required to provide their consent. Those psychotics who were deemed incapable by the Board on the basis of records provided by the referring agents were not required to provide consent. Finally, there was no provision whatsoever requiring consent if someone was deemed to be a mental defective.
- *An expansion of the system that could identify and refer people for sterilization.* The sources of cases to be brought before the Board were now to be referred not only by asylum and institutional directors, but medical directors of any Mental Hygiene Clinic could also bring patients forward for consideration.
- *A widened set of protections for professionals involved in eugenic operations.* In the revised Act, protection from subsequent litigation included surgeons, the "person who consents" (which presumably included the director of the institution or hygiene clinic when the sterilization was involuntary), anyone who referred a patient, anyone who examined a patient, or any Board member (Government of Alberta, 1937). This last provision clearly indicates that, at some level, the government understood that what was being proposed was not going to be acceptable to at least some of the people who would be caught in its new, more comprehensive, eugenic net.

The implications of these changes for almost anyone experiencing mental health or social problems were significant, given the shift from heritability to risk. However, the implications of the consent requirement changes for inmates of Michener were enormous in that they were automatically considered to be mental defectives simply by virtue of their incarceration in the institution.

Sterilization and IQ Testing

The identification and classification of mental disability has been and continues to be highly contentious and riddled with ambiguities. In particular, the parameters of what was once characterized as "mentally defective" have been notoriously difficult to ascertain, shifting with differing definitions, disciplinary factions, the development of new categories of disability, and the economies and politics of differing testing instruments (Trent, 1994). The standardized IQ testing used to discern and categorize intelligence has been strongly critiqued as culturally problematic, too narrow in its concept of intelligence, and an artificial way in which to rank people along mathematical scales and norms, rather than a valid indicator of capacity (Gould, 1981).

Concerns about standardized testing are worrisome enough even under ideal conditions. However, the methods used to discern mental defect at Michener were hardly ideal, as the story of Leilani Muir attested. In her lawsuit against the Alberta Government, which involved an extensive and painstaking examination of the records relating to her history before and after her time at Michener, it became clear that Ms Muir had never been tested before her admission. Indeed, it was unclear from the admission forms whether any medical personnel had examined or signed off on any actual examination before or as part of Ms Muir's admission. Apparently, she was referred by a Mental Hygiene Clinic and the institution assumed that she would have received psychometric testing there, while the clinic assumed that her testing would occur at the institution. In short, testing for mental defect before her internment seems simply have been missed (*Muir v. Alberta*, 1996). Several years after admission, Leilani Muir did receive a psychometric assessment that scored her as having an IQ of 64, placing her well under the 70-point cut-off that the Eugenics Board claimed to use as its determinant of defectiveness. In the trial the courts dismissed this low score as inaccurate, and a test administered at the time of the trial found her score to be "well within the normal range" at more than 90 points.

The inaccuracy of her Michener tests can be attributed to a number of causes, including that Ms Muir, like many other inmates, was heavily and inappropriately medicated when tested, that she had not been well educated during her years in the institution, and that she had suffered the ill effects of sensory and intellectual deprivation within the institution. Thus, her scores were depressed in great part as a result of the conditions of her internment (*Muir v. Alberta*, 1996). In addition, the court found that the scoring of the tests to inform the decision on whether to sterilize Ms. Muir were arbitrary; her IQ scores showed borderline scores on at least one of three scales, meaning that she would only have barely fit within the range deemed "appropriate" by the Board for sterilization without consent, even if the tests had been properly administered.

That psychometric testing within the institution may have been inadequate or improperly administered as a matter of course is quite possible. Ex-worker Jim Sullivan worked as a student during the summers of his second and third years of university, and on graduation he came to work at Michener full time. He said:

> Oh yes, I worked as the senior psychologist when I was just recently graduated. I had a bachelor's degree in child psychology ... I had never given a WISC-R and I was a senior psychologist. I had seven people working under me. I learned fast!

The WISC-R, or Wechsler Intelligence Scale for Children (Revised), is a psychometric test that incorporates several subtests that together provide verbal, performance, and general IQ scores for children. It would be highly unusual for someone not certified as a psychologist to administer such testing, and in Alberta, even in 1974 when Jim began his new position, a bachelor's degree would in no way qualify someone to call themselves a psychologist or to administer psychological testing of this nature. In reflecting on his possible role in assisting the eugenic process, Jim said:

> Certainly when I tested a few of the School Age girls, 'cause they'd be about that right age – 11, 12, 13 – we did not know we were doing it for sterilization. We were never told that. We were never told there was going to be a eugenics board or anything ... We would be given a roster of people to screen for IQ, only IQ. Nothing else ... It was below 70 as I recall. And what they miss, of course, is these kids had been invariably culturally deprived for years.

Jim's description echoed some of the concerns raised in the Muir trial about IQ testing for the Eugenics Board: an inexperienced tester, a testing instrument that was itself not a real indicator of capability, and of course, children being tested who were doomed to fail because of their Michener experiences. In addition, we get a sense of the routinized quality of that testing. In Jim's description, children deemed ready for the IQ screening were those who were also ready for adult sexuality and hence ready to be considered for eugenic "repair."

A final concern about the use of psychometric testing to determine mental defectiveness as an objective guideline for sterilization is that, by the time of its heightened operations in the 1950s and 1960s, the Eugenics Board seemed to have disposed of even that flimsy safeguard and was making judgments based on feelings rather than numbers. Muir's lawyers discovered several cases among the files where what little due process was in place was ignored in favour of insubstantial evidence. In her judgment, Justice Veit noted:

> Despite the fact that the Eugenics Board claimed to have an IQ cut-off point of 70, persons above that level were approved for sterilization; some of those persons had conditions such as spinal meningitis, hearing defects, or had been accused of criminal offences. (*Muir v. Alberta*, 1996, p. 38)

A telling example of the judgment process was the case of a young deaf teen. His IQ had been tested at 76; nevertheless, the Board approved his case and he was subsequently sterilized. The record shows that, in addition to "intelligence," the Board took the child's poor work ethic and frequent masturbation into account to aid its decision. In the Muir case Dr Margaret Thompson, a geneticist who was a member of the Board that had approved the sterilization of this boy, was called as an expert witness. In her examination, she explained the decision, testifying that

> social success is a factor to be taken into account in a sterilization decision. When the school reported that he was a poor worker, [Dr Thompson] concluded that despite all the information that he was a nice quiet boy, he was not really functioning in society. She said that she was being protective of him when she decided to have him sterilized. (*Muir v. Alberta*, 1996, p. 30)

As additional evidence in the Muir trial, Thompson acknowledged that she, as a Board member, had also approved the sterilization of male children with Down syndrome even though it was clearly known at the time that male Down syndrome children are unlikely to be fertile. Her response was that it did no harm and that sterilization was important to "make assurance sure" (*Muir v. Alberta*, 1996, p. 30).

Surveillance and Sterilization

A final troubling aspect of the 1937 amended Sterilization Act lay in the addition of the Mental Hygiene Clinics[1] as new sources for identifying and recommending individuals for processing by the Eugenics Board. The first permanent Mental Hygiene Clinics were established in 1929 in Edmonton and Calgary as an offshoot of the earlier mental health surveys conducted by Clarence Hincks; their original mandate was to identify and prevent juvenile delinquency (Dechant, 2006). Throughout the 1930s, an additional six locations across the province were established, offering weekly or bi-weekly clinics, and in 1934 the implementation of a travelling clinic once yearly to northern locales was added (Dechant, 2006). Clinics were typically minimally staffed by a psychiatrist and a social worker, and they saw both adults and children in the community who were either self-referred, or more typically, referred by family physicians or teachers. The operations of the clinics were described by Mr E. J. Kibblewhite, who was an appointed member of the Eugenics Board from 1969 to 1972, as follows:

> The psychiatrist in every case interviews the patient and relatives and guardians where this is possible, and does what examining seems indicated in the physical, neurological and psychiatric fields. The social worker assists in the interviews and does any psychological and mental testing work required, and in a certain number of cases, outside investigation work. (Kibblewhite as cited in Dechant, 2006, p. 44)

Although the intention and undoubtedly much of the work of the clinics was needed and helpful to the citizens of a developing and often harsh society, the mandate of these clinics to engage in significant testing and examining of citizens, coupled with the investigative work of social workers in people's homes, produced a significantly broadened capacity for surveillance across the province. In addition, at least in the case of the Red Deer Guidance Clinic, the relationship to the institution whose inmates were most likely to come under the eugenic lens was quite intimate, since the director of the Clinic at Red Deer visited the Michener Centre once weekly as a consultant on inmate cases (LeVann, 1954, 1967–1968). In addition, the Eugenics Board on occasion made special tours of the Guidance Clinics for educational and planning purposes, as part of their duties and as directed by the minister of health (c.f. LeVann, 1961–1962; McCullough, 1940).

Under the amended Sterilization Act, the new mandate of these clinics to locate and present individuals for consideration by the Alberta Eugenics Board had tremendous effects. Following the passing of the 1937 amendment, the Eugenics Board's annual reports began to include notations about the role of Guidance Clinics in locating and referring people for Eugenics Board considerations. From these notations, which were admittedly not reported every year, we learn that over a 28-year period, 47% of all cases referred to the Eugenics Board for approval came through the provincial Guidance Clinics (see Table 9.1). More importantly, over the decades of the clinics' capacity to refer, the percentage of all cases they referred steadily increased so that for approximately the last 15 years of the Eugenics Board operations, the clinics referred fully 70% of cases. Thus, at least part of the steady increase in "successful" cases that occurred over the duration of the eugenics program can be attributed to this heightened capacity of the clinics to bring the broader community into the purview of the Eugenics Board.

The annual reports for PTS Michener that included information about the number of Guidance Clinics referrals invariably concluded with the phrase, "although some of these had been institutionalized prior to presentation," indicating some of the collaboration and overlap that existed between the institution and the clinics. The mandate of the clinics was to both refer children for admission to institutions, including Michener, and to follow up on the children when and if they were returned to community life. Thus, the heightened powers of the clinics served not only to increase the numbers of children and young adults referred for sterilization but also contributed to the tremendous population growth that occurred in the institution during the 1950s to 1970s. The clinics became a lens onto the community and a funnel into the institutions.

Table 9.1 Cases Referred by Guidance Clinics, by Gender, for Selected Years

Year	Number of Cases Passed	Referred by Guidance Clinic	Percentage Referred	Male	Female	% Male
1940	114	16	14	6	10	38
1941	117	34	29	11	23	32
1945	121	36	30	12	24	33
1946	106	23	22	9	14	39
1947	91	13	14	4	9	21
1949	109	31	28	8	23	26
1954	81	41	51	25	16	61
1956	72	50	69	28	22	56
1957	128	63	49	24	39	38
1959–60	102	76	75	35	41	46
1961–62	111	76	68	35	41	46
1963–4	106	76	72	36	40	47
1963–64	125	88	70	37	51	42
1967–68	82	60	73	23	37	38
Totals	1,465	683	47	293	380	43

Source: Department of Mental Health Annual Reports, 1940–1968.

There was one final amendment made to the Act in 1942 which broadened the range of the Eugenics Board further by expanding on the qualities of individuals who would be deemed appropriate for eugenic consideration. The new Act included people with "neurosyphyllis with deterioration *not* amounting to psychosis ... epilepsy with psychosis *or* mental deterioration or ... Huntington's Chorea" (Government of Alberta, 1942). While people with epilepsy and syphilis could be considered, they still were required to provide their consent. However, consent was not required from individuals with Huntington's chorea, with or without psychosis; these people composed a new group who could be sterilized without their consent. Thus, at a time when the excesses of Nazi racial hygiene were already becoming known in the Western world, the province increased its eugenic action to take in new categories of people, including those who were less psychologically compromised by their conditions than previously considered appropriate. Finally, the inclusion specifically of people with syphilis reflects a continuing focus not necessarily on heritability but on the sexual morality of people the state saw as appropriate to be surveilled and contained through the Sexual Sterilization Act.

The Eugenics Board

The Board appointed to oversee and implement the practical side of the Sterilization Act has been strongly critiqued for its methods and practices. Douglas Wahlsten (1997), a behavioural geneticist at the University of Alberta who has written about the Leilani Muir trial and the Alberta Eugenics Board, argued that the Board was able to operate outside of the courts and public scrutiny for several reasons. First, appointment to the Board was made by the government through the University of Alberta, without any outside checks and balances and without a need for public announcements (Wahlsten, 1997). In practice, the appointment process was less important than one might imagine, as Dr J. M. MacEachran, a professor and chair in philosophy at the University of Alberta, was appointed as the original Eugenics Board chair and he remained in that position for the better part of 40 years. Besides MacEachran, the Board make-up remained largely unchanged for the duration of its operations, including a total of only 21 members over its 43 years (Grekul, Krahn, & Odynak, 2004; Wahlsten, 1997). The membership stability permitted a sustained climate of acceptance and enthusiasm for the eugenic project, accompanied by a strongly bureaucratic and routinized approach. In addition, Board meetings were not like a hearing, but were conducted behind closed doors, often without the individual present, and frequently on the isolated campuses of the institutions in which selection and operations took place. Finally, the Board make-up included the Michener superintendent, which posed a conflict of interest, because the man responsible for deciding the reproductive fate of these children was also a person interested in controlling that reproduction within his institution (Wahlsten, 1997). An additional conflict concerning the specific membership of Leonard J. LeVann arose from the fact that biological materials extracted from inmates during sterilization surgeries fed directly the research that LeVann was conducting with geneticist and fellow Eugenics Board member Margaret Thompson, whose ideas about ethics and eugenics were expressed in her expert witness testimony during the Muir trial, cited earlier (*Muir v. Alberta*, 1996; Wahlsten, 1997).

That the Board was and remained enthusiastic about its work and committed to the goals of sterilizing Alberta's "unfit" can be read in the minutes of a meeting in late February 1972. Here, the Board chairman, Dr R. K. Thomson, "spoke briefly to the members in regard to the proposed repealing of the Sexual Sterilization Act at the next sitting of the Legislative Assembly" slated to take place on June 2 – just three months later (Thomson, 1972, p. 2). Rather than suggest a ratcheting back of operations, the chairman instead noted his views against the repeal and advised that he would be preparing a response to a letter received from the newly appointed director of the Division of Mental Health about the Board's objections. The Board went on, after this meeting, to schedule continuing regular meetings and approve sterilizations right up until the end of the Act's force.

Eugenic operations were not limited to vasectomies or tubal ligations; they occasionally and without any clearly provided medical reason included appendectomies, the removal of ovaries and testicles, and less frequently, the removal of uteruses (hysterectomies) or testicular materials for biopsy (MacEachran, 1960; *Muir v. Alberta*, 1996). In my examination of 128 randomly selected Alberta Eugenics Board meeting minutes, notations about the type of surgery were uniformly given without clarification or justification. Entries simply listed the type of operation to be performed – vasectomy (male sterilization by cutting the vas deferens), salpingectomy (female sterilization by cutting the fallopian tubes), orchidectomy (male castration by removing the testicles), or oophorectomy (female castration by removing the ovaries). Although explanations were absent, there were occasional clues as to the "social" reasons used to justify these additional surgeries. For example, in Case #4219, a young woman's mother requested that her sterilization include castration by oophorectomy in addition to sterilization, "as she finds if very difficult to look after [X] at the time of her periods" during the occasions when the daughter made home visits (Thomson, 1966, p. 2). Other social reasons could have included abnormal sexual behaviour or aggression, which presumably would be improved by reducing the hormone levels of the young people under consideration; in short, surgical castration was used to make the lives of caregivers easier.

While the Board minutes read in a highly routinized, sparse, and matter of fact way, one can also occasionally tell that the surgeries themselves were not always carefully conducted. For example, on 9 June 1947, the Board discussed a woman who had had a salpingectomy performed earlier and who was now "about three months pregnant"; an examining physician had performed a laparoscopy and found that one of the tubes had not been touched, although the woman's sterilization operation report indicated that "both tubes were excised, cauterized with carbolic followed by alcohol, and then inverted." The Board ordered a second operation, to be followed up in subsequent hearings (MacEachran, 1947b, p. 1). Similarly, on 20 September 1957, the Board was presented with the case of a female who, despite having had her ovaries removed in a previous eugenic surgery, continued to menstruate. Using a rationale similar to that of Dr Margaret Thompson, who was cited above as justifying sterilizing young males with Down syndrome as "making assurance sure" (*Muir v. Alberta*, 1996, p. 30), the Board concluded:

> the operation had not been complete [and] after *careful consideration* [emphasis added], [the Board] directed that another attempt be made to remove both ovaries, and as a precautionary measure, a salpingectomy be performed at the same time. (MacEachran, 1957b, p. 2)

Despite the above claim, any description of the Board as entering into its decisions after "careful consideration" must be treated with some cynicism. With each case presented for consideration, the Board was to assess the individual's diagnosis, physical examination records, family history, personal history, school history, psychometric results, economic history, personality, previous illnesses, jail record, present illnesses, attitude, attitude of parent, reason for recommended sterilization, and any prior Board encounters (Park & Radford, 1998). However, the Board heard these cases in such a way that properly assessing any information would have been extremely difficult. More often than not, the case was presented without the attendance of the individual so that the Board saw only the file and assessments made by Guidance Clinic or institutional staff (Park & Radford, 1998). In addition, the meetings operated like a machine, taking a shockingly brief time to accomplish the Board's work. On 29 January 1948, the Board met at 10:00 in the morning at the Provincial Mental Hospital at Ponoka, approving six vasectomies, one orchidectomy/castration, and 10 salpingectomies; they then broke at 12:00 for lunch and drove an hour down the road to the Provincial Training School, where they reconvened at 3:00 in order to approve a further two vasectomies, three orchidectomy/castrations, and four salpingectomies, adjourning at 5:00 (MacEachran, 1947a). Thus, in four hours of meeting time, the lives of 24 individuals were "carefully considered" at an average of 10 minutes per case. The speedy consideration of files was typical.[2] On 23 April 1954 the Board decided 10 cases in 1 hour and 15 minutes, or 7.5 minutes per case (MacEachran, 1954); on 9 October 1963, the Board approved eight salpingectomies, two vasectomies, and one oophorectomy/castration in a meeting that lasted 2 hours and 15 minutes, or 12.3 minutes per case (MacEachran, 1963); and in another session, on 8 October 1968 at Michener, 10 cases were heard and approved in only 9 minutes per case (Thomson, 1968). Bear in mind that, during all these meetings, time was taken to sign forms in connection with the cases, consider and approve previous meeting minutes, and set times of subsequent meetings so that the time for considering files was fitted in around bureaucratic minutiae.

The meeting minutes provided commencement and adjournment times, a listing of Board members present and absent, locations of the meetings, notations about who would act as secretary for the meeting, indications of which surgeon would be appointed to perform the surgeries, and simple lists of case numbers and names presented. There was no discussion of the cases themselves, no indication of the presence or absence at the hearings of the individuals whose cases were being presented for decisions, nor was there mention of the kinds of considerations that went into the decision making about individual cases. Where there *was* discussion recorded, it centres on administrative matters, such as acknowledging letters of thanks from institutions for Board visits, schedules for upcoming meetings, decisions about sending flowers for sick or retiring colleagues, discussions about equity in assigning surgeons to perform operations, or special requests, such as the one on 8 June 1956 by a parent wanting to have the surgery done closer to her home in Edmonton, with an ensuing lengthy discussion about recouping surgery costs (MacEachran, 1956).

The bulk of the minutes consisted of lists of cases presented, followed by lists indicating whether the cases were *Passed Clear* (approved, without consent required), or *Passed Pending Consent of the Patient, Consent of Patient and Husband,*[3] *Patient and Mother, or Patient and Father.* These lists of cases presented and processed were depressingly uniform; I reviewed minutes of 128 meetings of the Eugenics Board, and not once was a case *not* passed. There was one distinctive difference, however, in terms of whether the surgeries are *Passed Clear* or they are passed subject to receiving consent from the patient or a guardian. When the meetings were held at Michener, the lists read *Passed Clear* with unwavering uniformity, reflecting that Michener inmates were not required to provide consent because they were de facto considered to be mentally defective. A rare exception to this rule provides us with some insight into how the Act was interpreted and how distinctions between labels of "psychosis" or "mental defect" were applied. A female whose case was presented at a meeting held at the Alberta Mental Hospital in Ponoka was passed for a salpingectomy but with the following notation:

Passed subject to consent of patient, with condition that if upon recovery consent is not given, the patient should be re-tested and, should the psychometric examination indicate mental deficiency, the patient then be represented to the Board prior to discharge. (MacEachran, 1957a, p. 1)

In this instance, because the inmate was in a psychotic state at the time of the hearing, she could not legally be approved without consent, could not in fact

provide that consent herself, nor could she be tested accurately for mental defect and be operable without her consent. To deal with this quandary, the Board
made the provision that, if she recovered from her psychosis, she would be
asked whether she consented to sterilization. If she did not consent, then an IQ
test might take care of the matter. If she scored below 70, her case would then
be reheard so that she could be Passed Clear and operated on without her consent before discharge. Clearly, the Board used IQ scores as a serious – and cynical – mechanism for eugenic decision making and action.

A final and important aspect of the lists provided by the Eugenics Board is
that they show how Alberta's eugenic actions were highly gendered, with female
surgeries significantly overrepresented (see Figure 9.1). Because of its captive
population of individuals deemed mentally defective, Michener became the primary feeder institution for eugenic consideration (Grekul, Krahn, & Odynak,
2004), so it would follow that the eugenic numbers would be in keeping with the
gender ratios in the institution. However, the institution consistently housed
more males than females (see Figure 9.2.), perhaps because boys presented more
alarming behavioural challenges in their communities. The overrepresentation
of females in the eugenic population thus takes on more weight when contrasted
against the overrepresentation of males in the actual Michener population.

The gendered aspects of the Eugenics Board's actions were multiple. In addition to the numbers of surgeries performed, the numbers of cases presented to
the Board favoured females over males. There are a number of speculative reasons for this gendered eugenic culture. First, the maternal feminist UFWA
leadership played a strong early role in pushing for eugenic legislation, in great
part because of their gendered roles in government. The responsibilities of
UFWA women for family, health, and social welfare portfolios as ministers and
members of Parliament, in the courts as magistrates, and in the communities
as doctors and social workers, contributed to their enthusiasm for eugenics as
a solution to social issues. It also brought them into contact with women whose
family problems and unwanted pregnancies were deeply burdensome, and
these gendered foundations informed the program from its beginnings. Similarly, those nurses and social workers who performed family histories and assessments for the Mental Health/Guidance Clinics that acted as clearinghouses
for the eugenic cases saw women as the means of containing "taint" and its
ensuing social ills. Grekul (2008) has argued that women who came into contact with the eugenic machine were targeted for moral reasons. Thus, women
whose families were plagued by poverty or addiction issues were chosen because they were "overly" fertile in the community, or women who were on the
borderline of mental defect but who could "pass" as normal in the community
were pinpointed as dangerous breeders, or women who had borne illegitimate

Figure 9.1 Operations performed on cases passed by the Eugenics Board, by gender, for selected years.

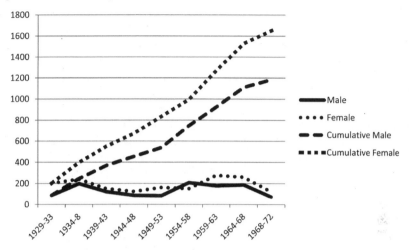

Sources: The Eugenics Board (1968); Grekul (2002).

Figure 9.2 Population of Michener by gender for selected years.

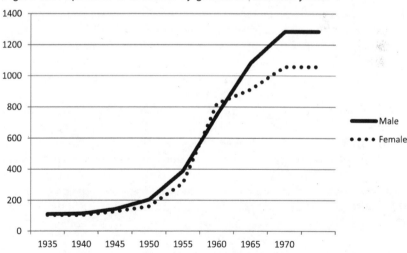

Source: Alberta Social Services and Community Health (1985).

children or who engaged in questionable or promiscuous sexual behaviour in the community were tagged as deviant (Grekul, 2008). These justifications also figured into decisions concerning Michener females, whose family back-grounds would certainly have been perceived as risk factors for future "bad breeding;" however, as will be heard in the narratives of survivors, sometimes sterilizations occurred at Michener to cover up gendered sexual activities within the institution.

Until now, my analysis of Alberta's eugenic activities has focused on the Sexual Sterilization Act, the records of Eugenics Board meetings, the Muir court case, and the annual reports to the minister of health. I now turn to survivors' descriptions as a way of understanding the process as it was experienced and to begin to convey the impact of these routinized and cynical actions.

Survivors' Descriptions of Sterilization

It moved me, when speaking with survivors, to note that although they were usually able to speak about their experiences of violence, abuse, and neglect with forthrightness, when it came to speaking about sterilization, there was much more shame in discussing what had been done to them. Of the 22 survivors, 9 did not disclose whether they had been sterilized, 2 were not sterilized, and the remaining 11 (6 females, 5 males) admitted to being sterilized during their time at Michener. I suspect that more than 11 of the survivors had been sterilized; however, several explicitly declined to speak about sterilization issues. Survivors were often not able to say how old they'd been when the operations occurred, in part because of the general timelessness of a history lived in monotony and deprivation, but also because some of them only came to understand that they had been sterilized after leaving Michener.

Ray Petrenko was an exception, as he remembered the process quite clearly. Ray recalled this mother and father coming to visit him, which was a memorable occasion in itself. They told him that he would be having an operation because "people in Michener Centre said that this had to be done because they didn't want people that were living in Michener Centre to have, to make little kids." Ray, who was 16 years old at the time, and probably old enough to understand what was happening to him, went on to say that he himself was not asked for his permission: "all we were told was that we were going to go on a trip, but they didn't tell me, they just told my Mom and Dad that this had to be done." He did recall being part of a formal Eugenics Board process, noting:

It was a Board that I remember that I went in front of, and they asked me how I liked it in the institution. You were afraid to say if you didn't like it because there were people from Michener there nudging you to say you liked it. I felt that I was being, I felt I was being pushed ... and I didn't know until I moved out of Red Deer that this board was put together by the government, and it was a sterilization board.

Ray also remembered being coached before going into the meeting as to what he should say: "we were told to say that everything was fine, that you were treated properly." From Ray's narrative, we get a glimpse into how hearings were conducted. Children and young adults were occasionally brought before the Board but were given little information about what the hearings' purpose was. They were then asked a series of questions that, because of the Board's composition, the presence of Michener staff, and the location of the hearing on the Michener sites, would have been very difficult to answer honestly, and would not have invited inmates' questions in return.

A few weeks later, Ray and a number of other inmates were told they "were going on a trip" and then taken to the Clinical Building on the Michener campus for admission and surgery. While Ray did not recall any examination or testing before the Board hearing, he clearly remembered the pre-surgery medical examination he underwent, because he was processed by a woman doctor:

I had never seen a woman doctor, because I'm a guy, before. I felt kind of embarrassed because where she was examining me before the surgery – I had to take off my underclothes and she examined the testicles and all that. I couldn't, you know, at that time I knew that my body was private and I felt embarrassed ... it was scary because I didn't know why I was being examined because I wasn't sick or nothing. But, when you got to be sixteen, that was the rule, I guess.

It was only later, while still in the institution that Ray began to understand what had happened to him. He said, "eventually [my friend] and I, and other people, would talk about it by ourselves, you know." Eventually, he pressed his parents for information, and after some time they admitted to having consented to his sterilization. Ray said, "But I don't blame my parents that I'm – doctors said that people with disabilities had to have this sterilization done."

In a similar vein, Sandra Karnak described her sterilization occurring without any meaningful preparation. She had the flu when she was 13 years old and was sent to the infirmary for care. While there, she described, "they kept me in that room and had me doped up and then they shaved me ... they put me out, and I don't remember after that."

Ex-worker Jim Sullivan concurred with Ray's and Sandra's descriptions of inmates not being properly told or prepared for the sterilization operation:

When these guys would end up being sterilized, they wouldn't have any notion of
what that would really mean. Afterwards, they would say, "they fixed me and they
never told me," but nothing before [the surgery].

From both Ray and Jim's descriptions, it appears that although there was a
culture of formal dishonesty and silence before the sterilization process, for
some of the inmates there was also an underground knowledge about sterilization, at least after the fact when young inmates began to put the pieces together.
These two bodies of competing understanding – on the one hand, a cloak of
secrecy, and on the other, a covert knowledge – undoubtedly contributed to a
culture of shame and fear.

For some, the secrecy and confusion surrounding sterilization has continued.
Gerta Muller described her surgery in similar terms as Ray, but she remained
unclear even today as to whether she had a hysterectomy or oophorectomy,
saying, "I don't know exactly. I'll never know exactly either." Nevertheless, she
does know that she cannot bear children. She also noted that "they gave me the
operation because I don't walk very well," but this speculative explanation only
came to her long after the fact, from her physician in the community.

For others, although there was some discussion before sterilization, it was
couched in indirect terms or stated as an inevitability. For example, ex-worker
Evelyn said that most of the people she dealt with on the Low Grade ward where
she worked did not menstruate because they were given a hysterectomy as
"standard practice, as soon as you were thirteen, I do remember on our ward ...
the charge nurse arranged for some young girl to go for a hysterectomy." In this
narrative, yet again, we hear how bodies were manipulated to facilitate the ease
and efficiency of care for workers, particularly when Low Grades were involved,
and how this became a routine and inevitable part of treatment.

Harvey Brown's story shed further light on the routine quality of sterilization in the institution. Harvey was sterilized at 15 years of age. When asked
whether he had known about the surgery prior to its occurrence, he said, "No,
not really. Well, they were going to tie my cords." He explained that while he
was told that his "cords" would be tied, at that young age he had no idea what
that actually meant in either the short or long term. Harvey did not go in
front of the Eugenics Board. Instead, he said, "they told my dad what was going to happen when I was 13 years old, when I first moved in," and in turn, his
father presented this information to him as something that could be neither
refused or deferred. Harvey did not need to attend any hearing concerning
his sterilization because his father had already signed the forms giving consent during his admission to Michener; in his case, sterilization was written
into his internment. This consent on arrival was true in Leilani Muir's case as

well. On admission, Ms Muir's mother signed a form that stated, "I am agreeable that sterilization be performed on my child Leilani Marie Scorah if this is deemed advisable by the Provincial Eugenics Board" (*Muir v. Alberta*, 1996, p. 9). At no other point in Ms Muir's institutionalization and sterilization process was her mother required to provide any further agreement or consultation; the deed was done as a routine part of the admission process (*Muir v. Alberta*, 1996).

The routinization of sterilization decisions, taken almost as an inevitable part of being a Michener inmate, is reflected in the following comments from Donna Bogdan:

> They said that we're going to have an operation, and I didn't quite understand what they meant by sterilization or anything. They never went into detail. So all of us had to go in to a Eugenics Board. They were the ones that made the decision. They sterilized us and that was that. Everybody had to go through it. It was routine. They said, "You're going to get your appendix out" or something. I wasn't sure, I didn't understand. I thought, well, that was the routine that was done.

Donna's mention of the appendectomy reflects what witnesses said during the preparation for the Muir trail: repeatedly, people described being deceived by being told they were having routine appendectomies, rather than that they would be undergoing eugenic surgery (*Muir v. Alberta*, 1996).

In terms of inmates' acquiescence to the surgeries, given the sensitivity of many preteens and teenagers about their bodies and sexuality, it is not surprising that these young people would find it difficult to ask questions or seek clarification. As well, given the oppressive culture of everyday life in the institution, the inability of these children to question authority or imagine having a voice in their own affairs should not be surprising. Finally, when we consider the unbridled authority of the Eugenics Board and its colluding relationship with the institution's administration, we can be sure that the climate in which these operations occurred was indeed unassailable and incomprehensible.

Finally, it should be noted that even parents were not always sure what was happening in terms of sterilization. When Gerta Muller left the institution and was discussing participation in one of the sterilization lawsuits against the government, she spoke with her parents about what they had known about her surgery. Her mother told her that although she had consented to the surgery, she said, "well, we thought it was about your nerves." Gerta went on to say, "They didn't even know. Nobody knew." This was also apparent during my interview with Carl Semkow's mother, Mavis. Early in the interview, when I was collecting simple demographic information, she stated that Carl had not been sterilized at Michener. However, later on when I asked specifically about consent for sterilization, she expressed less certainty:

> I don't remember if I signed anything like that or not. I know they sent me papers to sign to have his teeth taken out ... but a paper for sterilization, I don't remember if I ever signed. I can only remember signing my name once when we took him up, but I'm not sure what that meant.

While Mavis's statement cannot be taken as saying that she did sign a release, it also demonstrates the lack of clarity involved in the institutional orders concerning consent, information, and transparency relating to the bodies of Michener inmates. In the end, both alternatives in Mavis's story – consent form signed or not – are equally plausible.

Sterilization and Sexuality

That sexuality – and particularly, *female* sexuality – was policed through eugenic surgeries was made clear in the final judgment of the Leilani Muir case for unlawful sterilization, where Justice Viet argued that

> in some cases, the board authorized the hysterectomy or oophorectomy in order to eliminate menstruation in females; according to the language of one typical case, the female trainees were "difficult to handle and to keep clean during menstrual periods." These operations were also ordered where female trainees masturbated or had lesbian tendencies. (*Muir v. Alberta*, 1996, p. 38)

Sterilization was often scheduled at the time of puberty, as survivors' narratives attested and as ex-worker Evelyn described. However, it also appears that in some cases, particularly among High Grade inmates who were more likely to become sexually active, sterilization was done in response to sexuality rather than simply to prevent it. Gerta Muller described a disturbing story:

> This girl, [X], she was caught and raped ... she was telling us the story and we were laughing and snickering, not that we didn't believe her, but we thought it was funny. I mean, from Ward 9, the boys were bullies. That's why she got the operation, because she got pregnant.

In Gerta's story we hear how the sexual assault of a young woman in care was not responded to with protection or assistance but instead with erasure. Further, by sterilizing her, any subsequent abuses would have been able to go underground. In essence sterilization increased the vulnerability of this girl, as it would hide at least some of the effects of sexual abuse.

Jim Sullivan provided a more global perspective on the intersections between sterilization and the covering up of pregnancies in the institution:

> There were pregnancies, but they were well-hidden. I say that from a word-of-mouth standpoint. You often heard of that, they would be very quickly moved over to the infirmary and it was always some minor surgery – abortion and sterilization. It's pure conjecture on my part only because it was all over, we heard it everywhere.

Although Jim's description was distanced in tone, Sandra's description was much more personal. Recall that Sandra was only 13 years old when, experiencing flu-like symptoms, she was sent to the infirmary. While there, she was rushed to surgery. Clearly, at some point, someone informed her that she had been pregnant before her surgery. She described the aftermath of her surgery:

> I asked and asked the supervisor, "Was I really pregnant, or what?" She said, "Yes." I asked, "Was it a girl or boy?" and they wouldn't tell me. I know who the father was, but I couldn't tell. I couldn't tell him anything because he couldn't see the kid.

In Sandra's story there is much that is difficult to consider. A young girl, barely at the age of puberty, living in intolerable and socially isolated conditions, becomes pregnant. Then, without any formality or consultation, she loses not only the baby but any hope of having future children, all under the guise of social improvement and care. Finally, in a culture of secrecy and deceit, the entire experience is erased, and she is left with no one to speak with about it. It is also important to note that the unsavoury connection between sexual abuse inside the institution and sexual sterilization did not necessarily end with the repeal of the Sterilization Act. In one instance, 13 years after the repeal of the Act, a "low-functioning" inmate who could not speak was "found to be 19 weeks pregnant during a medical examination" and was given an abortion three days later, all presumably without her consent (Monchuk, 1985c). It is unclear from the newspaper coverage whether parents, family members, public guardians were involved in this decision to provide an abortion. However, given the woman's non-verbal and intellectual assessment, it is highly unlikely that she would have been consulted on the decision to abort, just as she was not consulted on the sex that led to the pregnancy.

Despite the high profile of this case – it made it to the newspapers and led to an RCMP criminal investigation – there is little satisfaction to be had about how the case was handled. This inmate lived on an all-female, locked ward, and although the early investigation did not rule out the possibility that one of the six male staff members on that ward had perpetrated the sexual assault, no criminal charges were laid, reflecting an internal culture that made uncovering how such acts were perpetrated inside the institution extremely difficult (Monchuk, 1985d).

Sterilization After-Effects

If eugenic sterilization in Alberta in general, and among the Michener population in particular, really was motivated by concerns over heritability and taint, then people should have been released following sterilization. And indeed, sterilization – as was the clear intent of the original 1927 Sexual Sterilization Act – was supposed to be offered to inmates' parents or to inmates who were able to give their consent, as a condition for release back into the community (*Muir v. Alberta*, 1996). However, as often as not, sterilization bore little connection to freedom inside or outside the institution. Within the institution, even after being sterilized, survivors continued to be housed in gender-segregated and locked units, and their personal lives remained subject to surveillance and control. Sterilized inmates typically were not released back into the community because they were too highly valued inside the institutional walls as helpers and workers and in the broader community as an unpaid army of docile labourers (*Muir v. Alberta*, 1996). Thus, sterilization, although promised as such, was not a route to freedom. This fact was reflected among the survivors I interviewed. Of 11 people sterilized, none were released back into the community until many years later, when they left Michener as part of the deinstitutionalization movement.

These practices of continued internment not only show the exploitation of inmate labour that was endemic in the institution but also seriously undermine the genetic/eugenic rationale for sterilizing inmates. The eugenic operations at Michener thus were grounded in disability discrimination, disdain for these children's human and civil rights, and a sense of absolute control over these children's bodies as objects to be managed and used at will. The routine, unthinking, and disdainful treatment threaded throughout the eugenic process does not reflect a scientific set of attitudes but instead "degenerated into unscientific practices ... because the members of the board thought that it was socially appropriate to control the reproduction of 'these people'" (*Muir v. Alberta*, 1996, p. 32). In short, the processes of dehumanization that occurred within the institution also extended to the Eugenics Board's dealings with institutional inmates; these were simply creatures, not lives that mattered.

In her conclusion of the Muir case, the judge noted that not only was the surgery itself irreversible, but the emotional damage to Ms Muir was catastrophic and ongoing. This was true for the people with whom I spoke as well. For some, the violation of their ability to choose and to control their own bodies was paramount. Ray said, "I felt dirty inside because I figured that somebody had taken part of my body away from me." Echoing this, Sandra Karnak said, "I felt lost, like something had been taken away from me." For yet others, to have been lied to and to not have been asked for consent was foregrounded. To not have been able to choose, indeed, not to have even been asked, felt like the deepest violation.

For Harvey, though, the issue came down to children. He acknowledged that he wished he'd been asked, but he also noted that if he had been asked, he wouldn't have understood what he was giving up. Life in the institution had simply never provided him with an opportunity to understand human connection or family or to even vaguely entertain the possibility of being able to make a contribution. He said:

> Well, see now, it's a completely different story since I moved [out of Michener], since I live in the community ... I could probably, with some help, take care of a child. That's what makes my day, well it makes my whole day at WalMart when somebody comes up and asks for help, and I think I could have done that. I could have been a good father.

In Harvey's description we hear the real price of these high-handed decisions and actions. For Harvey and those who share his experiences, the possibilities of intimate human connection through creating and sustaining a new life remain compelling yet impossible desires.

Conclusion

The passive eugenic actions of institutionalization and segregation in Alberta were coupled with an enduring active eugenics program that lasted 44 years. Blossoming out of progressivist urges to improve the nation and provide women with the capacity to limit their family size, the eugenics movement also incorporated foundational notions of racism, sexism, imperialism, and, with the 1937 amendment to the Sexual Sterilization Act, virulent ableism. Once established, the Eugenics Board and the government that regulated it fostered an exceptionally cynical and routinized process of evaluation and approvals, working hand in hand with other government agencies, including the institutions and the network of Mental Hygiene/Guidance Clinics that funnelled citizens into the institutions and the eugenic machine. Of the almost 5000 cases put before the Board, fewer than 1% were not approved; and of those cases not requiring consent because of the mental defect provisions, almost all went on to surgery (Grekul, 2002). Cases were heard in consistently heartless circumstances, and the "good work" of the Board went on unimpeded and unchallenged long after the science of eugenics was well discredited. The human cost of this brutal system was tacitly acknowledged by the government itself when in 1995 the Muir lawsuit was launched. The government could have invoked a statute of limitations clause on the case, making it impossible for Leilani and her lawyers to go to trial. However, following significant public outcry after the state threatened to do so, it withdrew its objections and permitted the trial to go forward, in essence acknowledging its culpability (*Muir v. Alberta*, 1996). In 1999, after a number of subsequent successful class action lawsuits, the government made a formal apology for the statue and for the way it was implemented ("Alberta Apologizes," 1999).

When I discuss eugenics or teach it in my classes, most people seem truly horrified that such action could have occurred so recently in a modern, progressive nation state. They tend to be much less shocked when they learn of a system of institutions for people deemed to be "mentally defective" or intellectually disabled or mentally ill, at least until they are educated about the grim details of what passive eugenics in the form of institutionalization can look like. While it is not my intention here to underestimate the harms of active eugenic programs, it is also important to understand that the damage of long-term internment in places like Michener Centre also amounts to significant and sustained state-sanctioned abuse.

There has been no series of lawsuits and apologies relating to passive eugenics comparable to that achieved for active eugenics. Further, although the state has apologized for the eugenic program, even in the Muir court case and judgment, there is a clear sense that institutionalization for "some people" is acceptable or at least appropriate. A significant portion of the judgment against the state during the Muir trial rested on the notion that Ms Muir had been incorrectly deemed to be mentally defective, and thus both her internment and sterilization were particularly onerous. Indeed, the judgment included $125,000 to compensate Ms Muir for the incorrect assessment of her as a "moron, a high grade mental defective [because] this stigma has humiliated Ms. Muir every day of her life, in her relations with her family and friends and with her employers" (*Muir v. Alberta*, 1996, p. 3). In addition, she was awarded another $250,000 for "improper detention" that led to many travesties to her young person: loss of liberty, loss of reputation, humiliation and disgrace; pain and suffering, loss of enjoyment of life, loss of normal developmental experiences, loss of civil rights, loss of contact with family and friend, subjection to institutional discipline. (*Muir v. Alberta*, 1996, p. 4)

Finally, Ms Muir was awarded $250,280 for pain and suffering related to "wrongful sterilization." The weight of the settlement thus was based on Ms Muir's wrongful confinement and her stigmatization stemming from that wrongful confinement in an institutions for mental defectives, intimating that these aspects – being mistakenly institutionalized and subsequently stigmatized – were the worst things that had happened to her. On the one hand, that argument implied that it was inappropriate to intern people who are "like the rest of us" at places like the Michener Centre, but on the other hand, the question about the appropriateness of the institutional system itself remained unchallenged. This is dangerous thinking. The point surely must be that eugenics – in its active surgical forms or in the passive form of institutionalization and its attendant travesties – is unacceptable to inflict on anyone.

Chapter Ten

But That's All in the Past, Isn't It?

The last half of the twentieth century saw significant changes to services offered to people with intellectual disabilities in the West, as the result of a number of highly publicized exposés of institutional life. Several high-profile Americans consciously chose to take intellectual disability out of the closet and worked assiduously to change attitudes and practices concerning hiding children away in institutions. Television stars Roy Rogers and Dale Evans, whose wholesome family show ran from 1951 to 1957, entertained children and their parents with their exploits as modern-day cowboys and cowgirls who saved the weak, helpless, and good from crooks and bullies. Rogers in particular was an icon for families and a hero to children. He made more than 100 movies, and the Rogers/Evans television program was accompanied by a comic book series, a line of clothing, and a number of books and children's toys. The couple had a daughter, Robin, who had Down syndrome, and Evans published a bestselling book commemorating Robin's brief life, going on to open a school that offered a very public community-based training and educational program, the Dale Rogers Training Center (Dale Rogers Training Center, 2013; Trent, 1994). Rogers and Evans's pride and openness about their child had a tremendous influence on people's attitudes toward children with intellectual disabilities, as did the life of Rosemary Kennedy, older sister to US President John F. Kennedy. Despite her intellectual disabilities, Rosemary was very much a part of public life until she was "treated" with a lobotomy for moodiness and irritability at the age of 23 and subsequently institutionalized (John F. Kennedy Presidential Library and Museum, 2013). Despite her institutionalization, her life in the community before her internment inspired her sister Eunice to establish the Special Olympics and brother John to initiate a national enquiry into the state of mental health and special educational services, which was followed by sweeping legislative changes (Trent, 1994). Finally, Rosemary's other brother, Senator Robert

Kennedy, made a series of highly publicized, deeply critical tours of several institutions in 1965 (Blatt & Kaplan, 1974).

Robert Kennedy's tours were followed by a bitter debate in the senate between Kennedy, who was arguing for reform, and Nelson Rockefeller, who argued such expenses were a waste and that Kennedy's whirlwind tours had been sensationalist and did not represent the quality of care being provided to intellectually disabled children (Blatt & Kaplan, 1974). These tours and the subsequent debates inspired a particularly important project by Burton Blatt, a professor at Syracuse University, and his friend, photographer Fred Kaplan. Motivated by Kennedy's actions, and familiar with the conditions in his state's institutions through his work as a special educator, Blatt enlisted his partner to make several visits to institutions during which Kaplan took photographs through a camera hidden in the belt of his trousers. The resulting book, a harrowing 128-page photo essay, was self- published as *Christmas in Purgatory* in 1966,[1] and 1000 copies were produced and distributed by supportive parents' groups to legislators, journalists, and leaders in the nascent parent advocacy movement (Blatt & Kaplan, 1974). The impact was immense and contributed to a number of similar reports, in turn leading to investigations into abuses that fuelled the movement for change in the institutional systems.

The sea change in the 1950 and 1960s of attitudes toward institutionalizing intellectually disabled children seems to have been somewhat slower to start in Alberta than in the rest of North America. This sluggishness was in part caused by the politically and socially conservative leadership in the province. Alberta has experienced remarkably stable government, with only three changes in political leadership since the success of the UFA in 1921 and the opening of Michener in 1923. The originally progressivist leadership of the UFA reigned from 1921 to 1935, falling to the highly conservative Social Credit Party during the economic depression of the 1930s, which had hit Alberta farmers particularly hard. The Social Credit government reigned uncontested, and it was really only with the election of the Conservative Party in 1971 that real social and cultural shifts began to be implemented at the political level.

For its first eight years, the Social Credit government was led by William Aberhart, a Baptist minister, evangelist, and radio personality whose weekly radio shows throughout his tenure as premier promoted a potent mixture of social and political conservatism. On Aberhart's death in 1943, the leadership was taken over by his party secretary, Ernest Manning, another Evangelical Baptist preacher and radio personality, who led the party until late 1968, handing the reins over to placeholder Harry Strom, who saw the end of Social Credit rule in early 1971. During the 36 years of its reign, and particularly during the Manning decades, the party led the province virtually unopposed, and Alberta came to be characterized as the most politically and socially conservative province in the country. Although Manning's 25-year leadership included the period encompassing attitude change toward institutionalization outside of Alberta, it is perhaps unsurprising that he showed little enthusiasm for institutional and educational reforms for children with intellectual disabilities in his province. Manning's oldest son Keith[2] was a long-term resident of the Michener Centre (Pringle, 1997). As with many former inmates, it is not clear that Keith's admission was appropriate. In an autobiographical work on his political beginnings, Keith's brother, Preston, describes Keith as someone with a seizure disorder who on discharge from Michener lived in a group home, married, and worked for a living (Manning, 1992).

Whatever Premier Manning's personal feelings about institutionalization and sterilization might have been, he nevertheless came under considerable public pressure from parent groups, media, and, eventually, the general public to make improvements to services and treatment for people with intellectual and mental health disabilities. As a result, beginning in 1968, Manning's last year of leadership, he commissioned Dr W. R. N. ("Buck") Blair to engage in an investigation and evaluation of mental health services across the province. In addition to a number of prominent mental health postings, Blair had served as a member of the Eugenics Board for the last half of 1967, presumably resigning to take on the investigation. Perhaps because of his involvement on the Eugenics Board, or perhaps because he was a political appointee, Dr Blair's resulting reports did not propose changes to the Sexual Sterilization Act. Rather, he recommended only cosmetic improvements to the province's eugenic actions, suggesting the appointment of more medically and psychologically qualified personnel to the Board and in the clinics and institutions that referred people to the Eugenics Board, and asking that educational programs be implemented for Board members so they could keep up with current biological and social research concerning intellectual disability (Blair, 1969). However, the Blair Report, as it came to be known, *did* propose significant administrative and organizational changes to services for people with intellectual and mental health disabilities, including better coordination between services, departments, and agencies; better staff training; more research and evaluation; and, importantly, a move from centralized institutions to more community-based programs (Blair, 1969). Thus, even before the repeal of the Sexual Sterilization Act, the government was hearing and, at least in theory, considering information that indicated the end of the institutions should be near. Nevertheless, despite the fact that the official recommendations of the government's own commission urged the end of institutionalization yet failed to condemn involuntary sterilization, it was involuntary sterilization that ended fairly soon after the publication of the Blair Report, while the institutions have lingered.

Implications for the Current Alberta Context

While the Blair Report was perhaps the foundational critique of institutional-ization in Alberta, others were involved in critical investigations and evalua-tions of services for people with intellectual disabilities over the years. Dr Jean Pettifor, who helped found the Psychologists' Association of Alberta, spear-headed ethical protocols for psychological research and therapy, and advocated for community living during a lengthy career (Rutherford, 2013), worked for 24 years in the Guidance Clinics, until the repeal of the Sexual Sterilization Act, which initiated the dissolution of the Clinics. In an article reflecting on her decades of work as a leading psychologist in the province, she described the climate during these investigations and reforms in the following terms:

> During the 1960s there was much unrest in the government services in mental health, disabilities, child welfare and education, especially when journalists brought stories of neglect, incompetence and abuse to public awareness. We were directed to refuse access to certain journalists at our guidance clinic offices, although se-cretly we were glad someone was willing to publicize the deficiencies in the larger systems. (Pettifor, 2010, Reform section, para. 1)

That workers and administrators inside the system were resistant to change should not surprise; recall my discussion in the chapter on work and vocational training about how unionized employees, keen to sustain their jobs, have lob-bied against closing the institution in Red Deer, arguing publicly that to reinte-grate people to community would be cruel and irresponsible while failing to mention that jobs are on the line. With the 2013 government announcement that it intended to close Michener in April 2014,[3] the union distributed email petitions to its employees (including at my own university) and left them in public spaces like libraries and community halls for signature. On the petition, the union identified itself only as the collection point for signed petitions, while the form is headlined as an initiative of "Friends of Michener Centre," and there is no mention at all of jobs. Instead the petition makes an emotional appeal for Michener to remain "open for the vulnerable Albertans with severe develop-mental disabilities who have called Michener home for decades, which would allow them to live out their lives with peace, dignity and stability" (Friends of Michener Centre, 2013).

Workers and officials are not the only people who have been interested in sustaining the institution. It must be acknowledged that many parents and fam-ily members have also been supportive of institutionalization, and in Alberta many of them have worked very hard to improve the institution from within as a way to improve the quality of life of their family members but also to stave off wholesale closure. The Michener parents' group has been, perhaps ironi-cally, a consistently strong supporter of keeping the Michener Centre going. For the years that followed the significant deinstitutionalization of the 1970s and 1980s, and prior to the reorganization of the current board structure in the mid-2000s, the Michener Centre's board was parent-driven, and the board and its publications rallied significant internal support for keeping the institution operating. For example, in its April 1993 newsletter, the Parents' Association encouraged its membership to continue lobbying the government for Michener to remain open and to push the government to establish a parent-run board. The Parents' Association president asked parents to "keep contacting their MLAs with our view that Michener Centre must have a [parent] Board to se-cure for our loved ones a safe and happy place for them to live" (Keates, 1993, p. 2). The parents' group was successful, and rather than turn the running of the institution over to a non-partisan or a disability advocacy group, the Michener board became parent-driven until significant administrative and governance shifts concerning services for people with disabilities occurred at provincial and local levels in 2005.

For these parents, the goal has been to improve the lives of those remaining at the Michener Centre, and to that end, it must be acknowledged that much has been done. Beginning in 1954, the Parent-School Organization for Excep-tional Children (now known as the Society of Parents & Friends of Michener) began significant fundraising and worked to improve living conditions in the institution. As described earlier, these efforts included building a skating rink and a curling rink, and purchasing physiotherapy equipment, sports equip-ment, television sets for the day rooms, and a bus for field trips. In addition, the parents' group established a summer camp on donated lakefront property in a town near to Red Deer, which permitted a number of inmates to have breaks from the grind of institutional life. As well, during the deinstitutionalization movement, the Michener board decided to construct a number of bungalows to serve as group homes, built directly on the Michener campus. While establish-ing group homes on the isolated campus of a former institution under the same leadership that ran the institution may not be entirely in the spirit of commu-nitization, these efforts undoubtedly improved the lives of some children and adults living at Michener. Conversely, they also contributed to sustaining the institution through constant improvements and investments, and as such, they acted in contradiction to efforts to end institutionalization as an option for Albertans. Further, it is important to point out that these improvements oc-curred during the period that this book investigates, and while survivors did occasionally mention going out on day passes, their recollections of institu-tional life bore little resemblance to the happy portrayals on the Parent-School

Organization's website and in the archival Parent-School Organization news-letters, which show bucolic picnics and happy children using the recreational facilities. Thus, although these efforts were certainly laudable, the reality is that the changes they wrought were in many ways superficial, given the overwhelm-ing evidence of what daily life in the institution was like.

In the current debates over closing the Michener Centre, parents have fig-ured as key supporters of keeping the institution going, providing media inter-views and lobbying alongside the AUPE in the Keep Michener Open campaign. Family members have called the closure shameful, offering emotional but sometimes inaccurate arguments, such as those put forward by Peter Keohane, whose sister was interned in 1967. In the *Globe and Mail*, a nationally distrib-uted Canadian newspaper, Keohane asserted:

> The whole time she's been there, there's never been a fence. There's never been barbed wire. There's never been eugenics ... There's been a bunch of people who have struggled through life, trying to do the best for their families. (Wingrove, 2013, para. 9)

Keohane is correct in noting that there never has been barbed wire or fencing to restrict inmates' movements; locked units and buildings made such mea-sures unnecessary. However, there is ample evidence that eugenics was present and active during his sister's first six years of residency.

It is understandable that parents and family members who either placed their family members in Michener or who have had them remain there would want to minimize the darker aspects of Michener's history. In 2001 I attended a meeting with the former, parent-driven board of directors of the Michener Centre, dur-ing which I and two colleagues requested a tour of the facilities (see Appendix II). During that meeting, several of the directors in attendance expressed strong reservations about this research. These parents wanted to be sure I would not "create an inaccurate impression about the current nature of ... Michener," and they were concerned about "the effect of the project on the current progress at Michener" (Michener Board, 2001). It was only four years later, with a signifi-cant shift in philosophy and board membership to a government rather than parent-led leadership,[4] that I finally received permission to view the facility.

In response to the concerns raised by that earlier parent-run board, I feel it important to clarify that I do understand that the Michener Centre today is not run in the same ways as the institution described in this book. I also am con-vinced that the primary purpose and outcome of this book is not to impede any progress being made in terms of services for people with intellectual disabilities in Alberta or elsewhere. Rather, my goal in writing this history has been to highlight what did happen to people at Michener, because it is important to remember such things rather than hide them.

That being said, while Michener no longer houses a huge, abandoned, and abused population living under abject conditions, it does continue to exist and to admit new residents. Michener Services, as it is now called, houses approximately 230 adults with intellectual disabilities in "39 homes on a 300-acre [120 hectare] site in Red Deer. [It] also supports 10 other individuals in 2 off-site homes located elsewhere in Red Deer" (Alberta Human Services, 2013, para. 1). When the Alberta government had announced its intention to close Michener Centre by April 2014, the planned removal of the institution's residents did not include over 100 individuals living in group homes built on the campus during Michener Centre's deinstitutionalization efforts. With the new government leadership's decision in September 2014 to keep the centre open, not only will residents continue to live in group homes and on wards in more traditional campus buildings, but individuals who were moved out of Michener can now be readmitted.

The buildings on the Michener campus remain a resource that is difficult to find a good use for but that nevertheless compose a significant asset that many feel *should* be made useful in some way. For those community-living advocates who want to see the institution gone forever, the availability of these facilities represents something of a sword of Damocles; the threads of goodwill and progress achieved in terms of support for community living are thin, while the weight of the availability and continued utility of the old institutional buildings hangs heavily. These tensions are highlighted in a set of recent Michener board minutes (PDD Central Region Community Board, 2007). In one section, indicating a hope of improving and expanding the facility, there was significant discussion about upgrading and renovating older facilities, building new ones, and moving people from one residence to another on the campus. Elsewhere, reflecting that populations were actually decreasing and space was abundant, the papers discussed how Michener facilities were being rented to working homeless people as a way to provide them with affordable housing not available in the community. And finally, a concern was raised by a Michener board member who also served on the board of the Society of Parents & Friends of Michener, conveying that members of the parents' society were anxious about the loss of space at Michener and the decreasing number of admissions to Michener:

> Questions have been asked from Edmonton and Calgary why people cannot enter Michener Services since there is not enough places for people with developmental disabilities to live. (PDD Central Region Community Board, 2007)

In this comment, we can read that because of the inadequacy of meaningful resources supporting community living, pressures on the institution to house individuals with intellectual disabilities continue. Earlier, I discussed the effect that economic shifts have had historically on services for people with intellectual disabilities, where broader economic scarcity has often resulted in reduced supports and limited resources being apportioned to people with intellectual disabilities. These economic downturns have historically had the effect of making congregated care or institutionalization come to be seen as the most attractive option (Trent, 1994). In the case of Michener, leaving the bricks and mortar of the place standing means that there remains a too-easy alternative in the form of reinstitutionalization when the will and resources to support community living fall short.

Implications for the Broader Context

Excavating this institutional history not only allows us to understand the particular abuses that occurred at Michener or the risks attached to its continued existence but also illuminates what can happen within other institutions, and thus it raises concerns about what might be happening in such places today. In the first pages of *Christmas in Purgatory,* author Burton Blatt made a statement that has resonance for this aspect of Michener Centre's history:

> We have a deep debt of gratitude to those who permitted us to photograph that which they are most ashamed of. To reveal the names of the places we visited is, assuredly, an invitation to invite their instant dismissal. However, we have a much more forceful reason for not admitting to where we have been. These pictures are a challenge to all institutions for the mentally retarded in the United States. We are firmly convinced that in many other institutions in America we could have taken the same pictures – some, we are sure, even more frightening. (Blatt & Kaplan, 1974)

Blatt's statement implies that, in a sense, it does not matter where the picture, or in the case of this book, the stories come from, because institutions – all institutions – are prone to these horrors. Unfortunately, Blatt's assertion still resonates today. Large institutions housing people with intellectual disabilities, while certainly less common in developed countries than in the past, do continue to exist, and the conditions in these institutions are as hidden and often as brutal as those described in this book.

Many states in the United States continue to operate large institutions, including California, New Jersey, and Texas ("Texas Lambasted," 2008). Texas maintains 13 "state schools" for some 5000 residents that generally reflect the size and conditions that existed in Michener during the time of this study. The US Justice Department has accused the state of violating residents' rights to proper care, and there have been continued complaints about crowding, unsanitary conditions, unusually high injury rates, neglect, and even deaths while in care ("Texas Lambasted," 2008). Violence in these institutions seems to be endemic. In 2002, at Texas's Denton State School, a care worker beat resident Haseeb Chishty so severely that he became paraplegic and can neither feed himself nor use the bathroom. In the trial for the beating, worker Kevin Miller, who is serving a 15-year sentence for the crime, justified his actions, stating, "It got to the point it was fun beating him, torturing him" ("Texas Lambasted," 2008). Even this incident seems to have initiated little change in the institutions, however. In 2009, a horrific episode at one of the institutions exploded briefly into the public consciousness. Video footage was released by police showing that inmates at a state school in Corpus Christi, Texas, were being forced by staff to participate in a fight club for over a year on a regular basis. In one of the videos, a resident is seen

> trying to run away from his attacker and a large group of employees and residents track … him through the halls. When cornered, he wails and moans and tells the employees, "I will behave." (Hill, Rhee, & Ross, 2009, para. 3)

The staff member who had videotaped this footage was not a whistleblower concerned about this abuse, or at least not publicly. Rather, the cell phone of one of the staff members involved was found by someone else in the institution (it is not clear if this was a visitor or another staff member) who turned the phone over to police who then saw the footage. In their investigation, police were told by inmates that they had been threatened with imprisonment and beatings if they did not cooperate in the club; investigators also found that in a two-year period, "more than 800 employees [at the institution] had been suspended or fired for 'abusing facility residents'" (Hill et al., 2009, "More Than 800 Employees," para. 1). These incidents, and the widespread culture of institutional violence and apathy they represent, are reminiscent of the tolerance for violence and dehumanization that occurred in Michener for decades. It seems fair to say that the very nature of large institutions can engender a desensitized attitude by workers and inmates alike toward brutality and violence. Further, these conditions clearly lead many institutional workers to view inmates of such places as subhuman and hence undeserving of basic human dignity or rights.

When asked to speculate why these institutions, despite repeated exposure and outrage over conditions, continue to exist, Texas community advocate Jeff

Garrison-Tate replied, "Many of the institutions are large employers in small towns, and they often pay more than other jobs in rural areas. Lawmakers fear taking action that would lead to layoff" ("Texas Lambasted," 2008, "Trouble Closing Schools," para. 2). This position is clearly mirrored in the story of the Michener Centre, where opposition to closure has been vociferous among worker groups. However, the problem is deeper than simply that these places provide good career opportunities to local community members, although clearly this is an element in the continued existence of institutions. In addition, the dearth of reliable, affordable, and acceptable community living options remains an impediment to deinstitutionalization, and – as in the case of Michener – leaves the door open to potential reinstitutionalization. When interviewed about Texas's response to abuse allegations, State Representative Larry Phillips, who was appointed to chair a legislative committee studying the institutions, said, "Even if we said we wanted to close all state schools, the community resources aren't there at this time" ("Texas Lambasted," 2008, "Trouble Closing Schools," para. 3). Similar arguments about the paucity of community-based supports have been consistently raised by advocates for the Michener Centre's continued existence, including during the most recent debate over its closure. The risk with this argument is that, when the bricks, mortar, and employment opportunities of larger institutions remain in force and the resources for community inclusion are lacking, the temptation to sustain institutions remains strong.

This threat of continued or renewed institutionalization is what has motivated the writing of this book. Almost a century ago, the Michener Centre began its existence driven by the best of intentions for housing, educating, caring for, and rehabilitating children and youth with intellectual disabilities. Although it failed abysmally to deliver on its promises to those children and their families, it did succeed in growing wildly beyond its original vision as a result of political and economic expediency, bureaucratic silence and self-interest, and the apathy and prejudices of the general populous. This "success" produced terrible outcomes for its inmates in the form of crowding, understaffing, economic exploitation, social isolation, sensory and intellectual deprivation, neglect, and an almost inevitably abusive routine. These same factors and outcomes continue to exist in current institutions for people with intellectual, mental, and health-related disabilities. It is my hope that by exposing the insights and experiences of some of the survivors of life inside one institution that I will offer a compelling argument that such places should – indeed *must* – no longer exist.

Research Participants – Biographical Information

Institutional Survivors

Betty Dudnik lived on a farm outside a small town in Alberta with her parents and three siblings until she went to live at Michener for training when she was just seven years old. She stated that her parents could not handle her and manage the farm at the same time. Betty stayed at Michener until she turned 18, when she moved into a group home of her own choosing in a large Alberta city. A cousin of Betty's also lived at the Michener Centre. Betty declined to discuss sterilization.

Beverly Buszko was raised by her parents and lived with her three siblings in a large Alberta city. She contracted polio as a child and thus left school when she was only in grade five. Her parents had many problems of their own; Beverly described her father as a heavy drinker and stated that both parents were abusive to her. She entered the Michener Centre at 10 years of age and left in 1977, when she turned 18.

Bonnie Cowan lived with her parents and two siblings until she was 13 years old. Bonnie has a seizure disorder and limited verbal skills, and never attended school as a child. Her parents were convinced to institutionalize her because her mother was advised by the family doctor that Bonnie would be best served in a place where she could receive 24-hour, expert care. Bonnie left the institution at 18 years of age, in 1976. Her "interview" (written responses by her mother) did not indicate whether she was sterilized while at Michener.

Carl Semkow had cerebral palsy and intellectual disabilities, and he is now deceased. Along with his sister, he was institutionalized for 13 years. Carl's mother, Mavis, provided an interview about institutionalizing him and about his life. It is not certain from Mavis's interview whether Carl was sterilized.

Donald Graham is both blind and deaf. He completed grade three before entering Michener and has taken adult literacy classes since his discharge. He was nine years old when he moved to the Michener Centre from his small town several hours' drive away. His parents continued to visit while he lived in Michener, but he has lost touch with his two siblings. He was 23 years old when discharged in 1980. He declined to say whether he was sterilized in Michener.

Donna Bogdan is of Ukrainian heritage. Placed in an orphanage shortly after her birth, she lived there and in multiple foster placements until she was 16 years old, when she says Child Welfare placed her into the Michener Centre for training. She completed grade eight before her institutionalization. She lived in the Michener Centre until 1981, when she was 28 years old, and she was sterilized during her stay there.

Gene Forzinsky was raised by his Ukrainian parents in a small town in Northern Alberta until he was 15 years old. He experienced learning difficulties in school, repeating several grades. Eventually, his parents were convinced by doctors and social workers that the Michener Centre could provide Gene with an appropriate education. Gene spent four years at Michener, leaving in 1975 at 19 years of age. While in Michener, Gene was sterilized.

Gerta Muller's parents were first-generation German-Polish immigrants who farmed in a remote rural community in Alberta. Gerta attended school until she reached grade six, when she contracted polio. She missed several years of schooling while she was ill and recovering, and was not reintegrated into the regular school system because, as she stated, the school was unable to accommodate her mobility needs. She was admitted to the Michener Centre at the age of 25 in 1972, and was discharged at the age of 27 in 1974. She did not participate in the decision to admit her to the institution, and during her stay she was involuntarily sterilized.

Guy Tremblay is Metis. He lived with his three siblings and his parents in a small town in Saskatchewan until, at a very young age, he suffered severe head injuries in a motor vehicle accident. As a result, Guy spent most of his remaining childhood years in various hospitals and received only sporadic schooling. He was moved to the Michener Centre when he was nine years old, and left at the age of 39, in 1986. While living at Michener, Guy was sterilized.

Harvey Brown was raised by a single father along with his four siblings in a small town in Alberta. He described his early life as extremely poor, and his father as a man who struggled to support and care for his family. In school, Harvey experienced difficulties in learning, and he completed only grade six. He was admitted to Michener in 1965 at the age of 13 and discharged in 1971 at the age of 19. He was involuntarily sterilized while there.

Janice Holmes's sister wrote her "interview." Janice lived in a small Alberta city and attended the public school system for four years. She lived with her family until she was 11 years of age, at which point her mother decided that the institution would be better for her, in part because she felt overwhelmed with caring for Janice. She lived in the institution for 26 years, leaving in 1986 when she was 37 years old. She was sterilized while living at Michener.

Jim Molochuk was born to first-generation Ukrainian immigrants and lived as a child in a large Alberta city. He experienced learning difficulties in the public school system, which he attended until grade three, when he was removed from school and left much to his own devices. Both his parents were working to support their large family, and they were offered few resources to support Jim in his training or development. One day, when he was bottle-picking in an alley near his home, he experienced a seizure. His parents were persuaded by social workers on Jim's case to admit him to the Michener Centre because of health concerns and so that he could receive a proper education. He was admitted to the institution in 1949, when he was 12 years old, and he left in 1974 at the age of 37. He was involuntarily sterilized during his years at Michener.

Laura Smith was raised, along with her four siblings, by her father, who was a widower. While at Michener, Linda lived for nine years in Alberta School Hospital (ASH) and in a group home on the Michener Campus for a further 11 years. In 1990, when she was 29 years old, her father and her sister purchased a home for her and removed her from Michener Centre. During her years of living in the ASH facility on Michener Campus, Laura was sterilized.

Louise Roy is Metis and was raised until her early teens by her mother, who Louise described as a heavy drinker "who didn't want me." The family was impoverished and lived in a medium-sized city. Louise attended school until she was "12 or so" and then was admitted to the Michener Centre, where she stayed for 11 years, leaving when she was 23 years old. She declined to discuss sterilization.

Mary Korshevski, who is Ukrainian, lived with her two siblings and her widowed mother in a small city in Alberta. She attended school until grade five, when she contracted polio. As with Gerta Muller, Mary spent many years hospitalized and that prevented her from attending any further schooling. On Mary's discharge from the hospital, her mother found it impossible to maintain her own job and care for Mary. Her family doctor convinced her mother that the Michener Centre would provide Mary with training and care. Mary entered the institution at age 15 and left it when she was 36 years old, in 1976. While in Michener Centre, she was sterilized. Mary was accompanied during her interview by her long-term roommate and supporter, Edna.

Michel Aubin considers himself to be French Canadian, and he grew up in Alberta. His mother is First Nations and his father came from Quebec. He grew up in small-town Alberta, with his parents and two brothers. Michel began to experience seizures in his early teens, and he also began to experience some social problems because of being excluded from the public school system. Caught stealing chickens at 13 years of age, he was sent to live at Michener. After five years there, he moved to Deerhome, where he stayed another 14 years. Michel also had a cousin who lived many years at Michener. He declined to say whether he was sterilized while in the Michener Centre.

Paul Anjou is Metis and lived with his parents and two siblings until he was seven years old and entered the Michener Centre. He had attended school in the community for a couple of years but was expelled because of his "bad temper" and his difficulties in learning. His parents farmed in a rural area of Alberta and the pressures of farming proved too much for them. Paul spent 18 years at Michener, leaving in 1985 at 25 years of age. By then, his parents had moved away, and he lost touch with his family. He did not speak about sterilization during his interview.

Ray Petrenko is of Ukrainian origin. He grew up in a large Alberta city with his parents and siblings. At school, he was identified as a "slow learner" and experienced difficulties keeping up with his peers. He noted that the school and the family doctor convinced his parents that the Michener Centre would be a good place for him to gain an education. He entered Michener at a young age; however, he was not given schooling but instead began to work in various aspects of the institutional economy for the balance of his stay. He was sterilized at 16 years of age. After leaving Michener in mid-adulthood, Ray took adult literacy classes and now fills an active and important leadership role in disability advocacy issues both at the provincial and national level.

Sam Edwards lived with his divorced mother, who was a school principal, in a small central Alberta town. When he was 11 years old, his teacher complained about classroom misbehaviour and referred Sam and his mother to the Guidance Clinic. Sam's mother, Dorothy, was convinced to admit him but shortly after began to express misgivings about the institution's practices and about Sam's treatment there. Less than a year later, she pulled Sam out of the institution and began a complaint process against Michener through the provincial ombudsman. On her death, she left Sam numerous documents relating to this episode in their family history.

Sandra Karnak lived with her Ukrainian-born, working-class parents and her brother in a small southern Alberta town until she was 12 years old. She described her mother as a woman with a drinking problem who was violent and difficult to live with. She recalled a fairly ordinary early childhood until she "became sick and had to go to the hospital for a long time" before her admission to Michener. She lived in the Michener Centre from 1968 to 1974 when she turned 18. She was involuntarily sterilized during her stay at the Michener Centre.

Sean Hoskins lived with his mother at his grandparents' home in a large Alberta city for most of his childhood. He occasionally saw his father and stepmother, who lived not far away in a smaller town. He attended school until grade six and then was left to his own devices. He got into some trouble stealing clothing off clotheslines and was sent to the Michener Centre when he was 12 years old. One of Sean's brothers also spent time at the institution. Sean left Michener at the age of 19, in 1978. He declined to speak about sterilization.

Tammy Burns lived with her parents and two siblings in a medium-sized Alberta town until she was 18 years old. In 1971, she was admitted to the Michener Centre because her "mom thought [she'd] get more stimulation and have more friends." She has a seizure disorder. She now lives in a supported home in the community, having left the institution at 33 years of age in 1986. Tammy's interview was written by a caregiver. She declined to answer questions concerning sterilization.

Mother of Institutional Survivor

Mavis Semkow is the mother of two children who were institutionalized for many years at the Michener Centre. Mavis's background is Anglo-Saxon, and her ex-husband's background is Polish. Mavis described her early years as a mother as quite stressful; she lived in considerable poverty and continues to do so. As well, her husband was a heavy drinker and quite violent. As a result, Mavis's marriage was an on-and-off-again affair, and for much of her two children's early years, Mavis was a single parent. She described being persuaded that a Michener placement would be the "best thing" for her two children. It is also possible that the social worker involved in Mavis's case suspected neglect or incompetence; in either case, Mavis placed her children in Michener when they were 13 and 11, respectively. The children remained there for 13 years, until Mavis was able to facilitate their return to a community home. Mavis indicated that neither of her children was sterilized while in Michener but also noted that she was not sure about some of the details concerning consent for procedures to be undertaken in the institution.

Former Institutional Workers

Evelyn Stephens worked at the Michener Centre as a summer intern. Her experiences there led her to getting involved in the Community Living movement and to a long career of advocacy for individuals with disabilities. She is on the faculty of a large university and is active on several boards relating to disability.

Jim Sullivan worked at the Michener Centre in multiple capacities. He began as a junior psychology undergraduate summer student, working on the wards, and over several summers he was progressively promoted. When he completed his BA, he worked as a senior psychologist in the institution for several years. He continues to work in the field of disability in the community and is an educational psychologist and administrator.

Coral James worked at the Michener Centre for a year and a half as a young woman. She worked as an IA (institutional aide) on several wards. She went on to obtain a graduate degree in education and works currently as a consultant to the Edmonton School Board.

History, Power, and Access to Knowledge

In 2005, when Alberta celebrated its centennial as a Canadian province, the official commemorations deployed images of wholesome families, wide-open spaces, explorers, homesteaders, ranchers, and oilmen. This was history in revision and remembrance; depictions of humble, hard-working, and decent White folks facing the challenges of a wild country, civilizing the unruly land, and building communities were used to represent the true history of the province. Silence has prevailed concerning many other memories that could have been invoked as part of the history of taming the West. This book sheds light on one particular set of memories that have been excluded from dominant recollections of Alberta's past. These are the memories of a small numbers of survivors who were institutionalized as "mental defectives" in the province, many of whom were involuntarily sterilized as part of the Alberta government's long-enduring eugenics program.

These survivor narratives are specific to one institution, the Provincial Training School (PTS), known at times as the Alberta School Hospital and finally as the Michener Centre. However, the practices of institutionalization and segregation they described reflect broader discourses and practices that operated across Europe and North America during the twentieth century relating to science, eugenics, and fitness for citizenship. As such, these memories mirror similar marginalized histories, including those of the disabled people who provided the template and experimental population for the Jewish Holocaust in Germany (Kuhl, 1994) and of the survivors of psychiatric institutionalization and abuse in most Western countries throughout the nineteenth and twentieth centuries (Pfohl, 1978). These are important memories to access, not only for those who survived, but for those who, because of innocence or ignorance, may repeat the horrors of institutionalization, perpetrated in the name of human betterment and human service against people deemed to be inferior or problematic.

The Role of Oral History

In social research, telling people's stories and reconstructing memories has become a legitimate research strategy. In discussing sociological health research, Arthur Frank (2002) has argued that narratives open the possibility of claiming one's personal memories as legitimate and telling one's own experiences as a counter-narrative to the dominant medical model. In that dominant model, patients (or in this case, inmates) are conceived as little more than their diseases or conditions, and patients' subjective knowledge is regarded as irrelevant to the understanding or treatment of illness and disability (Frank, 2002; Sakalys, 2000). The power of narrative to reclaim knowledge by making memories public thus offers individuals an opportunity to bear witness to their experience, to affirm personal perspectives on illness and disability as real and legitimate, and to challenge dominant health care ideologies (Balshem, 1993; Charmaz, 1990; Frank, 2002; Kleinman, 1988; Sakalys, 2000). In addition, these narratives offer a politicized reading of relations of power, offering the patient an opportunity to authenticate harms suffered and drawing on the perspectives of subordinated individuals to expose the workings of power and domination within the medical encounter (Balshem, 1993; Sakalys, 2000). Mike Bury (2001) notes that narrative and memory work are not limited only to those who are ill; a politics of narrative can be used by a broad range of people who have been harmed or marginalized by powerful institutions.

The individuals who initiated this oral history project, many of them Michener survivors, understood the importance of telling marginalized memories. Ray Petrenko, who survived more than 20 years of institutional life, was a central motivator in getting this project started. During his interview, he noted:

> I feel that it's time the people listen to our stories and I think that eventually if you can get this [project] going ... hopefully this will help, this tape [recording] will help to educate people, so something like this will never happen again, so people with disabilities will never be abused again.

Ray added another element to the theoretician's arguments for the power of narrative and memory reclamation. In his analysis, not only does retelling and remembering have the power to legitimate the individual's memories and perspectives but reclaiming these memories by telling them from the perspective of the survivor also has two other strengths. First, this memory work conveys a cautionary tale against institutionalization both past and future by showing us what life inside these pastorally situated buildings was like for those who lived within their walls. Second, it produces an emancipatory message of empowerment for individuals with disabilities by evidencing that history from survivors' perspectives matters.

Disability scholar Susan Wendell (1996) has argued that memory work from the perspectives of individuals with disabilities is crucial to the construction of an emancipatory disability history. By this Wendell means that the distanced and purportedly objective knowledge constructed by historians, sociologists, and other scholars often falls short. In the recent past, researchers have begun to expose the systematic institutionalization, degradation, and eugenicization of disabled individuals that occurred in the West during much of the twentieth century (Dowbiggin, 1995; Jones, 1999; Kevles, 1995; Kuhl, 1994; McLaren, 1986, 1990; Park & Radford, 1998; Proctor, 1995; Radford, 1994). However, most of these histories have not drawn on the accounts of those who, having survived these practices, can tell us about the intimate mechanisms of disability oppression at its most profound level. Emancipatory history that comes from the positions or standpoints of survivors draws on the assertion that telling one's memories serves to name hurts, describe exploitation, acknowledge power relations, and remember history as it occurred for those most oppressed by it, rather than reproducing memories that serve dominant interests.

Offices of the Public Guardian

While the value of reclaiming memories from the perspectives of those who have suffered most is inarguable, such memories are not easy to access. This difficulty was abundantly clear at several junctures in conducting the research for this book. An example of the difficulties encountered in accessing individuals rests in the guardianship arrangements of institutional survivors. Many individuals with intellectual disabilities, including many of those individuals released from the Michener Centre in the Community Living movement of the 1970s and 1980s are under public guardianship arrangements. For many Michener survivors, these arrangements came about as a result of their institutionalization, as many Michener residents became legal wards of the institution during their internments. Some were individuals whose parents or other family members had died, leaving the institution with sovereign authority over the inmates. Others were individuals whose families had abandoned them to the institution, handing legal authority over them to the Michener Centre administration at the time of institutionalization. Finally, some, because of lengthy internments under extreme conditions of deprivation, had learned little about managing their daily affairs in the outside world; as such, these people needed assistance in managing their financial and legal matters on release. Thus, for many ex-inmates – and, in the current context, for adults with intellectual disabilities who have never been institutionalized – there is some need to provide legal safeguards as they have been deemed to be unable to make decisions about their legal situations. A solution was created for this dilemma through the formation of Offices of the Public Guardian, which were established by the Government of Alberta to provide "decision-making mechanisms for individuals who are unable to make personal, non-financial decisions for themselves" to ensure the rights of these individuals are protected (Government of Alberta, 2005a, para. 1).

In the early stages of the project, when I approached several Offices of the Public Guardian to seek permission to recruit research participants, this role of protection seemed to operate more as obstruction; my offers to provide information sessions, and my requests to send former inmates calls for participation were consistently denied, either through active refusal or, more typically, through lack of follow-through. Inevitably, such denials were accompanied by claims that the office was protecting Michener survivors from the trauma of having to relive their experiences. However, one can also speculate on reasons other than paternalism for keeping these individuals from telling their stories; in "protecting" individuals from telling painful memories, one government office fails to facilitate access to individuals who might have negative things to say about another government office, in effect protecting the dominant, and sanitized, memory of Alberta's eugenic history. These actions also effectively denied these individuals the right to refuse or agree to tell their own marginalized memories of life in the institution.

The protectionism of the Public Guardian Office also has meant that, in this research project, the most marginalized survivor voices have been silenced, because only the survivors who were able to act as their own legal guardians have been able to tell their memories. Public guardianship orders primarily affected individuals who were deemed to be less independent and less intellectually capable, meaning in turn that individuals who avoided public guardianship were those deemed most capable while in the institution and on deinstitutionalization. Thus, the survivor memories that are being told in this research come from individuals who are their own legal guardians and who speculatively would have been deemed to be more capable and intelligent than many other inmates during their institutionalization. In turn, this means that the stories of these research participants may reflect experiences in wards that were less oppressive than average. In the Michener Centre, residents were segregated in wards according to hierarchies of disability from High Grades to Low Grades, and it is likely that the participants in this project enjoyed better living conditions within the institution than others who were perceived as less intellectually competent, both during their time in the institution and once they were released back into the community.

Accessing the Institution

The ability of privileged and powerful social actors to obstruct an emancipatory history of the Michener Centre has been evidenced in numerous ways throughout this project. In 1999, early in the research, I spoke with the then-current manager of planning and communications at Michener Centre, asking about the status of the institution and whether the Michener Centre would be willing to provide access to their on-site archives. I will return to the question of the archives later. As to the current institutional status, she informed me that although officially the Michener Centre "discourages" admission and supports communitization, there were still at that time a few admissions every year and a total population of almost 550 residents, all adults committed for long-term residency (at writing, this number hovers around 125) (personal communication, May 19, 1999). She also expressed that, tying in with the Michener Centre's role as one of the largest employers in the area, the board at that time would have liked to have increased admissions (personal communication, May 19, 1999). In other words, although there was a large grassroots movement during the 1960s to 1990s seeking to close such institutions, the Michener Centre continues to exist and until recently expressed an interest in strengthening its role, on the one hand, as an institution for disabled people and, on the other, as a major employer of non-disabled people. Finally, she noted that Michener itself had been wanting to write another history of the centre (an official government history of the Michener Centre was produced in 1985), this time with a focus on how the centre acted as a career stepping stone for many Albertans schooled as mental deficiency nurses (MDNs) in a two-year training program that ended in 1973, just as Michener was winding down its eugenics program (personal communication, May 19, 1999). When asked about the eugenics program at Michener, her response was not to deny that such things had ever happened; it would be impossible to do so in light of several high-profile court cases successfully launched against the Alberta Government for unlawful and involuntary sterilization (Grekul et al., 2004; *Muir v. Alberta*, 1996; Wahlsten, 1997). Rather, the communications manager stated, "That wasn't Michener Centre. That was the provincial government. We just went along with it because we had to. In fact, we'd be happy to have the truth told" (J. Mason, personal communication, August 30, 1999).

In light of Michener's stated ambitions to expand its operations, and its desire to produce its own sanitized memories, it is not surprising that the institution was reluctant to cooperate in the survivors' oral history project. In the spring of 2001, I and two research collaborators appealed to the Michener Centre board of governors, asking for a tour of the grounds. I had never seen the facilities where the survivors' experiences took place and I thought it would be useful to see the hallways, dormitories, solitary confinement cells, medical examining rooms, and other spaces that figured so poignantly in the survivors' stories. We were asked to attend a board meeting held on the Michener campus. There are two noteworthy points concerning this request: first, the Michener Centre is a public institution, funded by public dollars, and it is in theory neither an asylum nor a prison. It is a "care facility," and as such, members of the public are not typically barred from being on the campus. In fact, in the past two decades, a number of recreational facilities, including a theatre, a swimming pool, and a gymnasium, have been built on the Michener campus, and these are open to the general public. Thus, our request was more of a courtesy than a require- ment. A second point concerns the makeup of the Michener board at the time. The board was composed of nine members, all of them acting as volunteers. These individuals, from various districts across Alberta, included small busi- ness owners, management consultants, volunteers, members of philanthropic societies, and, in some cases, sitting members of other disability advisory com- mittees reporting to government. Thus, not only did these board members represent qualities of ideal citizenship, but they were also individuals who had been selected by the government for service on the board because of their high moral and social standing.

Our request to the board was not well received. After what seemed like an interminable wait in a cool, dark, echoing hallway, we were invited in to present our request to a stone-faced audience. When we finished, one board member noted that he "had some concerns about the project particularly in relation to its potential to continue to create an inaccurate impression about the cur- rent nature of ... Michener," while another indicated "history is important but ... how [would] the project be placed in the context of the society at the time?" (Michener Board, 2001). Each of these responses implied that, although history might be good to know, this history would not be: this history would instead pose a threat to the desired, official memory and to the legitimacy of the insti- tution in the present moment. In other words, echoing Ray Petrenko's earlier insights, these individuals also understood the political potential of memories from the margins. Predictably, some weeks later we received a polite letter bar- ring our access to the Michener campus.

In 2003, the board of the Michener Centre was disbanded and handed over to the governance of the Persons with Developmental Disabilities (PDD) Central Region Community Board, which is a volunteer-run board. A request to this new board resulted in a visit to the Michener grounds in October 2005; we were accompanied at all times while being provided a tour of showcase areas, and although we were provided access to some of the older buildings, we were not given a tour of areas like the behaviour support unit, where patients with disciplinary issues were managed. Our impression was that Michener, despite its then almost 350 residents, was for the most part a bucolic ghost town but that its administrators remained committed to keeping what remained of its active operations going. Indeed, despite a sustained struggle for closure of the institution, in September 2014, the Conservative government announced its intention to keep Michener open.

Privacy and Protectionism

A final example of how the powerful are able to restrict or erase undesirable memories relates to my efforts to access Michener's archives, including daily record logs, proceedings of sterilization hearings, minutes of disciplinary committees for staff members, budgets, lists of escape attempts and resulting actions, admissions, and experimental treatment records, all of which pertained to the survivor narratives. I sought these records not to substantiate or disprove the claims in survivor narratives but instead to understand how the centre handled such incidents on a routine institutional basis. In 1999, when I first spoke with the communications manager at Michener, many of these records were housed primarily at the institution itself, and I was not provided access to these privately held records. The reasons for holding these records privately rather than surrendering them to the public archives can only be speculated on; however, according to provincial privacy legislation, in Alberta hospitals and school records are considered to be non-government files, and they are not required to be transferred to the public archives (L. Miller, personal communication, October 14, 2006). Unfortunately, on 18 June 2003, lightning struck the administration building at the Michener Centre, and the ensuing fire resulted in the loss of these irreplaceable materials.

Not all the records for Michener were housed at the institution, however, and although it is not entirely clear which records were held at Michener, many of the institutional records have been transferred into the public archives of the Province of Alberta. Although one might hope that the partial surrender of the institutional documents to the provincial archives would result in easier access to Michener's historical records by researchers and claimants against the institution, this has not been the case. In 1996, the province implemented the Freedom of Information and Protection of Privacy Act (FOIP), designed to "to allow any person a right of access to the records in the custody or under the control of a public body subject to limited and specific exceptions" (Government of Alberta, 2005b, p. 11). Any records archived after 1996 are subject to the Act, while materials archived before the law came into effect are not protected by FOIP. In practice, this means the few files from the Michener Centre that were placed into the public archive before 1996 are fully open to citizens and researchers. However, the vast majority of the files were archived after the protectionist law was enacted.

In a similar vein to the question of whose memories were being protected when we early on sought access to the grounds of the Michener Centre, the question of whose privacy is being protected with the FOIP laws bears some scrutiny. In effect, when individuals seek information that is FOIP protected, they must make an application to the government for clearance, after which the archivist then painstakingly goes through each record that is requested, whiting out any names that are in the record and writing in the phrase "Section 17(1)" where each name would have appeared. Obviously, this is a very time-consuming process. It is also a very expensive one. My first request to the FOIP officer was for one daily record book taken from each ward within the Michener Centre, selected proceedings of staff meetings taken during two sample years, some records of medical experiments conducted on-site over one year, and some assorted correspondence. It should also be noted that, because applicants are not able to view the contents of the files and boxes before making requests, my selections were quite arbitrary, and quite thin; I fully expected to return for additional materials based on the results of this first Request for Access. Mercifully, the archivist did not immediately fill my request but instead sent a fee estimate for this first round of archival materials. That initial estimate totalled more than $13,000, hardly an amount that could be called accessible. I believe I can be forgiven for speculating that FOIP is designed not to provide citizens with access to historical materials but instead to protect public bodies from citizens' (and particularly marginalized citizens') access to these institutional records. This process restricts access, forcing one to engage in what amounts to little more than a fishing expedition rather than an informed choice that could come from browsing the files oneself, a process which is exacerbated by the prohibitive costs attached to that fishing.

In the end, the memories accessed in this oral history project have been highly constrained: I was able to reach only people who are articulate enough, and free enough, that they could engage in the research process without the barriers of protection by their guardians. Until recently, I was able only to see the hallways and exteriors of the buildings where the survivors lived. I was able to view just a fraction of the archival materials, and that was because a sympathetic woman in the provincial archives saw the importance of accessing the institution's hidden memories and began working with me in creative and accommodating ways. Nonetheless, despite all these barriers, it is undeniable that 22 interviews with institutional survivors, several hundred pages of archival material, and several collaborating interviews with ex-workers from the Michener Centre have tapped into a rich vein of silenced and de-legitimated memories. These materials contain the promise of constructing a new, emancipatory set of memories relating to institutionalization, allowing us to understand that the official memory of the Michener Centre is not the only version. Instead, survivor narratives permit us to understand that although the institutionalization of people with disabilities may have seemed like benign paternalism and well-intentioned, if faulty, social engineering from the outside, the centre instead resulted in systematic deprivation, isolation, violence, dehumanizing treatment, and wilful exploitation for those who were unfortunate enough to find themselves on the inside. Further, it seems almost certain that making these survivor narratives public holds the potential to not only rewrite the history of the institution but also change the ways that people think and perhaps act concerning institutionalization. We can make these speculations in part because of the consistency with which the powers that be have acted to protect their own versions of the past; if survivors' memories had no such potential, then those in power would not be so concerned about silencing or erasing them.

It is important to understand the methods of the interviews and archival collections, and to understand something of the perspective taken in analysing these materials. This book draws on qualitative, semi-structured interviews with 22 former inmates of the Michener Centre. Research participants were recruited through a variety of agencies that provide services and supports for individuals with developmental disabilities in Alberta, as well as through snowball sampling and a response to calls for participants on a local radio program. As noted earlier, the individuals who participated in this research are their own legal guardians, which is not necessarily representative of Michener ex-residents. This fact may mean that those who were able to provide an interview are more independent and perhaps more capable than other possible interviewees. In turn, this may also mean that the stories these people told reflect more positive experiences than those of the individuals who were unable to participate, which is a sobering thought. Life in the institution was harsh, even for those fortunate enough to be assigned to a High Grade ward.

The use of narrative methods, it has been argued, is particularly important in accessing excluded memories, because narrative research relies on the voice of the subject to determine the narrative's frame of reference (Booth & Booth, 1996). The interviews took a narrative form, beginning with the question, "Tell me how you came to live in Michener Centre," and then probes were used to explore schooling experiences, daily routines, privacy and personal space issues, employment practices, enjoyable experiences, social isolation, family matters, discipline, and, of course, sterilization experiences. Narrative research approaches are able to mitigate the problems of acquiescence bias that some researchers have noted in interviews with individuals with developmental disabilities (Heal & Sigelman, 1995). Contrary to Heal and Sigelman's thesis, I found that individuals interviewed for this project were quite prepared to refuse to answer questions and were also keen to correct misconceptions or hold their ground on points of importance. Almost all the individuals interviewed for this project were very verbally sophisticated and were able to provide face-to-face interviews up to an hour and half long. However, two of the individuals who participated provided written narratives that were produced in collaboration with family members or workers. These "interviews," while used in the research project, provided less information, particularly about institutional abuses or the brutality of daily life inside. This lack of detail may reflect the more limited verbal skills of these participants, or it may reflect the views of those who acted as intermediaries in writing these survivors' stories. In other words, these co-written data were much thinner than the interviews and perhaps echoed the perspectives of the workers and family members as much as those of the individuals themselves.

For most interviewees, regardless of their role in the institution, discussing the institution and its practices was perceived as an upsetting, but necessary and important, political and personal act. For some of the survivors, in particular, the interview process appeared to be quite frightening; the legacy of institutionalization meant that many of the interviewees expressed fears about disclosing incidents that happened in the institution, about "telling on" those who still seemed to exercise considerable sway over these individuals, and about angering family members who might have had some part in institutionalizing them, even though many years have passed since they left the institution. Although all participants were assured that they need not answer questions, and were told that they could withdraw from the research at any time, and despite the fears many participants expressed about speaking out, none of these individuals withdrew or refused their participation. Most participants expressed a sense of duty when reporting their experiences, reflecting their political motivations for participating. At the time of the interviews, individuals were promised anonymity in reporting research results; as a result, pseudonyms have been used for all research respondents.

In addition to the survivors who provided their own stories, or whose stories were provided in collaboration with workers and family members, the interviews included one mother who had placed two children in the institution and who subsequently struggled to have them returned to community living as adults. In this interview, the narrative centred more on the mother's decision to institutionalize her children and the factors that played into that decision, rather than on understanding of the conditions of her children's institutionalization. Despite the lack of information about practices within the institution, the information she provided nonetheless shed light on aspects of the institutionalization process that are important to this study. Finally, interviews were conducted with three former employees of Michener Centre, drawing on their recollections of the daily practices within the institution. These interviews were not collected as a means of confirming the stories of survivors, although in some ways, the inclusion of interviews with employees and the archival work was intended as a pre-emptive strategy against possible charges of false memory syndrome and acquiescence bias that might be levelled against survivors' recollections. Rather, these interviews were collected to provide multiple perspectives on daily life and to enrich my insights into the institution's practices.

The Inclusion of Archival Data

As noted earlier, initially the Michener history project was designed to draw on oral histories of institutional survivors, stemming from a consideration that oral histories permit insider perspectives that are best positioned to provide a counter-narrative to dominant historical narratives (Goodley, 1996). Centring the study on personal histories was also seen as critical because, as Elizabeth Bredberg (1999) has argued, much of disability history has been taken from the perspective of the institutions (such as clinical and medical practice) that were most oppressive to persons with disabilities, or when they have been from an explicitly emancipatory perspective, they have continued to focus on institutional practice without including the voices of the individuals most affected by those practices. Indeed, although researchers have begun to expose the systematic institutionalization, degradation, and eugenicization of disabled individuals that occurred in the West during much of the twentieth century (Dowbiggin, 1995; Jones, 1999; Kevles, 1995; Kuhl, 1994; McLaren, 1986, 1990; Park & Radford, 1998; Proctor, 1995; Radford, 1994), most of these histories exclude accounts from those who, having survived these practices, can tell us about the intimate mechanisms of disability oppression at its most profound level.

Thus, I felt considerable ambivalence in expanding the research beyond survivors' narratives, because doing so possibly runs the risk of disrespecting or further marginalizing the survivors' voices. It is important to stress that the decision to expand data sources was not made because of any inconsistencies in or doubts about the survivor narratives – I have never doubted that these stories are honest reflections of shared experiences. However, it is also true that triangulating data sources has been something of a concession to the imagined skepticism that such histories may engender among others. The Michener survivors' narratives are, like many other survivor narratives, filled with hidden and shocking stories of physical, sexual, economic, psychological, medical, and legal abuse, and like other survivor stories about these kinds of abuse, the potential for discrediting these memories is high. From Sigmund Freud, whose patients' reports of sexual abuse from male relatives were so discounted as to form the basis of his theory of oedipal desire and penis envy, to current debates over false memory syndrome that continue to keep vulnerable individuals from disclosing the harms done to them, relatively powerful social actors have consistently had the capacity to discredit and silence the memories of those in the margins. Individuals with intellectual disabilities may be especially vulnerable to discrediting strategies precisely because they are so devalued and stigmatized. For example, researchers have argued that individuals with intellectual disabilities are particularly prone to persuasion by researchers and therapists, particularly when claims of abuse have been involved (Ahlgrim-Delzell & Dudley, 2001; Finlay & Lyons, 2002; Heal & Sigelman, 1995; Scharnberg, 1996), and some have argued that this susceptibility to influence has led to false accusations simply to please interviewers and investigative workers (Ahlgrim-Delzell & Dudley, 2001; Scharnberg, 1996). In many ways, these discrediting claims are as dangerous to the construction of an emancipatory disability history as are the obstructionist actions encountered in the Michener history project. Thus, despite possible methodological and ethical disadvantages, I have opted to include multiple, triangulated data sources as a pre-emptive strategy; these methods will, I hope, preclude any possibility of powerful and interested parties from discrediting the Michener survivors' oral histories.

Finally, in light of the research and discourse on acquiescence and the skepticism that has been levelled against the claims of individuals with intellectual disabilities, it is important to consider the relative social value of these two groups. Individuals with intellectual disabilities, because of their social positions and their economic, cultural, and social capital, are vulnerable to discrediting. Conversely, those who enjoy economic, social, cultural, and intellectual dominance have been able to tell their own histories, to obstruct the telling of marginal memories, and to be relatively immune to both scrutiny and discrediting. Although there has been considerable speculation on the motives of vulnerable individuals and on the veracity of their narratives, there has been virtually no discussion of the false memory syndromes of the powerful institutions and social actors who seek to prevent marginalized histories from becoming known. Most certainly, it is time to for such a discussion to begin. In the meanwhile, however, by including archival materials and interviews with workers who have also survived the institution, I hope not to undermine these survivors' stories but to validate them.

Notes

1. Introducing the Michener Centre

1 The institution has had many names. It opened as Provincial Training School, but with the construction of an adult facility on the campus in the 1960s, the institution went under two names: Deerhome, for the adult facility, and Alberta School Hospital, for the children's side of the campus. In 1977 the institution finally was renamed the Michener Centre, in honour of locally born Roland Michener, a popular athlete and eventual governor general of Canada.

2 Although the general descriptor for inmates was *mental deficiency*, six classifications for admission to the institute were possible at that time: a child could be admitted on the grounds of being an idiot, an imbecile, a moron, constitutionally inferior, psychopathic, or mentally deficient and psychopathic (Alberta Social Services and Community Health, 1985).

3 In Canada, the terms *intellectually disabled* or *individuals with intellectual disabilities* are used, while in the United Kingdom *learning disabled* is more typical. In this book, when referring to current practices or situations, I will use the Canadian contemporary terminology.

4 Named for the address (Tiergartenstrasse 4) in Berlin of the bureaucracy in charge of registering, transferring, and murdering those with chronic mental illness or epilepsy, and long-term inmates of asylums and hospitals (Burleigh, 1994, 1997; Kuhl, 1994; Trent, 1993).

5 Only in 1972 did the Government of Alberta pass a law that removed the necessity of families paying for their children's internment in government institutions for the "handicapped" (Government of Alberta. Department of Social Services and Community Health, 1972–73).

6 "Sense training" stems from the late-nineteenth-century theories of Eduard Seguin and was based on the understanding that cognitive development could be

stimulated through heightened sensory experiences. As was noted earlier, Seguin's program was based on the conviction that cognitive impairments could be cured.

7 During this period, the children's side of PTS changed its name briefly to Alberta School Hospital to differentiate itself from Deerhome, the adult side.

8 As noted earlier, the annual reports for the years 1923 to 1968 are quite extensive, including records of admissions, paroles, the diagnostic categories of residents, training programs for staff and residents, accounts of farms produce, payments received, deaths, and so on. From 1969 forward, the annual reports are reduced to one or two pages.

9 Norway, Sweden, Finland, France, and Denmark all passed negative eugenics laws during the 1930s, England and parts of America and Canada passed comparable laws during the 1910s and 1920s, and of course the ascendance of eugenics programs during much of the first half of the twentieth century is well documented.

2. Entering the Gulag, Leaving the World

1 For a brief biographical sketch of all participants, please see Appendix I.

2 Admissions continued until recently. Some of these are aging ex-residents with deteriorating health who have no community care networks and who thus have "no place else to go" but the Michener Centre (Michener Centre Communications Officer, 1999).

3. Dehumanization as a Way of Life

1 Inmates, regardless of their age or whether they lived on the children's or the Deerhome side of the campus, were called *children*.

2 I explore this topic more fully in Chapter Eight.

3 Spatial arrangements did little to prevent same-sex relationships, perhaps because such connections were seen as less eugenically threatening. Nevertheless, surveillance within the units operated to make it challenging to engage in any kind of sexual or romantic activities.

4 As noted in Chapter One, these categories continued to be used in the annual reporting until 1968, the final year that annual reports of a detailed nature were produced by the Michener Centre.

5 In 1998, the Federal Court of Canada began the process to repeal this requirement (Kohn, 2008). In that same year, having passed a basic capacity test (four simple questions about location, age, and name) that was asked of all citizens, 97 residents of the Michener Centre were permitted to vote for the first time in their lives (Lozeron, 1988).

4. Ordinary and Extraordinary Violence

1 The real family name of both parties was quite unusual, and the initials of both people were given in the Incident Reports. These facts led me to an online search, where a recent obituary for the wife described her and her husband's lengthy contributions to life at the Michener Centre.

2 It is worth mentioning that Time-Out or Isolation Rooms are experiencing something of a comeback, particularly in the public school systems, as evidenced by a number of lawsuits launched by parent and advocacy groups against schools that have used these time-out rooms excessively (Fantz, 2008). This comeback is accompanied by language fitting the operant conditioning paradigm, where rooms are to be "used when a student needs to be temporarily separated or removed from the environment where he/she is behaving in appropriately until he/she can demonstrate appropriate behaviour" (New Brunswick Education, 2002). Further echoing the language of behaviourism, the use of these rooms is to be "systematically, planned, delivered, supervised, and evaluated to determine effectiveness with individual students ... by keeping accurate records of ... behaviors that led to the use of time-out ... [and] ... behaviors observed in the time-out room that led to the use of time-out" (New Brunswick Education, 2002).

3 In reality, most of the recommendations set out by the Accreditation Council in 1971 do not seem to have been followed at the Michener Centre. These standards included informed consent for research, access to personal belongings and clothing, residents' input on disciplinary policies in the institutions, payment for employment, training in managing money, privacy in terms of sending and receiving personal mail and visits, strict controls on the use of restraints, accommodation for heterosexual relationships, planned daily activities, regular outdoor access, freedom of movement, and a wide range of other human rights. The recommendations run to 158 pages, and they read contrary to almost everything evidenced in the record and in survivor narratives (Joint Commission on Accreditation of Hospitals, 1971).

4 All interviewees were asked to talk about whether they had been close to or afraid of any workers.

5 Ponoka Hospital was a long-term mental institution situated in the small town of Ponoka, Alberta, approximately an hour's drive from Red Deer, where Michener was situated. Like Michener, Ponoka was also a feeder institution for the province's involuntary sterilization machine.

6. Broken Promises: Education in the Institution

1 Children below the age of five did not come into the institution through the school system or as a result of not being provided with appropriate educational services

but were admitted through paediatricians, Guidance Clinics, public health workers, and family members (Ballance & Kendall, 1969).

2 It is telling that although the superintendent published his own "research" in academic journals as another avenue for legitimating the academic reputation of the institution, none of these articles pertain to education but instead focus on medical experimentation, a subject that will be explored in the chapter on eugenics and experimentation.

3 This is another instance of the institutional record standing in stark contrast to the oral histories obtained for this book. As is noted in the chapter on work, inmates consistently reported that they were not paid for their work, for the most part, and that when they did earn money, they had no control or access to it.

7. Training, Exploitation, and Community Dependency

1 *Villa* was the term used to describe several relatively small wards that housed between 30 and 40 of the most advanced High Grade children on the Michener Centre campus.

2 The Nazis frequently referred to disabled, impoverished, and racialized groups as *useless eaters* (Burleigh, 1994).

3 "Stellar" Rehabilitation Services continues to operate in the Red Deer area as a social enterprise, "a business that manage[s] operations and redirect[s] surpluses towards the social and environmental goals of the community" (Bubel, 2008). A 2008 viewing of its webpages indicated that supervisory workers for their bottle exchange were being sought at a rate of between $11.78/h and $12.08/h, which would have been a fairly low rate of pay in the oil-rich Alberta economy. There was no indication of the pay rate for non-supervisory workers.

8. Bad Medicine: Drugs, Research, and Ethics

1 As Janice's sister speculated in her write-up, and as Evelyn indicated in her interview, it is quite possible that inmates who bit themselves did so as a result of sensory deprivation, as a way of self-stimulating.

2 An anonymous reviewer of this book, with presumably some expertise in the administration of these kinds of medication, indicated that all "these medications in the amounts specified would be almost certainly fatal within a few a few days if not immediately" (Anonymous, personal communication, October 9, 2013). It is possible the poor training of mental deficiency nurses may have contributed to mistakes in charting doctors' order.

3 I use the term *resident* in this singular instance, to reflect the assertion made in the Muir trial transcripts by Justice Joanna Veit that there was considerable favouritism

in the institution. She described that, in particular, Keith Manning, the premier's son, was able to have a room of his own, keep a radio, and wear his own clothing during his many years at the Michener Centre (*Muir v. Alberta*, 1996).

4 In current monographs describing this drug, it would appear that the side effects attached to its use are not inconsequential and include gastric upset, dry mouth, tongue rolling, drooling, blurred vision, nocturnal confusion, hyperactivity, and more, including a warning concerning death from cardiac proarrhythmia.

5 The general consensus remains that Down syndrome males are extremely unlikely to be fertile, although there have been very rare cases of verified paternity (cf. Sheridan et al., 1989 and Pradhan et al., 2006).

6 It is not stated in Thompson's article why this young, pregnant woman was having a hysterectomy. However, the Eugenics Board did mandate eugenic operations on pregnant females, and this may have been such an instance.

7 An infamous example of unethical human research is the Tuskegee Syphilis Study conducted by the United States Public Health Service from 1932 to 1972 on impoverished African American men in Tuskegee, Alabama. In this study of almost 400 men testing positive for syphilis, the original purpose was to follow the course of syphilis to outline its effects and to examine the effectiveness of early treatments, such as mercury-based ointments (Reverby, 2009). However, the study quickly deteriorated. The men involved in the longitudinal research were never informed of their diagnoses, nor despite the discovery of penicillin and its effectiveness in treating syphilis in 1947, were they ever treated with antibiotics. The project ended with a leak to the press in 1972; however, these men were observed over several decades, deceived about their diagnosis, and never treated for their disease. In exchange, participants received regular health check-ups, hot meals, family health visits, cash incentives, and money for burials. Because they believed they were receiving free medical care as part of the study and trusted the officials leading the medical trials, and also because of their poverty, social marginalization, and limited resources, the men did not seek alternative treatment. It is known that not only did these men suffer and die unnecessarily, but they also infected wives, their non-marital sexual partners (who were not followed or informed by the researchers), and their children, many of whom died untreated as well (Reverby, 2009).

9. Eugenics and Sexuality

1 The Mental Hygiene Clinics were renamed in the mid-1930s to Guidance Clinics, perhaps because of the unsavory, eugenic associations with "hygiene."

2 In her evaluation of the full set of Eugenics Board files, Grekul (2002) did a comprehensive count of all cases and meetings of the Board during its decades of operation, concluding that each case considered took an average of approximately 10 minutes.

3 Of my random sampling of 128 sets of meeting minutes, there is not one case of a patient and his wife giving consent, so that none of the cases involved males whose female partners were charged with the responsibility of approving their steriliza-tion, reflecting the gender biases of the time and the gendered qualities of the cases and surgeries put before the Board.

10. But That's All in the Past, Isn't It?

1 The strong public reaction to the book led to a 1974 reissue, published by Allyn and Bacon. Now out of print but well worth reading, at this writing there was an electronic version available at http://www.bwgriffin.com/gsu/courses/edur7130/qualitative/12_Qual_Christmas_in_Purgatory.pdf.
2 Keith Manning's brother, Preston, went on to form the deeply conservative Reform Party of Alberta, which he eventually led at the national level before its absorption by the Conservative Party.
3 The proposed April 2014 closure did not occur and was deferred until the end of 2014. In the meantime, the reigning Conservative Party saw a leadership change and election in which Michener became a key issue, with several candidates vow-ing to revisit the question of closure should they succeed in winning the leadership vote (Henton, 2014).
4 The Michener board, run under the government department Persons with Developmental Disabilities (PDD) Central Region Community Board, includes residents who act as self-advocates, perhaps representing a major shift in gover-nance and, it is hoped, a new understanding about who should be making deci-sions concerning Michener Centre and its continued existence.

Bibliography

Abnet, C.C., Qiao, Y.-L., Dawsey, S.M., Dong, Z.-W., Taylor, P.R., & Mark, S.D. (2005). Tooth loss is associated with increased risk of total death and death from upper gastrointestinal cancer, heart disease, and stroke in a Chinese population-based cohort. *International Journal of Epidemiology, 34*(2), 467–474. http://dx.doi.org/10.1093/ije/dyh375

Agamben, G. (2002). *Remnants of Auschwitz: The witness and the archive* (D. Heller-Roazen, Trans.) Brooklyn, NY: Zone Books.

Ahlgrim-Delzell, L., & Dudley, J.R. (2001). Confirmed, unconfirmed, and false allegations of abuse made by adults with mental retardation who are members of a class action lawsuit. *Child Abuse & Neglect, 25*(8), 1121–1132. http://dx.doi.org/10.1016/S0145-2134(01)00260-5

Alberta apologizes for forced sterilization. (1999). *CBC News.* Retrieved from http://www.cbc.ca/news/canada/alberta-apologizes-for-forced-sterilization-1.169579

Alberta Department of Public Health, Mental Health Division. (1938). *Annual report.* Edmonton, Canada: Author.

Alberta Department of Public Health, Mental Health Division. (1940). *Annual report.* Edmonton, Canada: Author.

Alberta Department of Public Health, Mental Health Division. (1946). *Annual report, Provincial Training School.* Edmonton, Canada: Author.

Alberta Department of Public Health, Mental Health Division. (1949). *Annual report, Provincial Training School.* Edmonton, Canada: Author.

Alberta Department of Public Health, Mental Health Division. (1961–1962). *Annual report.* Edmonton, Canada: Author.

Alberta Government Department of Public Works, Site Development Section. (Cartographer). (1971). Michener Centre North, Red Deer (Deerhome) [map].

Alberta Human Services. (2013). Services directly delivered by the community board: Michener Services. Retrieved from http://humanservices.alberta.ca/disability-services/pdd-central-directly-delivered-services.html

Alberta School Hospital. (1967). *Guide and information for parents: Michener Centre.* Red Deer, Canada: Department of Health.

Alberta Social Services and Community Health. (1985). *Michener Centre: A history, 1923–1983.* Edmonton, Canada: Author.

Alberta Teachers' Association. (2002). *A Brief history of public education in Alberta: Monograph.* Edmonton, Canada: Author.

Alberta Union of Public Employees (2013). AUPE News: Keep Michener Open ads air Monday. Retrieved from http://www.aupe.org/news/keep-michener-open-tv-ads-air-monday/

Albrecht, G. L. (1993). *The disability business: Rehabilitation in America.* Thousand Oaks, CA: Sage.

Amary, I. B. (1980). *The rights of the mentally retarded-developmentally disabled to treatment and education.* Springfield, IL: Charles C. Thomas.

Anonymous. (1976b, December 21). [Letter to Dr. Kathleen Swallow]. (GR1990.0212, Box 4a, Unusual incidents, Doc. 9, pp. 1–3). Provincial Archives of Alberta, Edmonton, Canada.

Armstrong, D. (1983). *Political anatomy of the body: Medical knowledge in Britain in the twentieth century.* Cambridge, England: Cambridge University Press.

Bailey, V. (1997). [Review of the book From idiocy to mental deficiency: Historical perspectives on people with learning disabilities, by D. Wright & A. Digby (Eds.)]. *Journal of Social History, 31*(2), 481–483. http://dx.doi.org/10.1353/jsh/31.2.481

Bank of Canada. (2014). Inflation calculator. Retrieved from http://www.bankofcanada.ca/rates/related/inflation-calculator

Ballance, K. E., & Kendall, D. C. (1969). *Report on legislation and services for exceptional children in Canada.* Ottawa, Canada: Council for Exceptional Children Canadian Committee.

Balshem, M. (1993). *Cancer in the community: Class and medical authority.* Washington, DC: The Smithsonian Scholarly Institution Press.

Barnes, C. (2003). What a difference a decade makes: Reflection on doing "emancipatory" disability research. *Disability & Society, 18*(1), 3–17.

Blair, W. R. N. (1969). *Mental health in Alberta: A report on the Alberta Mental Health Study 1968.* Edmonton, Canada : Human Resources Research and Development Executive Council – Government of Alberta.

Blatt, B., & Kaplan, F. (1974). *Christmas in purgatory.* Syracuse, NY: Human Policy Press.

Booth, T., & Booth, W. (1996). Sounds of silence: Narrative research with inarticulate subjects. *Disability & Society, 11*(1), 55–70. http://dx.doi.org/10.1080/09687599650023326

Brady, S. M. (2001). Sterilization of girls and women with intellectual disabilities: Past and present justifications. *Violence Against Women, 7*(4), 432–461. http://dx.doi.org/10.1177/10778010122182541

Bredberg, E. (1999). Writing disability history: Problems, perspectives and sources. *Disability & Society, 14*(2), 189–201. http://dx.doi.org/10.1080/09687599926262

Brown, D. J. M. (1968). *Memorandum concerning elopements.* Deerhome, Alberta: Michener Centre.

Brown, D. J. M. (1972). *Memorandum to senior nursing staff: Elopement procedure.* Deerhome, Alberta: Michener Centre

Bubel, A. (2008). *Starting a social enterprise in Alberta: Social enterprise series.* Edmonton, Canada : Western Economic Diversification Canada, The Business Link.

Burleigh, M. (1994). *Death and deliverance: "Euthanasia" in Germany c. 1900–1945.* Cambridge, England: Cambridge University Press.

Burleigh, M. (1997). *Ethics and extermination: Reflections on Nazi genocide.* Cambridge, England: Cambridge University Press. http://dx.doi.org/10.1017/CBO9780511806162.

Bury, M. (2001). Illness narratives: Fact or fiction? *Sociology of Health & Illness, 23*(3), 263–285. http://dx.doi.org/10.1111/1467-9566.00252

Canadian Medical Association. (1961). *Canadian Medical Association code of ethics* [transcribed from the original by A. K. W. Brownell & E. Brownell]. Retrieved from https://www.cma.ca/multimedia/CMA/Content_Images/Inside_cma/Ethics/Code-of-Ethics/1961.pdf

Canadian Medical Association (1970). Canadian Medical Association code of ethics [transcribed from the original by A. K. W. Brownell & E. Brownell]. Retrieved from http://www.cma.ca/multimedia/CMA/Content_Images/Inside_cma/Ethics/Code-of-Ethics/1970.pdf

Canadian National Committee for Mental Hygiene. (1921). *Mental hygiene survey of the province of Alberta.* Edmonton, Alberta: Author.

Carlson, E. A. (2001). *The unfit: The history of a bad idea.* Cold Spring Harbor, NY: Cold Spring Harbor Laboratory Press.

Catlin, D. H., Ahrens, D. B., & Kucherova, Y. (2002). Detection of norbolethone, an anabolic steroid never marketed, in athletes' urine. *Rapid Communications in Mass Spectrometry, 16*(13), 1273–1275.

Cavanaugh, C. (2012). *Mary Irene Parlby: The Canadian encyclopedia.* Ottawa, Canada: Historica Dominion Institute.

Charmaz, K. (1990). 'Discovering' chronic illness: Using grounded theory. *Social Science & Medicine, 30*(11), 1161–1172. http://dx.doi.org/10.1016/0277-9536(90)90256-R

Christian, T., & Barker, B. (1974). *The mentally ill and human rights in Alberta: A study of the Alberta Sexual Sterilization Act.* Edmonton, Canada: University of Alberta. Faculty of Law.

Cookson. (1974). Dr. Cookson's report. (GR1990.0212, Box 4a, Unusual incidents, Doc. 67). Provincial Archives of Alberta, Edmonton, Canada.

Crissey, O. L. (1937). The mental development of children of the same IQ in differing institutional environments. *Child Development, 8*(3), 217–220. http://dx.doi.org/10.2307/1125629

Dale Rogers Training Center. (2013). About Dale Rogers Training Center. Retrieved from http://www.drtc.org/about.htm

Dechant, G. (2006). *Winter's children: The emergence of children's mental services in Alberta, 1905–2005.* Calgary, Canada: Muttart Foundation.

Deerhome Ward Progress Notes. (1974). (GR1990.0212, Box 4a, Unusual incidents, Doc. 91). Provincial Archives of Alberta, Edmonton, Canada.

Digby, A. (1996). Contexts and perspectives. In D. Wright & A. Digby (Eds.), *From idiocy to mental deficiency: Historical perspectives on people with learning disabilities* (pp. 1–21). New York, NY: Routledge.

Donaldson, C. (1989, August 10). Michener virus spreads. *The Advocate.* [Newspaper article]. Doreen Befus Fonds. Red Deer and District Archives, Red Deer, Canada.

Dowbiggin, I. (1995). Keeping this young country sane: C.K. Clarke, immigration restriction, and Canadian psychiatry, 1890–1925 [Editorial]. *Canadian Historical Review, 76*(4), 598–627. http://dx.doi.org/10.3138/CHR-076-04-03

Dybwad, G. (1961). Rehabilitation for the adult retardate. *American Journal of Public Health and the Nation's Health, 51*(7), 998–1004. http://dx.doi.org/10.2105/AJPH.51.7.998

Edwards, D. (1970, April 20). [Letter to George McLellan, provincial ombudsman]. Copy in possession of Sam Edwards.

The Eugenics Board. (1968). *Report to the Department of Health: 1967–1968.* (Accession Number 69.252). Provincial Archives of Alberta, Edmonton, Canada.

Fantz, A. (2008). Children forced into cell-like school seclusion rooms. *CNN.* Retrieved from http://www.cnn.com/2008/US/12/17/seclusion.rooms/index.html?eref=rss_us

Farrar, C. B. (1942). Euthanasia (Editorial). *American Journal of Psychiatry, 99,* 141–143.

Finlay, W. M. L., & Lyons, E. (2002). Acquiescence in Interviews with People Who Have Mental Retardation. *Mental Retardation, 40*(1), 14–29. http://dx.doi.org/10.1352/0047-6765(2002)040<0014:AIIWPW>2.0.CO;2

Foucault, M. (1977). Intellectuals and power: A conversation between Michel Foucault and Giles Deleuze. In D. Bouchard (Ed.), *Language, counter-memory, practice: Selected essays and interviews by Michel Foucault* (pp. 205–217). Oxford, England: Basil Blackwell.

Foucault, M. (1982). The subject and power. *Critical Inquiry, 8*(4), 777–795. http://dx.doi.org/10.1086/448181

Foucault, M. (1988a). Technologies of the self. In L. H. Martin, H. Gutman, & P. Hutton (Eds.), *Technologies of the self: A seminar with Michel Foucault* (pp. 16–49). Amherst, MA: University of Massachusetts Press.

Foucault, M. (1988b). *Madness and civilization: A history of insanity in the age of reason*. New York, NY: Vintage Books.

Foucault, M. (1990). The history of sexuality. (Vol. I). *An introduction*. New York, NY: Vintage Books.

Foucault, M. (1994). *The birth of the clinic: An archeology of medical perception*. New York, NY: Vintage Books.

Foucault, M. (1995). *Discipline and punish: The birth of the prison*. New York, NY: Vintage Books.

Frank, A. W. (2002). Why study peoples' stories? The dialogical ethics of narrative analysis. *International Journal of Qualitative Methods, 1*(1), 1–9.

Friends of Michener Centre. (2013). *To the legislative assembly of Alberta, in the legislature assembled* [Petition]. Retrieved from http://www.keepmicheneropen.com

Friesen, E. (1976a, August 10). Incident Report – John Wickstrom – Deceased. (GR1990.0212, Box 4a, Unusual incidents, Doc. 65). Provincial Archives of Alberta, Edmonton, Canada.

Friesen, E. (1976b, August 10). Incident Report – John Wickstrom – Deceased. (GR1990.0212, Box 4a, Unusual incidents, Doc. 64. Provincial Archives of Alberta. Edmonton, Alberta.

Garrett, M. E. (1976, December 29). [Letter to Mrs. & Mrs. X, Edmonton, Alberta]. (GR1990.0212, Box 41, Unusual incidents, Doc. 8). Provincial Archives of Alberta. Edmonton, Alberta.

Gearheart, B. R. (1972). *Education of the exceptional child: History, present practices, and trends*. Lanham, MD: University Press of America.

Geissler, C. A., & Bates, J. F. (1984). The nutritional effects of tooth loss. *American Journal of Clinical Nutrition, 39*(3), 478–489.

Goddard, H. H. (1912). *The Kallikak family: A study in the heredity of feeble-mindedness*. New York, NY: Macmillan.

Goffman, E. (1961). *Asylums: Essays on the social situation of mental patients and other inmates*. Garden City, NY: Doubleday Books.

Goldfarb, W. (1943). The effects of early institutional care on adolescent personality. *Journal of Experimental Education, 12*, 106–129.

Goodley, D. (1996). Tales of hidden lives: A critical examination of life history research with people who have learning difficulties. *Disability & Society, 11*(3), 333–348. http://dx.doi.org/10.1080/09687599627642

Gould, S. J. (1981). *The mismeasure of man*. New York, NY: W.W. Norton and Company.

Government of Alberta. (n.d.). *Guide and information for parents: Alberta School Hospital, Red Deer* [Pamphlet]. Edmonton, Canada: Author.

Government of Alberta. (1928). The Sexual Sterilization Act. *Chapter 37*, 117–118. Retrieved from Our Future, Our Past: The Alberta Digitization Project website: http://www.ourfutureourpast.ca/law/page.aspx?id=2906151

Government of Alberta. (1937). An Act to Amend the Sexual Sterilization Act. *Chapter 47*, 181–183. Retrieved from Our Future, Our Past: The Alberta Digitization Project website: http://www.ourfutureourpast.ca/law/page.aspx?id=2906151

Government of Alberta. (1942). An Act to Amend the Sexual Sterilization Act. *Chapter 48*, 179–180. Retrieved from Our Future, Our Past: The Alberta Digitization Project website: http://www.ourfutureourpast.ca/law/page.aspx?id=2958575

Government of Alberta. (2005a). Office of the Public Guardian (OPG). Retrieved from http://humanservices.alberta.ca/guardianship-trusteeship/office-public-guardian .html

Government of Alberta. (2005b). Freedom of Information and Privacy Protection Act. Retrieved from http://www.qp.alberta.ca/1266.cfm?page=F25.cfm&leg_type= Acts&isbncln=9780779762071

Government of Alberta. Department of Social Services and Community Health. (1972–1973). *Annual report: Services for the handicapped (Alberta School Hospital/ Deerhome, Red Deer)*. Edmonton, Canada: Author.

Government of Canada. (1872). An Act Respecting Public Schools 1872. In P. Dunae (Ed.), *The Homeroom: British Columbia's History of Education Web Site*. Retrieved from http://www2.viu.ca/homeroom/content/topics/Statutes/1872act.htm

Government of Northwest Territories. (1901). *The School Ordinance* C.O. 75, s. 1. (Chap. 29, pp. 1–44). Retrieved from http://207.167.4.168/wp-content/uploads/ 2011/03/chapter29.pdf

Grekul, J. (2008). Sterilization in Alberta, 1928–1972: Gender matters. *Canadian Review of Sociology, 45*(3), 247–266. http://dx.doi.org/10.1111/j.1755-618X .2008.00014.x

Grekul, J., Krahn, H., & Odynak, D. (2004). Sterilizing the "feeble-minded": Eugenics in Alberta, Canada, 1929–1972. *Journal of Historical Sociology, 17*(4), 358–384. http://dx.doi.org/10.1111/j.1467-6443.2004.00237.x

Grekul, J. M. (2002). *The social construction of the feebleminded threat: implementation of the Sexual Sterilization Act in Alberta, 1929–1972* (Unpublished doctoral dissertation). University of Alberta, Edmonton, Canada.

Haggerty, A. D. (1967). The effects of long-term hospitalization or institutionalization upon the language development of children. *Journal of Genetic Psychology, 94*(5), 205–210.

Haigh, D. J. B. (1976). Memorandum Re: Patient "X" (pp. 1): Psychiatrist, Alberta Social Services and Community Health. (GR1990.0212, Box 4a, Unusual incidents, Doc. 40). Provincial Archives of Alberta. Edmonton, Alberta.

Heal, L. W., & Sigelman, C. K. (1995). Response biases in interviews of individuals with limited mental ability. *Journal of Intellectual Disability Research, 39*(4), 331–340. http://dx.doi.org/10.1111/j.1365-2788.1995.tb00525.x

Hehir, T. (2002). Eliminating ableism in education. *Harvard Educational Review, 72*(1), 1–33.

Henton, D. (2014, June 5). Tory leadership won't halt closure of Michener centre, minister vows. *Calgary Herald*. Retrieved from http://www.calgaryherald.com/news/alberta/Tory+leadership+halt+closure+Michener+centre+minister+vows/9908197/story.html

Hill, A. M., Rhee, H., & Ross, B. (2009). Mentally disabled forced into "fight club" at Texas home. *ABC News: The Blotter*. Retrieved from http://abcnews.go.com/Blotter/mentally-disabled-forced-fight-club-texas-home/story?id=7556740

Hincks, C.M. (1927). Canadian National Committee for Mental Hygiene. *Canadian Medical Association Journal, 17*(1), 551–554.

Hollander, R. (1989). Euthanasia and mental retardation: Suggesting the unthinkable. *Mental Retardation, 27*(2), 53–61.

Hubert, J. (2000). Introduction. In J. Hubert (Ed.), *Madness, disability and social exclusion: The archeology and anthropology of 'difference'* (pp. 1–8). New York, NY: Routledge.

Hughes, B. (2002). Bauman's strangers: impairment and the invalidation of disabled people in modern and post-modern cultures. *Disability & Society, 17*(5), 571–584. http://dx.doi.org/10.1080/09687590220148531

Jaffe, E. D. (1967). A study of the effects of institutionalization on adolescent dependent children. *Israel Annals of Psychiatry and Related Disciplines, 5*, 169–181.

John F. Kennedy Presidential Library and Museum. (2013). Rosemary Kennedy. Retrieved from http://www.jfklibrary.org/JFK/The-Kennedy-Family/Rosemary-Kennedy.aspx

Joint Commission on Accreditation of Hospitals. (1971). *Standards for residential facilities for the mentally retarded*. Chicago, IL: Accreditation Council for Services for Facilities for the Mentally Retarded.

Jones, R. L. (1999). The master potter and the rejected pots: Eugenic legislation in Victoria, 1918–1939. *Australian Historical Studies, 29*(113), 319–342. http://dx.doi.org/10.1080/10314619908596105

Jordan, T. E. (1993). *The degeneracy crises and Victorian youth*. Albany, NY: State University of New York.

Juniper Ward Record. (1982, December 30). (GR1996.0337, Box 2. ASH. Dec 82-May 83. Doc. 19). Provincial Archives of Alberta, Edmonton, Canada.

Juniper Ward Record. (1983a, February 15). (GR1996.0337, Box 2. ASH. Dec 82-May 83. Doc. 66). Provincial Archives of Alberta, Edmonton, Canada.

Juniper Ward Record. (1983b, February 6). (GR1996.0337, Box 2. ASH. Dec 82-May 83. Doc. 56). Provincial Archives of Alberta, Edmonton, Canada.

Juniper Ward Record. (1983c, March 3). (GR1996.0337, Box 2. ASH. Dec 82-May 83. Doc. 78). Provincial Archives of Alberta, Edmonton, Canada.

Kaplan, A. (1964). *The conduct of inquiry: Methodology for behavioral science*. San Francisco, CA: Chandler Publishing Company.

Keates, D. P., Parents Organization. (1993, April). News from the Parents Organization. *Michener Messenger, 2*.

Kevles, D. J. (1995). *In the name of eugenics: Genetics and the uses of human heredity* (3rd ed.). Cambridge, MA: Harvard University Press.

Kleinman, A. (1988). *The illness narratives: Suffering, healing and the human condition.* New York, NY: Basic Books.

Koegler, S. J. (1976a, September 14). [Letter to Richard Short, Director, Services for the Handicapped]. (GR1990.0212, Box 4a, Unusual incidents, Doc. 51). Provincial Archives of Alberta, Edmonton, Canada.

Koegler, S. J. (1976b). [Report on accidental deaths.] (GR1990.0212, Box 4a, Unusual incidents, Doc. 37). Provincial Archives of Alberta, Edmonton, Canada.

Kohn, N. A. (2008). Cognitive impairment and the right to vote: Rethinking the meaning of accessible elections. *Canadian Journal of Elder Law, 1*(1), 29–52. Retrieved from http://www.law.syr.edu/media/documents/2009/1/Kohn__Cognitive_ Impairment__Right_to_Vote_Final_PDF.pdf

Kuhl, S. (1994). *The Nazi connection: Eugenics, American racism, and German national socialism.* New York, NY: Oxford University Press.

LaJeunesse, R. A. (1996). *Political asylums.* Edmonton, Canada: The Muttart Foundation.

Lane, M. (1873, June). Sense-perception, or object teaching. *The California Teacher: California Department of Public Education, Official Organ of the Department of Public Instruction, X*(12), 412–418.

Langford, N. (1997). *Politics, pitchforks and pickle jars: 75 years of organized farm women in Alberta.* Calgary, Canada: Detselig Enterprises Ltd.

Lee, R. (1980, October 28). Legionnaire's disease suspect at Michener. *The Advocate.* [Newspaper article]. Doreen Befus Fonds. Red Deer and District Archives, Red Deer, Canada.

Lee, R. (1981, October 21). Mother of city murder suspect objected to son visiting victim. *The Advocate*, p. A2. [Newspaper article]. Doreen Befus Fonds. Red Deer and District Archives, Red Deer, Canada.

Leithead, G. (1976, September 6). [Report Re: [Child's name]'s Mother to Dwayne Simmon, Relief Manager, Adult Activation Division]. (GR1990.0212, Box 4a, Unusual incidents, Doc. 52). Provincial Archives of Alberta, Edmonton, Canada.

Leonard, T. C. (2003). "More merciful and not less effective": Eugenics and American economics in the progressive era. *History of Political Economy, 35*(4), 687–712. http://dx.doi.org/10.1215/00182702-35-4-687

Lozeron, J. (1988, October 22). 97 residents to cast ballots after historic Michener enumeration. *The Advocate*, p. B2.

LeVann, L. J. (1950). A concept of schizophrenia in the lower grade mental defective. *American Journal of Mental Deficiency, 54*(April), 469–473.

LeVann, L. J. (1953). A clinical survey of alcoholics. *Canadian Medical Association Journal, 69*, 584–588.

LeVann, L. J. (1954). *Annual report, Provincial Training School, Red Deer.* Edmonton, Canada: Department of Public Health.

LeVann, L. J. (1956). *Annual report: Provincial Training School, Red Deer*. Edmonton, Canada: Department of Public Health.

LeVann, L. J. (1957). *Annual report: Provincial Training School, Red Deer*. Edmonton, Canada: Department of Public Health.

LeVann, L. J. (1959). Tripluoperazin dihydrochloride: An effective tranquillizing agent for behavioural abnormalities in defective children. *Canadian Medical Association Journal, 80*, 123–124.

LeVann, L. J. (1959–1960). *Annual report: Provincial Training School, Red Deer*. Edmonton, Canada: Department of Public Health.

LeVann, L. J. (1961a). *Annual report: Institutions for mental defectives (Provincial Training School, Red Deer; Deerhome, Red Deer)*. Edmonton, Canada: Department of Public Health.

LeVann, L. J. (1961b). Thioridazine (Mellaril) A psycho-sedative virtually free of side-effects. *Alberta Medical Bulletin, 26*(4), 144–147.

LeVann, L. J. (1961–1962). *Annual report: Provincial Training School, Red Deer*. Edmonton, Canada: Department of Public Health.

LeVann, L. J. (1962a). *Annual report, institutions for mental defectives*. Red Deer, Canada: The Provincial Training School and Deer Home.

LeVann, L. J. (1962b). Chlordiazeepoxide, A tranquillizer with anticonvulsant properties. *Canadian Medical Association Journal, 86*, 123–125.

LeVann, L. J. (1963a). *Annual report, institutions for mental defectives (Provincial Training School, Red Deer; Deerhome, Red Deer)*. Edmonton, Canada: Department of Public Health.

LeVann, L. J. (1963b). Congenital abnormalities in children born in Alberta during 1961: A survey and a hypothesis. *Canadian Medical Association Journal, 89*, 120–126.

LeVann, L. J. (1964). *Annual report: Institutions for mental defectives (Provincial Training School, Red Deer; Deerhome, Red Deer)*. Edmonton, Canada: Department of Public Health.

LeVann, L. J. (1965). Congenital abnormalities in children born in Alberta during 1962: a further communication. *Alberta Medical Bulletin, 30*(3), 145–155.

LeVann, L. J. (1967–1968). *Annual report: Institutions for mental defectives (Alberta School Hospital, Red Deer; Deerhome, Red Deer)*. Edmonton, Canada: Department of Public Health.

LeVann, L. J. (1968a). *Annual report on institutions for mental defectives (Alberta School Hospital, Red Deer; Deerhome, Red Deer)*. Edmonton, Canada: Department of Public Health.

LeVann, L. J. (1968b). A new butyrophenone: Trifluperidol a psychiatric evaluation in a pediatric setting. *Canadian Psychiatric Association Journal, 13*(3), 271–273.

LeVann, L. J. (1969). Haloperidol in the treatment of behavioural disorders in children and adolescents. *Canadian Psychiatric Association Journal, 14*(2), 217–220.

LeVann, L. J. (1970a, March 20). [Letter to Dorothy Edwards]. Copy in possession of Sam Edwards.

LeVann, L. J. (1970b). Clinical experience with Tarasan and thioridazine in mentally retarded children: A comparative double blind study. *Applied Therapeutics, 12*(5), 30–33.

LeVann, L. J., & Cohn, R. E. (1972). Clinical evaluation of Norbolethone therapy in stunted growth and poorly thriving children. *International Journal of Clinical Pharmacology, Therapy and Toxicology, 6*(1), 54–59.

Lippke, R. (2004). Against supermax. *Journal of Applied Philosophy, 21*(2), 109–124. http://dx.doi.org/10.1111/j.0264-3758.2004.00267.x

Low, S. E. (1939). *Auditor's report of the administrator of estates of the mentally incompetent.* (70.414 File 1854). Provincial Archives of Alberta, Edmonton, Canada.

Lozeron, J. (1976, August 20). ASH elopement blamed on staffing shortages. *The Advocate*, p. 13. [Newspaper article]. Doreen Befus Fonds. Red Deer and District Archives, Red Deer, Canada

MacEachran, J. M. (1947a). The minutes of the provincial Eugenics Board meeting, January 29. (GR1988.0211, Box 1, Item 1E, Doc. 4). Provincial Archives of Alberta, Edmonton, Canada.

MacEachran, J. M. (1947b). The minutes of the provincial Eugenics Board meeting, June 19, Provincial Mental Hospital, Ponoka. (GR1988.0211, Box 1, Item 1E, Doc. 5). Provincial Archives of Alberta, Edmonton, Canada.

MacEachran, J. M. (1954). The minutes of the provincial Eugenics Board meeting, April 23, Provincial Training School, Red Deer. (GR1988.0211, Box 1, Item 2A, Doc. 7). Provincial Archives of Alberta, Edmonton, Canada.

MacEachran, J. M. (1956). The minutes of the provincial Eugenics Board meeting, June 8, Provincial Training School, Red Deer. (GR1988.0211, Box 1, Item 2B, Doc. 18). Provincial Archives of Alberta, Edmonton, Canada.

MacEachran, J. M. (1957a). The minutes of the provincial Eugenics Board meeting, May 27, Provincial Mental Hospital, Ponoka. (GR1988.0211, Box 1, Item 2B, Doc.16). Provincial Archives of Alberta, Edmonton, Canada.

MacEachran, J. M. (1957b). The minutes of the provincial Eugenics Board meeting, September 20, Alberta School Hospital, Red Deer. (GR1988.0211, Box 1, Item 2B, Doc. 16). Provincial Archives of Alberta, Edmonton, Canada.

MacEachran, J. M. (1960). The minutes of the provincial Eugenics Board meeting, May 27, Provincial Training School, Red Deer. (GR1988.0211, Box 1, Item 2C, Doc. 22). Provincial Archives of Alberta, Edmonton, Canada.

MacEachran, J. M. (1963). The minutes of the provincial Eugenics Board meeting, June 8, Provincial Mental Institute, Edmonton. (GR1988.0211, Box 1, Item 3A, Doc. 34). Provincial Archives of Alberta, Edmonton, Canada.

MacLachlan, I. (2005). Personal correspondence: Census population for urban centres in Alberta. *Census of Canada*, Various years. Ottawa, Canada: Statistics Canada.

MacLean, R. R. (1960). *Annual report: Deerhome, Red Deer*. Edmonton, Canada: Department of Public Health.

MacNicol, J. (1992). The voluntary sterilization campaign in Britain, 1918–39. *Journal of the History of Sexuality, 2*(3), 422–438.

Manning, E. (1958). *Schedule II amending The Disabled Persons Pension Act*. Edmonton, Canada. Retrieved from http://www.ourfutureourpast.ca/law/page .aspx?id=2908339

Manning, P. (1992). *The new Canada*. Toronto, Canada: Macmillan Canada.

Martindale, C. (1983a, August 12). Senior patient says her only complaint is the food. The Advocate, p. C1. [Newspaper article]. Doreen Befus Fonds. Red Deer and District Archives, Red Deer, Canada.

Martindale, C. (1983b, August 15). Work a privilege afforded to few. *The Advocate,* p. B3. [Newspaper article]. Doreen Befus Fonds. Red Deer and District Archives, Red Deer, Canada.

Martindale, C. [ca. 1984]. Lack of privacy for severely retarded – But do they care? The Advocate. [Newspaper article]. Doreen Befus Fonds. Red Deer and District Archives, Red Deer, Canada.

Maulik, P. K., & Harbour, C. K. (2013). Epidemiology of intellectual disability. In J. H. Stone & M. Blouin (Eds.), *International Encyclopedia of Rehabilitation*. Retrieved from http://cirrie.buffalo.edu/encyclopedia/en/article/144/#s9.

McAlister, W. (1924). *Superintendent's 1923 report to the government of the province of Alberta*. Red Deer, Canada: Provincial Training School.

McAlister, W. (1926). *Provincial Training School, Health Department - Superintendent's report for 1926*. Alberta: Red Deer.

McCarthy, M., & Thompson, D. (1996). Sexual Abuse by Design: An examination of the issues in learning disability services. *Disability & Society, 11*(2), 205–218. http:// dx.doi.org/10.1080/09687599650023236

McCullough, D. L. (1938a). *Annual report, 1938: Provincial Training School*. Red Deer, Canada: Government of Alberta.

McCullough, D. L. (1938b). *Annual report: Provincial Training School, Red Deer, Alberta*. Alberta, Canada: Red Deer.

McCullough, D. L. (1940). *Annual report, 1940: Provincial Training School*. Red Deer, Canada: Government of Alberta.

McKinney, L. (1919). *Sessional Paper No. 27 - A Return to an Order of the House dated Feb. 11 1914 Re: Persons in the Asylums in the Province*. Edmonton, Canada: Government of the Province of Alberta.

McLaren, A. (1986). The creation of a haven for 'human thoroughbreds': The sterilization of the feeble-minded and the mentally ill in British Columbia. *Canadian Historical Review, 67*(2), 127–150. http://dx.doi.org/10.3138/CHR-067-02-01

McLaren, A. (1990). *Our own master race: Eugenics in Canada, 1885–1945*. Toronto, Canada: MacLelland and Stewart.

Michelin, L. (1999). Review recommends video, staff surveillance. *The Advocate*, p. A2. [Newspaper article]. Doreen Befus Fonds. Red Deer and District Archives, Red Deer, Canada.

Michener Board. (2001). Michener board minutes, May 17. Red Deer, Canada: Author.

Million, D. (2005). *Telling Secrets: Sex, power and narrative in the rearticulation of Canadian residential school history* (Unpublished doctoral dissertation, University of California Berkeley, Berkeley, California.

Moisander, P., & Edston, E. (2003). Torture and its sequel - A comparison between victims from six countries. *Forensic Science International, 137*(2–3), 133–140. http://dx.doi.org/10.1016/j.forsciint.2003.07.008

Monchuk, J. (1985a, November 22). Michener Centre reviews volunteer screening policy. *The Advocate*, p. A2. [Newspaper article]. Doreen Befus Fonds. Red Deer and District Archives, Red Deer, Canada.

Monchuk, J. (1985b). Michener resident's pregnancy under investigation. *The Advocate*. [Newspaper article]. Doreen Befus Fonds. Red Deer and District Archives, Red Deer, Canada.

Monchuk, J. (1985c, November 9). No Michener charges laid. *The Advocate*. [Newspaper article]. Doreen Befus Fonds. Red Deer and District Archives, Red Deer, Canada.

Monchuk, J. (1985d, November 25). Sex penalty angers parent. *The Advocate*, p. A2. [Newspaper article]. Doreen Befus Fonds. Red Deer and District Archives, Red Deer, Canada.

More than 260 Central Alberta AUPE members brave icy conditions to attend joint AGM. (2004, April 14). *AUPE News & Updates*. Retrieved from http://www.aupe.org/in_the_news/PR2004/apr1504.php

Muir v. Alberta (1996), 132 DLR (4th) 695 (Alta QB), Veit J.

Murphy, E. F. (1922). *The black candle*. Toronto, Canada: Thomas Allen Publisher.

New Brunswick Education. (2002). Time-out guidelines for New Brunswick schools. Retrieved from http://www.gnb.ca/0000/publications/ss/Time-outGuidelines-r.pdf

Nightingale Ward Record. (1982a, November 28). [Daily record book.] (Acc. 96.337, Box 1, Nightingale A, Doc. 6.). Provincial Archives of Alberta, Edmonton, Canada.

Nightingale Ward Record. (1982b, December 2). (GR1996.0337, Box 1. Nightingale A. Nov 82–June 83. Doc. 12). Provincial Archives of Alberta, Edmonton, Canada.

Nightingale Ward Record. (1982c, December 26). (GR1996.0337, Box 1. Nightingale A. Nov 82–June 83. Doc. 31). Provincial Archives of Alberta, Edmonton, Canada.

Nightingale Ward Record. (1983a, January 15). (GR1996.0337, Box 1. Nightingale A. Nov 82–June 83. Doc. 47). Provincial Archives of Alberta, Edmonton, Canada.

Nightingale Ward Record. (1983b, January 23). (GR1996.0337, Box 1. Nightingale A. Nov 82–June 83. Doc. 51). Provincial Archives of Alberta, Edmonton, Canada.

Noll, S. (1998). The sterilization of Willie Mallory. In M. Ladd-Taylor & L. Umansky (Eds.), *Bad mothers: The politics of blame in twentieth-century America* (pp. 41–57). New York, NY: New York University Press.

Oreopoulos, P. (2005). Canadian compulsory school laws and their impact on education attainment and future earnings. Retrieved from http://www.statcan.gc.ca/pub/11f0019m/11f0019m2005251-eng.pdf

Osgood, R. L. (2001). The menace of the feebleminded: George Bliss, Amos Butler, and the Indiana Committee on Mental Defectives. *Indiana Magazine of History*, 97(December), 253–274.

Park, D. C., & Radford, J. P. (1998). From the case files: Reconstructing a history of involuntary sterilisation. *Disability & Society*, 13(3), 317–342. http://dx.doi.org/10.1080/09687599826669

PDD Central Region Community Board. (2007). September 25 board meeting: Plain language minutes. Retrieved from http://humanservices.alberta.ca/documents/PDD/pdd-central-minutes-200709-plain-language.pdf

Pettifor, J. (2010). Reflections on respect and caring for persons with disabilities: My sixty-one years of Alberta history. *International Journal of Disability, Community and Rehabilitation, 9*(1). Retrieved from http://www.ijdcr.ca/VOL09_01/articles/pettifor.shtml

Pfohl, S. (1978). *Predicting dangerousness*. Toronto, Canada: Lexington Books.

Poore, C. (2007). *Disability in twentieth-century German Culture*. Ann Arbor, MI: University of Michigan Press.

Porteous, C. A. (1918). Some notes on the formation of the Canadian National Committee for Mental Hygiene. *Canadian Medical Association Journal, 8*(7), 634–639.

Porter, R. (1987). *A social history of madness: Stories of the insane*. London, England: Phoenix.

Porter, R. (1997). A simple fellow given to blowing at feathers exploited by his grasping brothers. [Review of the book From idiocy to mental deficiency: Historical perspectives on people with learning disabilities, by D. Wright & A. Digby (Eds.)]. *London Review of Books, 19*(9), 23–24. Retrieved from http://www.lrb.co.uk/v19/n09/roy-porter/a-simple-fellow-given-to-blowing-at-feathers-exploited-by-his-grasping-brothers

Pradhan, M., Dalal, A., Khan, F., & Agrawal, S. (2006). Fertility in men with Down syndrome: a case report. *Fertility and Sterility, 86*(6), 1865.e1861–1765.e1863.

Pringle, H. (1997). Alberta barren: The Mannings and forced sterilization in Canada. *Saturday Night, 112*(5), 30–40.

Proby, J. (1991, May 7). Michener drug dosage being reviewed. *The Advocate*. [Newspaper article]. Doreen Befus Fonds. Red Deer and District Archives, Red Deer, Canada.

Proctor, R. N. (1995). The destruction of "lives not worth living." In J. Terry & J. Urla (Eds.), *Deviant bodies: Critical perspectives on difference in science and popular culture* (pp. 171–196). Bloomington, IL: Indiana University Press.

Radford, J. P. (1994). Eugenics and the asylum. *Journal of Historical Sociology, 7*(4), 462–473. http://dx.doi.org/10.1111/j.1467-6443.1994.tb00076.x

Rafter, N. H. (1997). *Creating born criminals*. Chicago, IL: Illinois University Press.

Reid Crowther & Partners Limited. (Cartographer). (1977). City of Red Deer, East Red Deer Utility Trunks, 55th Street [Haul route map].

Reilly, P. (1991). *The surgical solution: A history of involuntary sterilization in the United States*. Baltimore, ML: The Johns Hopkins Press.

Rennie, B. J. (2000). *The rise of agrarian democracy: The United Farmers and Farm Women of Alberta, 1909–1921*. Toronto, Canada: University of Toronto Press.

Reverby, S. M. (2009). *Examining Tuskegee: The infamous syphilis study and its legacy*. Chapel Hill, NC: The University of North Carolina Press.

Richards, S. (2006, November). *Research on USP Marion: The first federal super max prison*. Paper presented at the American Society of Criminology conference, Los Angeles, CA.

Roche, P. (1994, January 8). Union fears Michener closure. *Red Deer Advocate*, p. B1.

Rooke, P. T. (1983). *Discarding the asylum: From child rescue to the welfare state in English-Canada (1800–1950)*. Lanham, MD: University Press of America Inc.

Rose, N. (1990). *Governing the soul: The shaping of the private self*. London, England: Routledge.

Rutherford, A. (2013). Profile: Jean Pettifor. *Psychology's Feminist Voices*. Retrieved from http://www.feministvoices.com/jean-pettifor/

RXList Inc. (2012). Mellaril. Retrieved from http://www.rxlist.com/mellaril-drug.htm

Sakalys, J. A. (2000). The political role of illness narratives. *Journal of Advanced Nursing, 31*(6), 1469–1475. http://dx.doi.org/10.1046/j.1365-2648.2000.01461.x

Sarraj, E. E., Punamaki, R.-L., Salmi, S., & Summerfield, D. (1996). Experiences of torture and ill-treatment and osstrauamatic stress disorder symptoms among Palestinian political prisoners. *Journal of Traumatic Stress, 9*(3), 595–606. http://dx.doi.org/10.1002/jts.2490090315

Savage, R. (2007). "Disease incarnate": Biopolitical discourse and genocial dehuman-isation in the age of modernity. *Journal of Historical Sociology, 20*(3), 404–440.

Scharnberg, M. (1996). Frailty, thy name is memory: An inverse witch trial in Denmark. *Issues in Child Abuse Accusations, 8*(3–4), 1–14.

Scheerenberger, R. C. (1983). *A history of mental retardation*. Baltimore, MD: Brookes Publishing Co.

Schell-Frank, D. (2000). *Education & international adoption: As our children grow*. Fort Collins, CO: Author.

Schizophrenia Society of Ontario. (2014a). Largactil (chlorpromazine). Retrieved from http://www.schizophrenia.on.ca/Schizophrenia-Psychosis/Medication-Resource-Centre/Typical-Antipsychotic-Medications/Largactil-(chlorpromazine)

Schizophrenia Society of Ontario. (2014b). Neuleptil (Periciazine). Retrieved from http://www.schizophrenia.on.ca/Schizophrenia-Psychosis/Medication-Resource-Centre/Typical-Antipsychotic-Medications/Neuleptil-(periciazine)

Schneider, H. J. (1996). Violence in the institution. *International Journal of Offender Therapy and Comparative Criminology, 40*(1), 5–18. http://dx.doi.org/10.1177/0306624X96401002

Schoen, J. (2001). Between choice and coercion: Women and the politics of sterilization in North Carolina, 1929–1975. *Journal of Women's History, 13*(1), 132–156. http://dx.doi.org/10.1353/jowh.2001.0034

Scott, J. (1985). *Weapons of the weak: Everyday forms of peasant resistance*. New Haven, London: Yale University Press.

Scull, A. (1984). *Decarceration: Community treatment and the deviant: A radical view* (2nd ed.). New Brunswick, NJ: Rutgers University Press.

Semanek, R. (1982). Accused killer would "do it again" psychiatrist says. *Red Deer Advocate*.

Sharpe, R. J., & McMahon, P. I. (2008). *The Persons case: The origins and legacy of the fight for legal personhood*. Toronto, Canada: University of Toronto Press.

Sheiham, A., Steele, J. G., Marcenes, W., Lowe, C., Finch, S., Bates, C. J., Walls, A. W. G. (2001). The Relationship among dental status, nutrient intake, and nutritional status in older people. *Journal of Dental Research, 80*(2), 408–413

Sheridan, R., Llerena, J., Matkins, S., Debenham, P., Cawood, A., & Bobrow, M. (1989). Fertility in a male with trisomy 21. *Journal of Medical Genetics, 26*(5), 294–298. http://dx.doi.org/10.1136/jmg.26.5.294

Skeels, H. M., & Dye, H. B. A. (1939). A study of the effects of differential stimulation on mentally retarded children. *Proceedings & Addresses of the American Association on Mental Deficiency, 44*, 114–136.

Slee, R. (2001). Social justice and the changing directions in educational research: the case of inclusive education. *International Journal of Inclusive Education, 5*(2–3), 167–177. http://dx.doi.org/10.1080/13603110010035832

Smart, B. (Ed.). (1985). *Michel Foucault:Critical assessments*. New York, NY: Routledge. http://dx.doi.org/10.4324/9780203405741.

Smith, J. D. (1985). *Minds made feeble: The myth and legacy of the Kallikaks*. Rockville, MD: Aspen Publications.

Soloway, R. (1990). *Demography and degeneration: Eugenics and the declining birthrate in twentieth-century Britain*. Chapel Hill, NC: University of North Carolina Press.

Stability at last. (1976, March). *Red Deer Advocate*. [Newspaper article.] Doreen Befus Fonds. Red Deer and District Archives, Red Deer, Canada.

St. Denys, N. (2003, April). Neil St. Denys Says Goodbye! *Michener Messenger*, 1–20.

Stevenson, H. W., & Fahel, L. S. (1961). The effect of social reinforcement on the performance of institutionalized and noninstitutionalized normal and feeble-minded children. *Journal of Personality, 29*(2), 136–147. http://dx.doi.org/10.1111/j.1467-6494.1961.tb01651.x

Sudnow, D. (1967). *Passing on: the social organization of dying*. Englewood Cliffs, NJ: Prentice Hall.

Sutherland, N. (1976). *Children in English Canadian society: Framing the twentieth century consensus*. Toronto, Canada: University of Toronto Press.

Swallow, K. (1975). Reference: 31035 (a) – Notifications Procedure: Director of Nursing. (GR1990.212, Box 3c, Elopements, Doc 1). Provincial Archives of Alberta. Edmonton, Canada.

Swallow, K. A. (1976, December 10). [Letter to Dr. S. J. Kroegler, Executive Director Regarding Penny Christien Simpson, Dec'd.] (GR1990.0212, Box 4a, Unusual incidents, Doc. 76). Provincial Archives of Alberta. Edmonton, Canada.

Texas lambasted over care of mentally disabled. (2008). *NBC News*. Retrieved from http://www.nbcnews.com/id/28036793/ns/health-health_care/t/texas-lambasted-over-care-mentally-disabled#.U5FLhygWAwY

Thomas, C. (2007). *Sociologies of disability and illness: Contested ideas in disability studies and medical sociology*. Basingstoke, England: Palgrave MacMillan.

Thompson, M. W. (1961). Reproduction in two female mongols. *Canadian Journal of Genetics and Cytology, 3*, 351–354.

Thompson, M. W. (1962). 21-trisomy in a fertile female mongol. *Canadian Journal of Genetics and Cytology, 4*, 352–355.

Thomson, R.K. (1966). The minutes of the provincial Eugenics Board meeting, September 13, Alberta School Hospital, Red Deer. (GR1988.0211, Box 1, Item 39B, Doc. 53). Provincial Archives of Alberta. Edmonton, Canada.

Thomson, R.K. (1968). The minutes of the provincial Eugenics Board meeting, October 8, Alberta School Hospital. (GR1988.0211, Box 1, Item 3C, Doc. 48). Provincial Archives of Alberta. Edmonton, Canada.

Thomson, R.K. (1972). The minutes of the provincial Eugenics Board meeting, February 22, Alberta School Hospital, Red Deer. (GR1988.0211, Box 1, Item 4, Doc. 1). Provincial Archives of Alberta. Edmonton, Canada.

Tileaga, C. (2007). Ideologies of moral exclusion: A critical discursive reframing of depersonalization, delegitimation and dehumanization. *British Journal of Social Psychology, 46*(4), 717–737. http://dx.doi.org/10.1348/014466607X186894

Trent, J. W. (1993). To cut and control: Institutional preservation and the sterilization of mentally retarded people in the United States. *Journal of Historical Sociology, 6*(1), 56–73. http://dx.doi.org/10.1111/j.1467-6443.1993.tb00040.x

Trent, J. W. (1994). *Inventing the feeble mind: A history of mental retardation in the United States*. Berkeley, CA: University of California Press.

Trent, J.W., Jr., (1995). Suffering fools. *Sciences, 35*(4), 18–22. http://dx.doi.org/10.1002/j.2326-1951.1995.tb03643.x

Unusual Incidents Report. (1975. June 4). (GR1990.0212, Box 4a, Unusual incidents, Doc. 98). Provincial Archives of Alberta. Edmonton, Canada.

Vallance, E. (1983). Hiding the hidden curriculum: An interpretation of the language of justification in nineteenth-century educational reform. In H. Giroux & D. Purpel (Eds.), *The Hidden Curriculum: Deception or discovery?* (pp. 2–27). Berkeley, CA: McCutchan Publishing.

van Rassel, J. (2014, June 27). Wildrose pledges to reopen Michener Centre, target $50 million for seniors. *Calgary Herald*. Retrieved from http://www.calgaryherald.com/news/politics/Wildrose+pledges+reopen+Michener+Centre+target+million/9981185/story.html

Wahlsten, D. (1997). Leilani Muir versus the philosopher king: Eugenics on trial in Alberta. *Genetica, 99*(2–3), 185–198. http://dx.doi.org/10.1007/BF02259522

Walmsley, J. (2000). Women and the Mental Deficiency Act of 1913: citizenship, sexuality and regulation. *British Journal of Learning Disabilities, 28*(2), 65–70. http://dx.doi.org/10.1046/j.1468-3156.2000.00042.x

Weikart, R. (2004). *From Darwin to Hitler: Evolutionary ethics, eugenics, and racism in Germany*. New York: Palgrave Macmillan.

Wendell, S. (1996). *The rejected body: Feminist philosophical reflections on disability*. New York, NY: Routledge.

Williams, B. (2004). Dying young, dying poor: A sociological examination among existential suffering low-socioeconomic status patients. *Journal of Palliative Medicine, 7*(1), 27–37. http://dx.doi.org/10.1089/109662104322737223

Wilson, H. G. (1940). *The annual report of the estates branch: Official guardian, administrator of estates of the mentally incompetent consolidated investment fund*. Edmonton, Canada: Department of the Attorney General, Government of Alberta.

Wingrove, J. (2013, March 15). Alberta's Michener Centre can't shake a sordid history. *The Globe and Mail*. Retrieved from http://www.theglobeandmail.com/news/national/albertas-michener-centre-cant-shake-sordid-history/article9848678/

Winzer, M. (2009). *From integration to inclusion: A history of special education in the 20th century*. Washington, D.C.: Gallaudet University Press.

Wittmeier, C. (1999, September 6). The final batch: Sterilization claimants may soon see taxpayer dollars, but not nearly what they've demanded. *Alberta Report, 14*, 12–13.

Wolfenserger, W. (1970). The Principle of normalization and its implications to psychiatric services. *American Journal of Psychiatry, 127*, 291–297.

World Medical Association. (2006). WMA Declaration of Geneva. Retrieved from
    http://www.wma.net/en/30publications/10policies/g1/ (Originally published 1948)
Young, S. N. (1998). Risk in research – from the Nuremberg Code to the Tri-Council
    Code: implications for clinical trials of psychotropic drugs. *Journal of Psychiatry &*
    Neuroscience, 23(23), 149–155.
Zemanek, R. (1982, September 10). Accused killer would "do it again" psychiatrist
    says. *The Advocate,* p. B2. [Newspaper article]. Doreen Befus Fonds. Red Deer and
    District Archives, Red Deer, Canada.

Index

Note: Page numbers in *italics* indicate figures and tables.

about, 26–7, 34; population distribution and, 152, *153*, *154*. *See also* industrialization
utility, 152–5. *See also* productivity

Vanderhoof, Mr (worker), 101
Vanderhoof, Mrs (worker), 99
Veit, Joanna: on absence of consent, 194; on favouritism in Michener, 256n3; on IQ testing, 204; on misuse of drugs, 185, 187–8; on sterilizations, 218, 221. See also *Muir v. Alberta*
Vicky (inmate), 120–1
villa: use of term, 256n1. *See also* High Grade wards
Vineland Training School for Feeble-Minded Boys and Girls (New Jersey), 20–2, 26
violence: biting self or others, 82, 88, 99–100, 180, 256n1; built-in type of, 110–12; culture of, 94–9, 103–6, 109–10, 122; evidence of, noticed by outsiders, 51, 58, 99–100, 106, 178–9; extraordinary type, *see* violence, extraordinary type; institutionalization of, 97–9, 104, 110–12; justification for, 62, 63; language for, 93–6; preventive quality of, 112, 114–17; resident-to-resident or to self, 99–100, 109–10; routinization of, 82–3, 93–9; sensory deprivation and dehumanization linked to, 82–4; social devaluation of terminally ill and, 54
violence, extraordinary type: invisibility of, 99–103; murder resulting in public enquiry, 106–8; as ordinary, 104–5; staff reporting discouraged, 103–6; survivors' stories of, 108–9; in Texas "state schools," 232–3. *See also* sexual assault

visitors: difficulties of, 55–6; policy on, 50–2, 54–5; professional persons, 189–90
vocational rehabilitation industry, 138, 151–2, 160
vocational training: agricultural type, 145, 147–8, 161; educational rhetoric and justification of, 9, 13–14, 162–3; escape opportunity in, 128; Foucault's cynicism about, 151–2; as High Grade option, 13; as semi-skilled labour, 138–9; unpaid labour outside Michener as, 164–6; utility and broader context of, 152–5. *See also* agriculture; economic exploitation; occupational training; productivity; work
volunteers, 107–8
voting rights, 91, 197–8, 254n5

wages (inmates): absent or miniscule, 158, 163, 164–5; held in trust, 165–6; records on, 256n3; standards on, 166
Wahlsten, Douglas, 208
wards: beds in, 69–70; climate of reprisal in, 101–5; daily reports on routine violence in, 94–5, 96; description of 1950s-style, 61–2; entrance hallway to, 64, *65*; escapes and, 127; exterior of, 59; hierarchies of disability reflected in differences in, 70–3, *71*, *72*, *73*, 74–5; inmates' work on, 158–60, 162; mechanized aspect of, 75; names for, 59; nursing stations of, 67–70, *69*, 83; sensory deprivation on, 81–2; spatial arrangements in, 63–6; transfers at adulthood, 4, 71–2, 133. *See also* day rooms; dehumanization; food; High Grade wards; hygiene; Low Grade wards; Side Rooms; time management